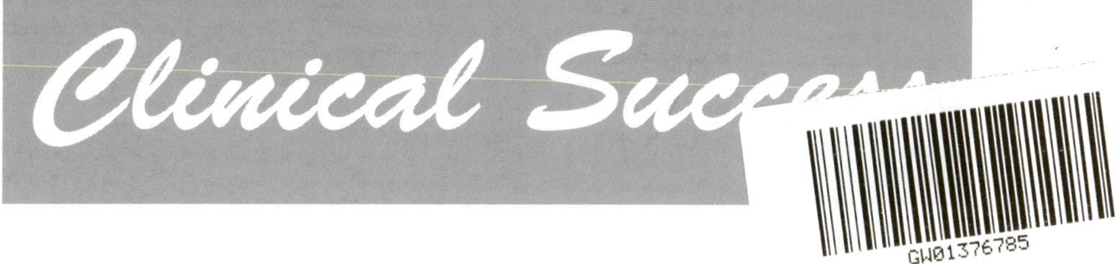

in

Endodontic
Retreatment

Stéphane Simon, DCD
Former Staff Physician
Department of Dental Surgery
University of Paris 7
Paris, France

Wilhelm-Joseph Pertot, DCD
Former Assistant Professor
Lecturer
Department of Dental Surgery
University of the Mediterranean Aix-Marseille II
Marseille, France

Foreword

Jean-Pierre Proust

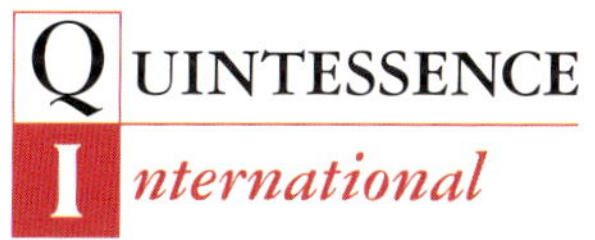

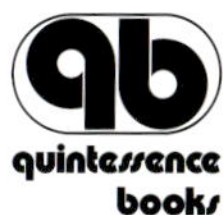

Paris, Berlin, Chicago, Tokyo, London, Milan, Barcelona,
Istanbul, São Paulo, Mumbai, Moscow, Prague, and Warsaw

First published in French in 2007 by Quintessence International Paris
La reprise du traitement endodontique

ISBN 978-2-912550-59-0

Quintessence International
11 bis, rue d'Aguesseau
75008 Paris
France

Design: STDI, Lassay-les-Châteaux, France
Printing and Binding: EMD, Lassay-les-Châteaux, France
Printed in France

Table of Contents

Foreword 5

1 **Endodontic Failures and Indications for Retreatment** 7

When to Retreat?
Preoperative Considerations: To Retreat or Not to Retreat?
Prior to Starting Retreatment
Taking a History
Radiographic Examination
Conventional Retreatment or a Surgical Approach?

2 **Removal of Existing Restorations** 21

Should Existing Restorations Be Removed Routinely?
Removal of Coronal Restorations
Removal of Restorative Material and Posts

3 **Access, Removal of Obturation Materials, and Negotiation of Canals** 43

Improving Access
Canal Anatomy and Clinical Implications
Removal of Obturation Material
Management of Fractured Instruments

4 **Management of Perforations** 89

Factors Influencing Prognosis and Type of Treatment
Materials Used for Perforation Repair
Perforations in the Coronal Third
Furcation or Strip Perforations
Perforations of the Pulp Chamber Floor
Perforations of the Middle and Apical Thirds of the Canal

5 **Treatment of Teeth with Open Apices** 109

Immature Teeth
Treatment by Apexogenesis
Treatment by Apexification
Management of Other Cases with Open Apices
Alternative Treatment Options

6 Prognosis and Retreatment 129

Endodontic Disease and Its Management
Assessment of Periodontal Health
Prognosis of Endodontic Treatment and Retreatment
Factors that Can Interfere with Healing
Endodontic Surgery: An Adjunct to Treatment

Bibliography 140

Index 141

Foreword

It is a great honor to be asked by Wilhelm Pertot and Stéphane Simon to write the foreword for this book. I like the fact that this book is clinically relevant and addresses the challenges that we, as dentists, face on a daily basis—indications for more retreatments than pulpectomies, difficulties of managing the sequelae of trauma, and the problems associated with fractured instruments.

The practical focus of this book makes it a worthy addition to the *Clinical Success* series published under the guidance of Jean-Marie Korbendau. Having been his student in 1963 to 1964, I remember with gratitude the rigorous practical and theoretic education he provided. Each week he asked us to present a written account of our clinical experiences, and he placed as much importance on the style as on the content. Unless clearly expressed, even the most important ideas become unintelligible.

This new book is devoted to the most time-consuming phase of endodontics—retreatment. The step-by-step guide shows the clinician how to overcome obstacles such as blockages, perforations, and immature apices. In addition it details how to successfully prepare and fill canals to prevent bacterial proliferation, thereby avoiding a subsequent bacteremia with its potential complications. The persistence of bacteria in the root canal system—away from the blood vessels that constitute the police force of our immune system—makes it necessary for us to place root fillings that wall off the bacteria and prevent further spread of infection.

Every day, I apply the same techniques outlined in this book as diligently as I can. In follow-up assessment with patients treated 6 months previously, I find they have been cured of unilateral sinusitis and headaches. Cardiac patients who need treatment for a devitalized tooth but are scheduled for immediate surgery cannot afford to wait 6 months to check if the lesion is healing; I am now convinced that root canal treatment for a devitalized tooth presents no greater risk than extraction, provided that the treatment is conducted in line with the recommendations presented in this book and with the best possible disinfection procedures in place.

This book is complete yet concise and easy to consult before appointments when you realize an alternative treatment option might be simpler (eg, extraction, implant). The authors guide the clinician through routine endodontic retreatment and its myriad complications including perforations, blockages, fractured instruments, and pulpal necrosis in immature teeth.

Whether you are a practicing clinician or a student, this book will aid in professional development. It offers a wealth of information accumulated by two practitioners who have acquired enormous practical experience in the field of endodontics. They have an extensive knowledge of the literature as well as a thorough understanding of the materials involved.

I am grateful for this opportunity to thank them for the invaluable contribution they have made in helping practitioners overcome the difficulties that are, alas, all too frequently encountered in endodontic retreatment.

Jean-Pierre Proust, PU-PH

Endodontic Failures

1

Indications for Retreatment

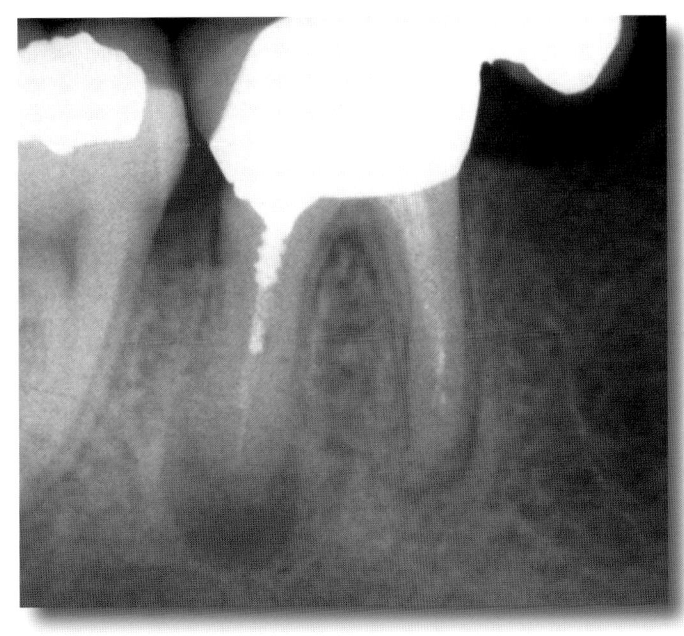

Endodontic treatment should fulfill a variety of objectives (Schilder, 1967 and 1974):

- Create a continuously tapering preparation from the crown to the apices
- Maintain the position of the apical foramen on the root surface
- Maintain the shape of the original canal as much as possible
- Keep the apical foramen as small as possible
- Use copious irrigation to ensure the root canal system is thoroughly cleaned and disinfected
- Obturate and seal the root canal system.

Although the procedures for endodontic treatment of a vital or necrotic pulp were first described decades ago, the number of unsatisfactory endodontic results remains rather high. Epidemiologic studies published over the past 20 years show that the number of inadequate treatments varies between 60% and 79%, with a failure rate (that is, cases where clinical symptoms or periapical lesions exist) of 22% to 63% (Boucher et al, 2002).

Endodontic retreatment can be defined as further treatment performed because the initial treatment was inadequate or the lesion failed to heal.

From a clinical standpoint, the four causes of failure are inherent within each stage of endodontic treatment (Ruddle, 2004):

- Inadequate access cavity due to failure to appreciate the anatomy of the tooth; this hampers visibility, which in turn results in the following:
  - Failure to detect accessory canals
  - Difficulty in correctly preparing the canal because of instruments further restricting visibility or difficulty in visualizing the entire canal system
  - Perforations in the coronal third of the tooth or in the pulp chamber floor
- Insufficient irrigation during canal preparation
- Improper use of instruments during preparation, which may result in the following:
  - Alteration of the canal trajectory, which can cause obstructions and eventual perforations
  - Blockages and subsequent loss of working length (obstruction by debris or a fractured instrument); this prevents irrigation of the whole root canal system
  - Widening of the apical foramen, making controlled obturation impossible
- An error in fitting the gutta-percha cone, resulting in moisture contamination, a fault frequently associated with inadequate preparation of the apex; however, obturation material extruded through the apex is not in itself an indication for either orthograde or retrograde retreatment.

From a biologic standpoint, endodontic failure can result from improper preparation, disinfection, or obturation of the root canal network. Reinfection of the canal system resulting from a poor coronal seal could also lead to endodontic failure.

Irrespective of the technical inadequacies or errors, all endodontic failures are directly associated with the presence of bacteria and their toxins in the root canal system; these irritants migrate into the periodontal tissues by any route possible (eg, apical foramen, lateral canals, accessory canals).

The goals of endodontic retreatment remain the same as the goals of the initial treatment: elimination of bacteria and prevention of further bacterial contamination by means of a well-obturated canal and a coronal seal. Achieving these goals ensures long-term success with little chance of relapse or reappearance of pathology (Figs 1-1a and 1-1b).

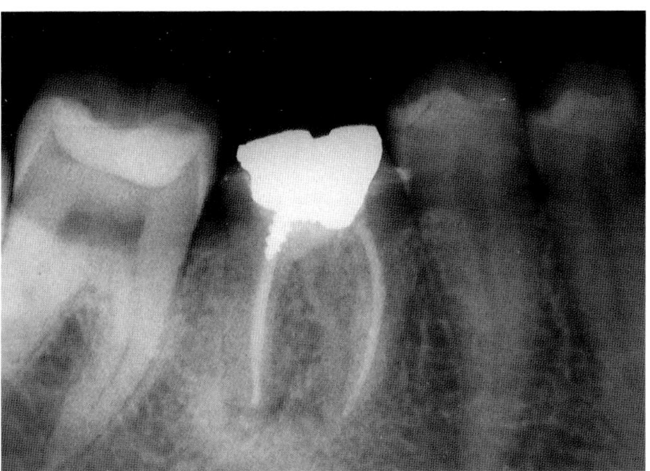

1-1a Preoperative periapical radiograph of a mandibular molar requiring endodontic retreatment prior to placement of a new crown.

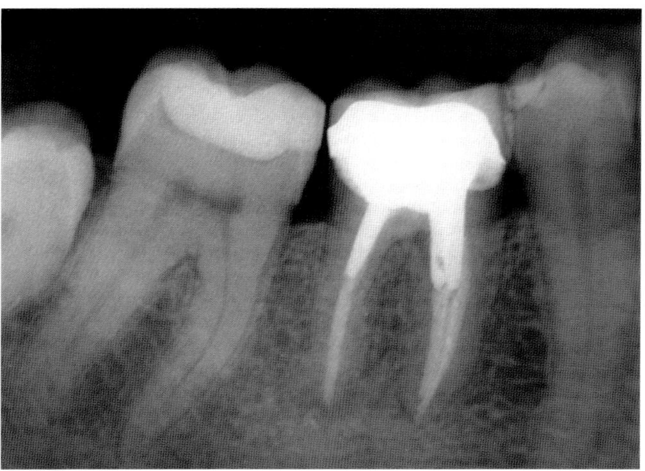

1-1b Periapical radiograph taken 9 years postoperatively. Good preparation and irrigation of the canal in conjunction with a good coronal seal ensures the longevity of the treatment.

Many endodontic failures can be attributed to inadequate training of the clinician and a lack of understanding of modern endodontic concepts and how to implement them. Resistance to change prevents many experienced practitioners from adopting new techniques, new instruments, and new materials; this, coupled with the misuse of unfamiliar equipment, contributes to a number of endodontic failures.

Endodontic treatment, when performed correctly, is predictable and enjoys a success rate above 95%. The same cannot be said for retreatment, in which access to canals can prove difficult, even dangerous, and in which negotiation of canals can be hampered by the following:

- Coronal restorations with large intracanal dowels
- Various canal filling materials such as hard and soft pastes, gutta-percha, or silver points
- Calcification of the apical portion of the canal as a result of inadequate preparation during initial treatment
- Iatrogenic causes including blockages, shoulders, ledges, perforations, and fractured instruments

Retreatment therefore necessitates the use of specific techniques and often proves complex and difficult.

When to Retreat?

A number of studies have shown that the decision to undertake endodontic retreatment is subject to both inter- and intrapractitioner variation. Agreement between practitioners on whether or not to retreat is rare (Aryanpour et al, 2000). The decision is often based on the individual practitioner's personal criteria rather than on a set of universally recognized, objective criteria (Pagonis et al, 2000; Kvist and Reit, 2002).

Although it would be very difficult to produce universal guidelines to identify cases that should be retreated, a consensus does exist regarding certain situations that require endodontic retreatment (Friedman, 2002).

After rigorous clinical examination to eliminate any possible causes of failure that are nonendodontic in origin (eg, cracks or fractures, food packing, occlusal trauma, sinusitis, trigeminal neuralgia), endodontic retreatment should be undertaken in the following cases.

Clinical symptoms

Retreatment is indicated when clinical symptoms persist after initial treatment. Patients generally complain of spontaneous pain of variable intensity that is exacerbated by occlusal problems or during mastication. There may be signs of swelling, an abscess, or a fistula. Radiographic evidence of a lesion is not always present (Figs 1-2a and 1-2b).

At a clinical level, the following apply:

- Immediate postoperative pain that subsides within days is not necessarily an indication that the treatment will fail in the long term. Periodontal inflammation after endodontic treatment or retreatment is a common occurrence and is not a cause for concern unless it persists.
- Sensitivity in occlusion does not necessarily imply endodontic failure but may simply indicate a high spot; if that is the case, symptoms will disappear once the high spot has been reduced.
- Complaints of pain in a treated tooth brought on by changes in temperature (particularly cold) should make the operator first suspect the pain is referred from an adjacent tooth or elsewhere. If this possibility is eliminated, other potential causes should be investigated; there may be untreated canals or contact between metallic elements and vital tissue, such as a silver point projecting through the apex, which can lead to pain.
- Pain or sensitivity on chewing could be related to a cracked tooth or root fracture. To avoid unnecessary endodontic treatment on such a tooth, the differential diagnosis must be considered after taking a thorough pain history, performing periodontal probing, assessing the occlusion, and taking a radiograph (Pertot and Simon, 2003).

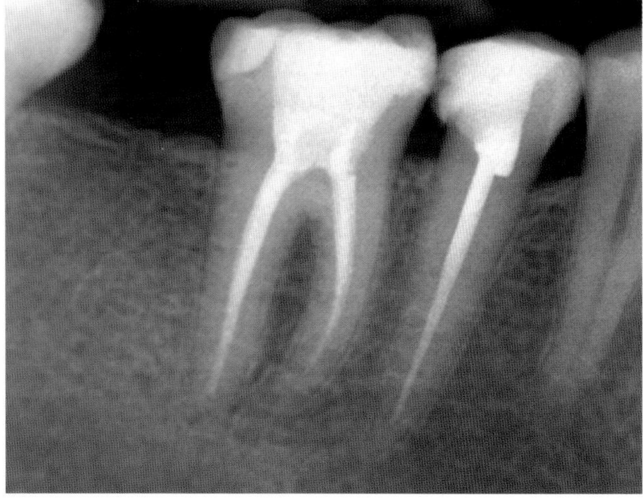

1-2a Periapical radiograph of a mandibular molar that is painful in occlusion; there is no radiographic evidence of a lesion.

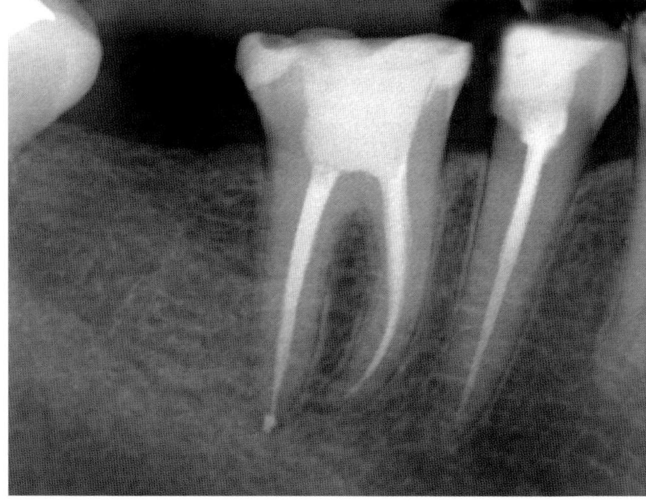

1-2b Postoperative radiograph. The pain subsided after endodontic retreatment.

Radiographic evidence

In the absence of clinical symptoms, many practitioners prefer not to retreat a tooth even if a periapical lesion is evident radiographically (Hulsmann, 1994). The development or persistence of a periapical lesion after a monitoring period of several months signals endodontic failure and is an indication for retreatment. A periapical lesion results from bacterial infection and therefore needs to be treated (Figs 1-3a to 1-3c).

The practitioner must first determine how much time has passed since the initial treatment and then, if possible, should compare previous radiographs to check if the lesion is in fact healing; this is particularly important if both the root filling and the coronal restoration appear to be adequate. Although the first stages of healing can be seen radiographically 3 months postoperatively with the formation of bony trabeculae, complete healing of large lesions may take several years.

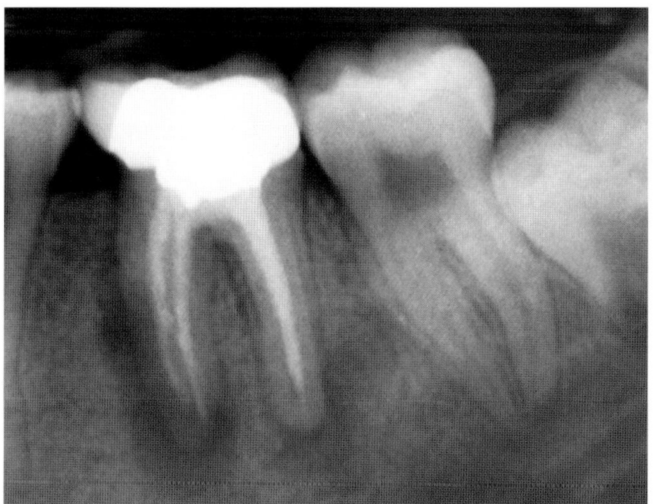

1-3a Preoperative radiograph of a mandibular molar with periapical lesions and severe resorption of the mesial root.

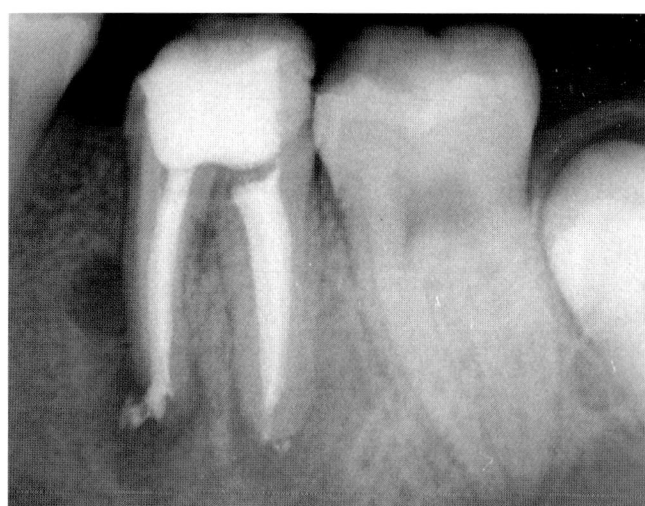

1-3b Immediate postoperative periapical radiograph.

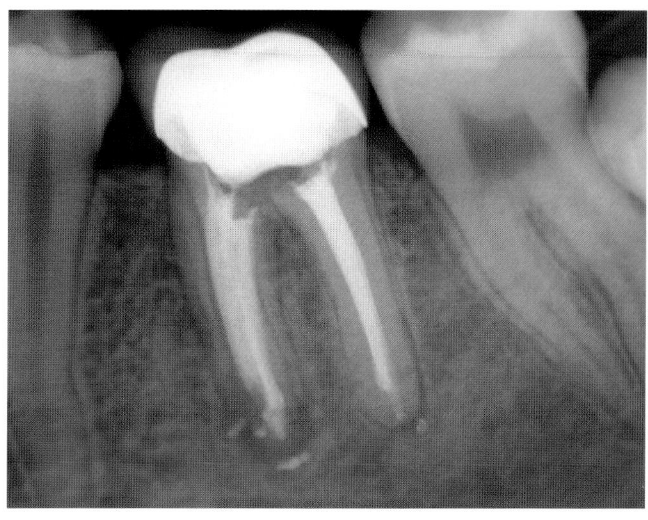

1-3c Clear evidence of healing, 1 year postoperatively.

Cases where new coronal restorations are planned

When a new coronal restoration is planned, radiographic examination is necessary to assess any previous endodontic treatment on the tooth; if deemed technically inadequate, the root filling should be redone as a preventive measure (Machtou, 1993) (Figs 1-4a to 1-4c). The absence of a radiographic lesion on a tooth with an inadequate root filling does not indicate the absence of bacteria in the canal network. Teeth whose canals have been contaminated by bacteria can remain asymptomatic as long as the balance between the body's defense system and the virulence of the bacteria is not altered. Disturbing this balance by instrumentation and crown preparation (impressions, post space preparation) can cause a lesion to develop where previously one did not exist (Figs 1-5a and 1-5b).

The objective of endodontic treatment or retreatment is to control the source of bacterial contamination, thereby tipping the balance in favor of the body's defense system. In retreatment cases where the canal cannot be negotiated to the apex, the use of rubber dam, correct tapering of the canal, and copious irrigation are usually sufficient to stimulate healing. *It is therefore important to retreat teeth with apparently inadequate root fillings even in the absence of clinical or radiographic signs of failure, in cases where new coronal restorations are planned.*

If no new restoration is planned, however, and if there is a healthy periodontium, a good coronal seal, and absence of clinical or radiographic symptoms, practitioners should refrain from retreating and should only monitor the tooth, even if the root filling is clearly unsatisfactory (unless medical reasons dictate otherwise).

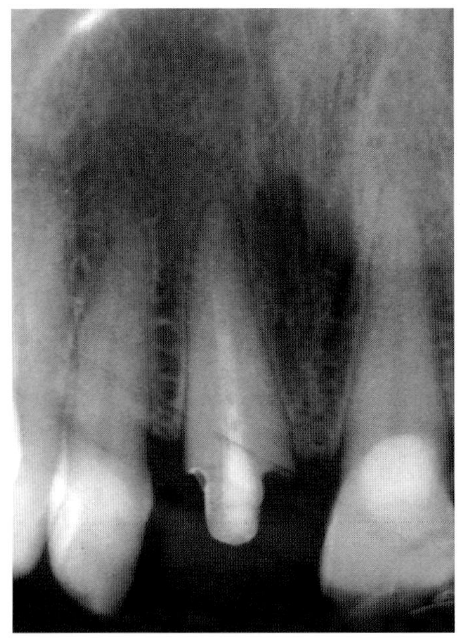

1-4a Preoperative radiograph of a maxillary incisor. A new crown is needed, but previous endodontic treatment is unsatisfactory. Retreatment is indicated even in the absence of any pathology.

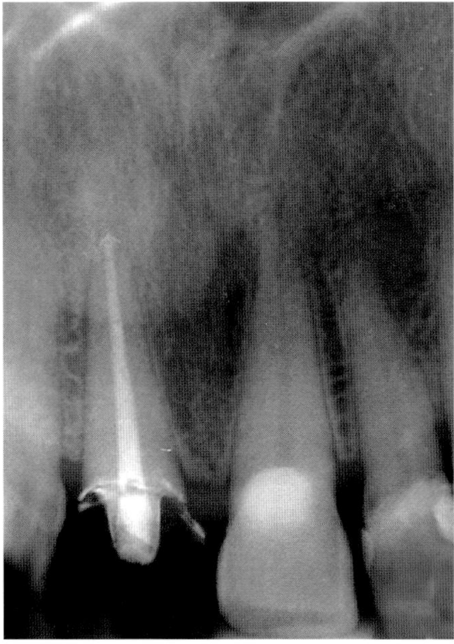

1-4b Immediate postoperative radiograph.

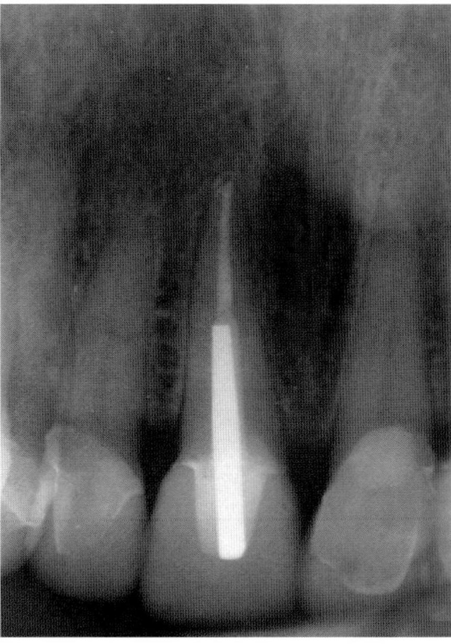

1-4c Radiograph taken 3 years postoperatively.

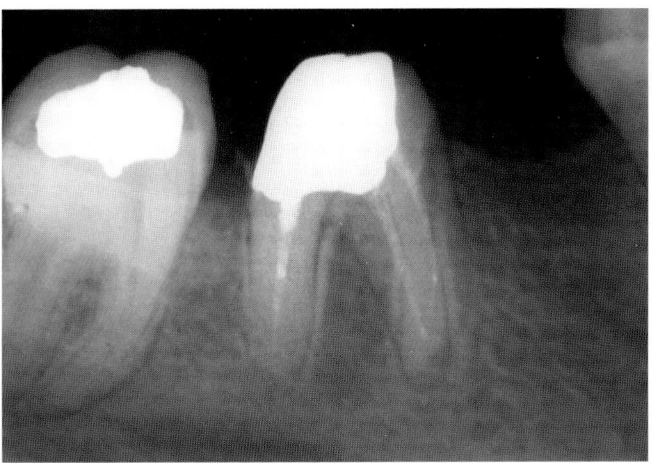

1-5a Preoperative radiograph of a mandibular molar. A new crown is required, but previous endodontic treatment is unsatisfactory. Retreatment was not completed because there were no clinical or radiographic signs of pathology.

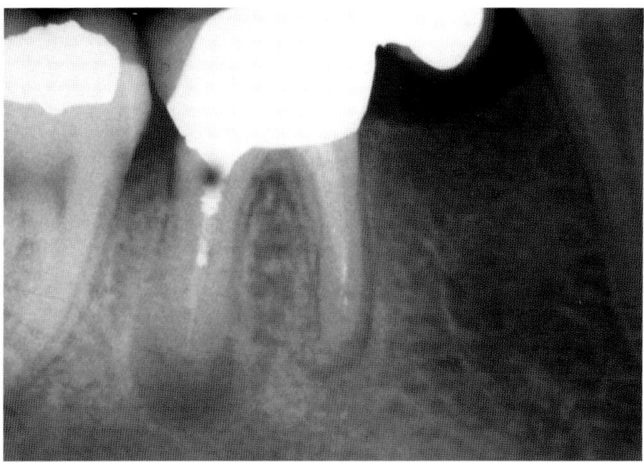

1-5b Radiograph taken 6 months after the crown was placed. A periapical lesion has appeared even though the root filling was undisturbed during crown preparation.

Cases where the coronal seal is deficient

Retreatment is indicated for any tooth where the access cavity has been inadequately sealed and has been open to the oral environment for a considerable period of time, even if the root filling seems adequate radiographically. Numerous studies over the past 10 years have demonstrated that if the coronal seal is deficient, bacteria can infiltrate and migrate down to the apex even when root canals are adequately filled. Although the reported time for this migration of bacteria varies from study to study, authors agree that the coronal seal is an important factor in the long-term success of root canal treatment. In vivo studies have shown that the first signs of periapical pathology can appear 4 months after treatment. These findings confirm the need to retreat all teeth where contamination has occurred and highlight the importance of restoring the tooth immediately after completion of endodontic treatment to ensure the best possible coronal seal.

For the same reasons, in complex cases where multiple teeth are prepared over several weeks, a good seal on temporary restorations is essential. After each root canal treatment, a definitive restoration must be placed as soon as possible. A provisional crown does not provide a good seal; bacterial contamination through the coronal aspect is inevitable until a definitive restoration is placed.

Preoperative Considerations: To Retreat or Not to Retreat?

Technologic advances in instruments and materials (eg, ultrasonic instruments for endodontic use), combined with magnification devices (loupes and microscopes), allow the clinician to achieve optimal results with retreatment. Nevertheless, except in cases where the need for retreatment is clear, many other factors must be taken into consideration before making the decision to retreat a given tooth or to consider alternative treatment options.

Is the tooth strategically important and what are the alternatives?

Once a root filling is deemed to have failed, the clinician should evaluate the importance of the tooth and assess alternative treatment options, exploring the advantages and disadvantages of each with the patient. Endodontic retreatment is not an end in itself. With the materials now available, experienced clinicians can expect to obtain good results in the retreatment of most teeth; it is, however, essential to consider the value of the tooth in the overall treatment plan. Thus, before making a decision on retreatment, the clinician should assess the strategic importance of the tooth, the periodontal condition, the occlusion, and any associated pathology (eg, perforation, resorption), and should evaluate the likelihood of a successful long-term restoration (Figs 1-6a to 1-6c).

Periodontal assessment

Any factors that may influence the long-term viability of the tooth should be ascertained by periodontal probing, assessment of tooth mobility, evaluation of the crown-root relationship, and identification of any bony resorption. Careful periodontal probing is necessary to evaluate the quality of the epithelial attachment, especially in cases with furcation

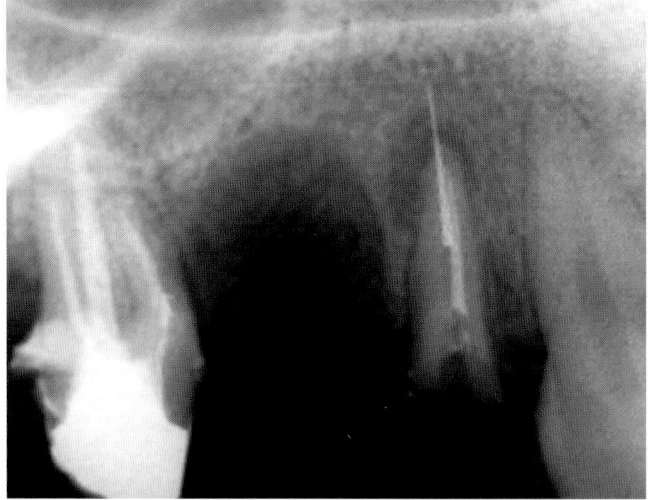

1-6a Preoperative radiograph of a maxillary premolar with a fractured instrument passing through the apex.

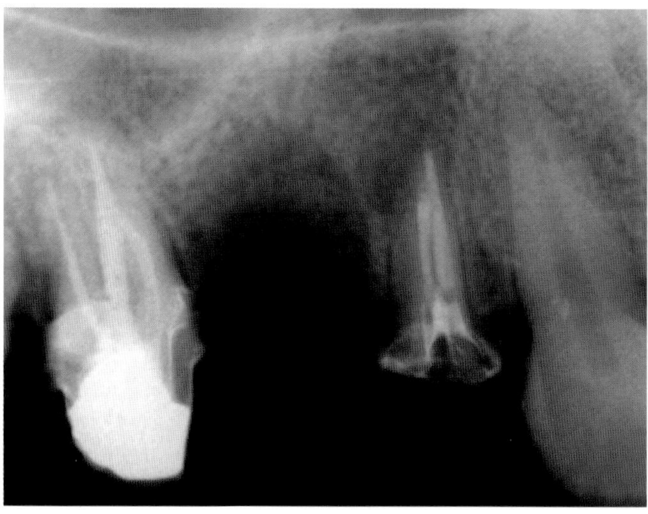

1-6b Immediate postoperative radiograph.

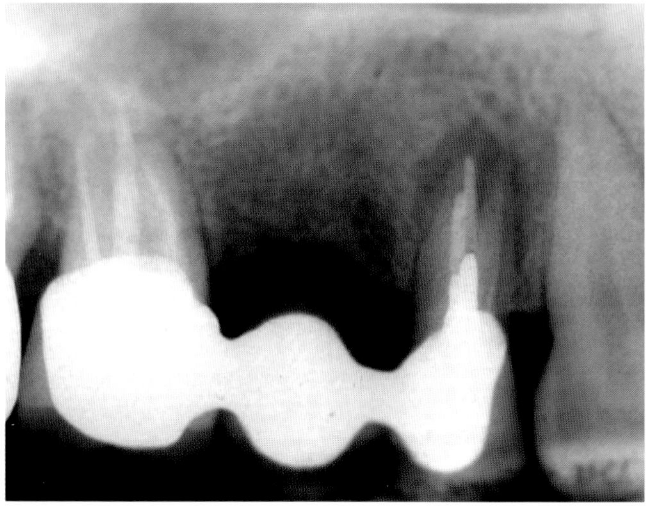

1-6c Radiograph taken 6 months later shows a root fracture. Using the already-weakened premolar as an abutment tooth for a fixed partial denture was arguably not the best course of treatment in this case.

lesions. A lesion of endodontic origin with no fistula has a favorable prognosis even when the lesion is large (Figs 1-7a and 1-7b). Conversely, a lesion that communicates with the oral cavity via a fistula, following destruction of the epithelial attachment, has a far less favorable prognosis (Figs 1-8a and 1-8b).

Periodontal probing, combined with an occlusal assessment and often a radiograph, is essential when considering a differential diagnosis of root fracture. Many retreatment procedures (both coronal and surgical) are performed unnecessarily because an undetected root fracture was the actual cause of the problems. A fairly consistent pocket depth around the tooth suggests the problem is likely to be of periodontal origin; an increase in pocket depth at a particular point suggests a fracture has occurred (Figs 1-9a to 1-9c).

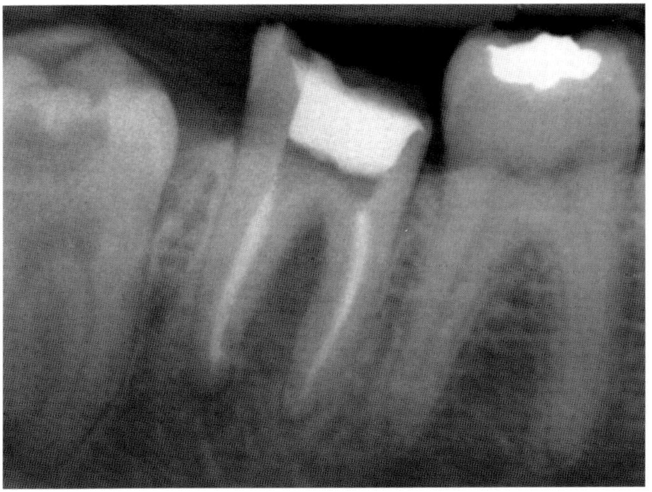

1-7a Preoperative radiograph of a mandibular molar with a furcation lesion. Periodontal probing revealed a healthy periodontium and no fistula.

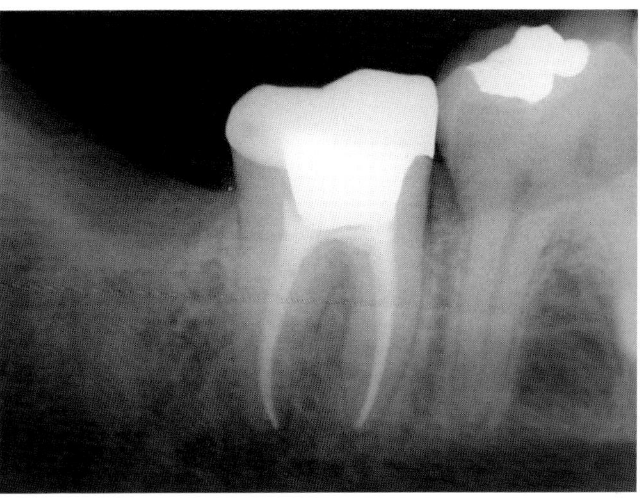

1-7b Radiograph 1 year postoperatively.

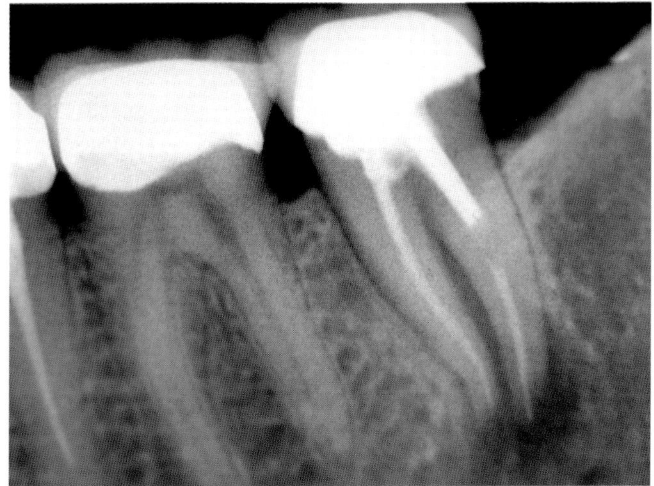

1-8a Preoperative radiograph of a mandibular molar with a furcation lesion. Periodontal probing demonstrated attachment loss and communication with the oral cavity via a sinus tract.

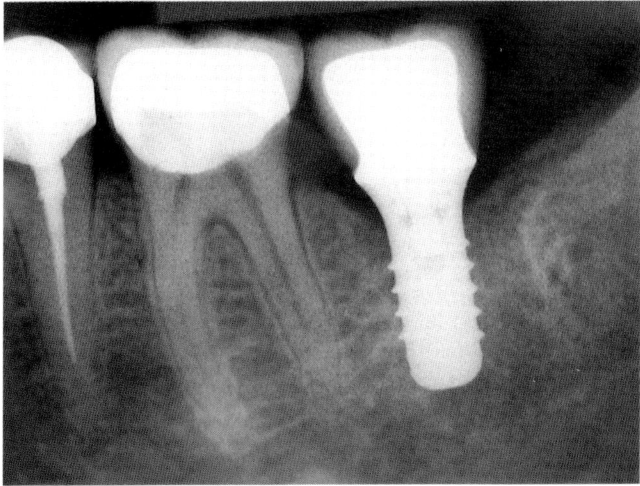

1-8b After discussion of treatment options and prognosis, the tooth was extracted and replaced with an implant.

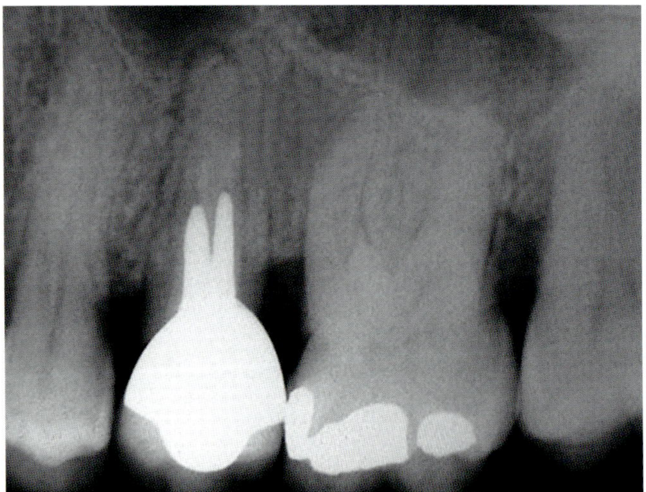

1-9a Preoperative radiograph of a maxillary premolar that was tender on occlusion. Previous endodontic treatment appears inadequate. The initial plan was to retreat this tooth surgically.

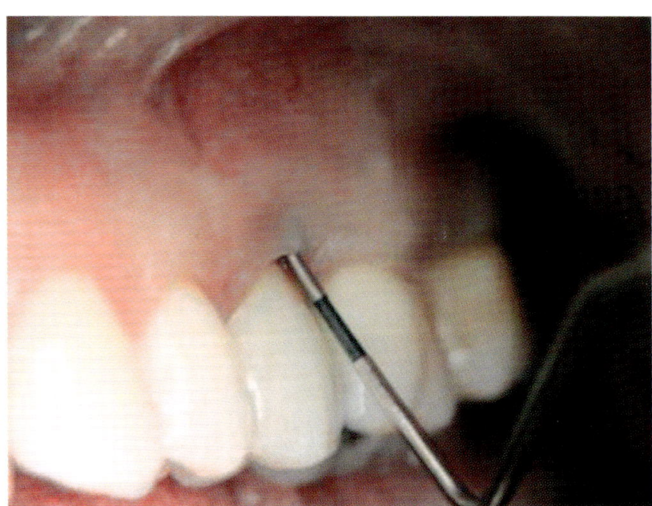

1-9b Periodontal probing revealed an area with loss of epithelial attachment. Considered in combination with the tenderness in occlusion, this suggests a root fracture.

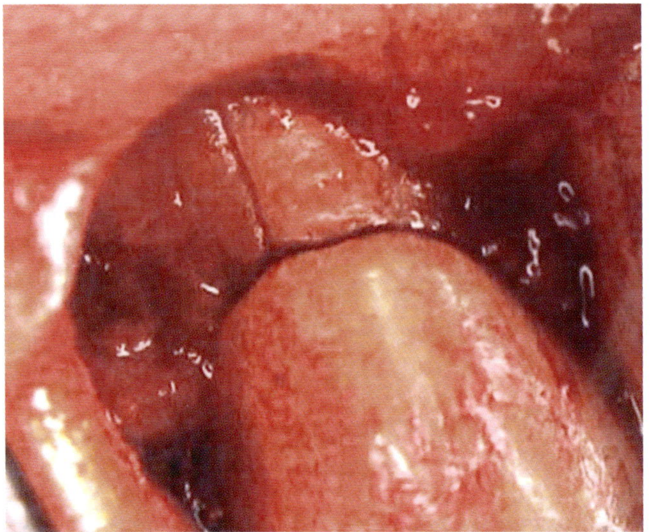

1-9c Raising a gingival flap confirmed the presence of a fracture.

Restorability of the tooth

The objective in treating a tooth endodontically is to allow it to remain as a functional unit in the arch. A tooth that has extensive caries or that has broken down and has little function or value in the overall treatment plan should not be restored. A tooth with a caries lesion that extends subgingivally may need periodontal intervention first to restore the biologic width. Where possible, crown lengthening should be completed prior to retreatment; this creates more favorable conditions for each stage of treatment. For the endodontist, the crown lengthening makes it easier to place a rubber dam clamp and allows the tooth to be restored before treatment; in this way the four-walled access cavity creates a reservoir for the irrigant. Crown lengthening also enables placement of a stable temporary dressing that is capable of resisting occlusal forces and preventing bacterial leakage. In the phase following endodontic treatment, the visibility gained by crown lengthening simplifies the placement of the final restoration. This helps to ensure long-term periodontal health and, above all, makes a good coronal seal possible.

Surgery time required and cost-benefit ratio

These factors must always be taken into consideration, irrespective of the treatment planned. This is particularly true for retreatment cases where duration of treatment may be long and the outcome is less predictable than with initial treatment. Unfortunately the technical difficulties of retreatment often mean that practitioners prefer to extract the tooth and replace it with an implant or a fixed partial denture rather than attempt to maintain the original tooth.

Patient demands

Endodontic retreatment can be time consuming, with a lower chance of success than initial treatment. It is therefore important to gain the cooperation of the patient, who should be fully informed about the entire procedure, the possible need for an adjunctive surgical procedure, and the risk of failure and subsequent extraction.

Operator skill and experience

In light of the factors discussed and the possible complications of retreatment, it may be appropriate to refer those patients in need of retreatment to endodontic specialists who have the expertise and equipment necessary to deal with complex cases. It is important, though sometimes difficult, to gauge the complexity of the treatment, to know one's limits, and to know when to refer.

Prior to Starting Retreatment

After considering treatment options and the indications for retreatment, the practitioner must investigate further before embarking on the clinical stages of retreatment. The resulting observations will help identify the cause of failure, bring to light any anticipated difficulties, and allow a treatment plan to be created that aims to overcome these obstacles. It is not always obvious from a simple radiograph what problems may occur; an apparently easy case can quickly become complicated and time consuming.

Taking a History

A thorough history from the patient provides useful information about the original clinical signs and symptoms (pain, edema, swelling, drainage) and about the previous treatment. If previous radiographs are available, they can be compared to recent films to assess changes in periapical pathology and help determine if any healing has taken place.

Radiographic Examination

Radiographs can provide only a fraction of the information needed; nevertheless, good quality films can be very valuable. Prior to starting endodontic retreatment, the clinician should have at least a conventional periapical film and an angled image taken using the parallax principle. In some cases a second angled film, taken from the distal aspect, allows an untreated canal to be identified or a fractured instrument to be located (Figs 1-10a and 1-10b).

Numerous retreatment failures have resulted from inadequate examination of radiographs, and therefore an underestimation of the difficulties of the case, before treatment is begun. Preoperative radiographs enable the clinician to accomplish the following:

- Assess root anatomy, look for the cause of failure, and determine if it can be rectified. Certain teeth with complex root canal configurations (eg, curved roots, C-shaped canals) can prove difficult to retreat. These cases can be further complicated by iatrogenic damage from the initial treatment (eg, fractured instruments, perforations).
- Examine the periapical area to identify any radiolucencies, detect any foreign bodies (eg, obturation material, fractured instruments), and assess the extent of any resorption.
- Assess the coronal restoration and evaluate the risk of damaging the tooth when removing the crown.
- Visualize the quality of the canal preparation and obturation and sometimes determine the nature of the obturation material. For example, a curved canal that has been obturated too short of the apex indicates a possible blockage and/or a calcified canal.
- Identify any fractured instruments and then assess the possibility of their removal.

Finally, it must be remembered that in addition to providing information, the radiographs play an essential role in establishing a medicolegal record. A preoperative radiograph of the tooth should be kept in the patient's files to demonstrate, should the need arise, the condition of the tooth before treatment. Without this it could be difficult after treatment to convince a patient that a fractured instrument or perforation was present before the retreatment was conducted.

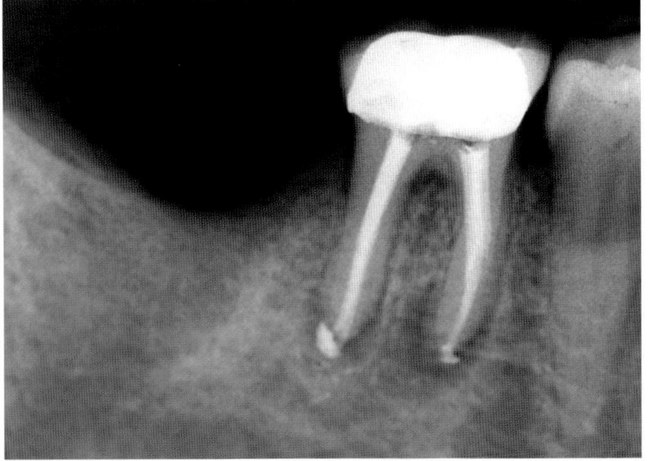

1-10a A periapical radiograph of a mandibular molar shows persistent periapical lesions, despite an apparently good root filling.

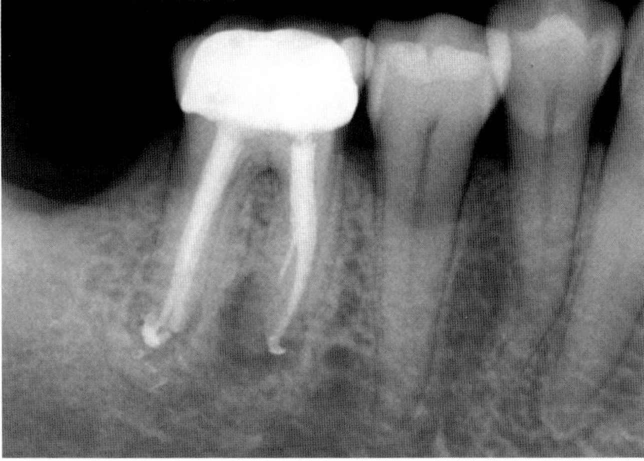

1-10b An angled radiograph reveals a fractured instrument in the mesial root. The radiograph shows the instrument lying in the mesiobuccal root; there may in fact be two separate apical foramina.

Conventional Retreatment or a Surgical Approach?

When planning endodontic retreatment, the option of a surgical approach must be considered. New technology and materials have been developed over the past decade that make surgical endodontic treatment more predictable. Nevertheless, except in cases where access is good and root canal anatomy is simple, retrograde treatment deals only with the apical portion of the canal, leaving the remainder unirrigated and unobturated. This technique could therefore prove to be ineffective at preventing further bacterial migration into the periapical tissues and eventually lead to failure of the retreatment. Thus, even when surgery is planned, orthograde treatment should be performed where possible, to ensure good irrigation and obturation of the coronal part of the canal.

A surgical approach is indicated in cases where iatrogenic damage has occurred in the apical third, thereby preventing repair of the defect by a conventional approach (tearing of the apical foramen, with or without extrusion of obturation material) (Figs 1-11a to 1-11d). In these cases, even when a surgical approach is indicated, conventional retreatment should be conducted first, whenever possible, to decontaminate the root canal system. Extrusion of material through the apex is not in itself an indication for surgical endodontics unless it

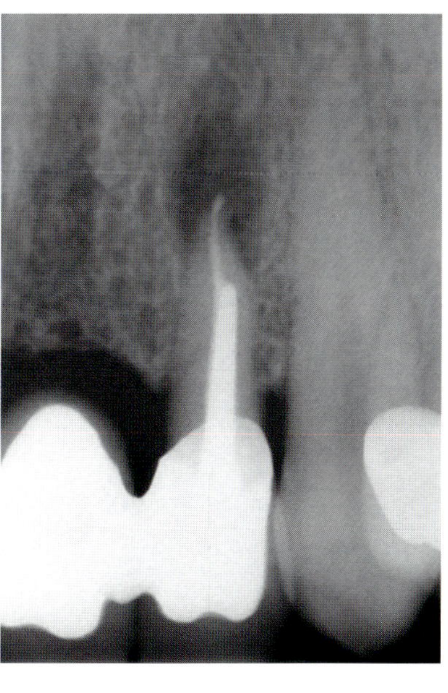

1-11a Preoperative radiograph of a maxillary lateral incisor that serves as an abutment for a fixed partial denture. A large post is in place and the apical foramen has been widened excessively.

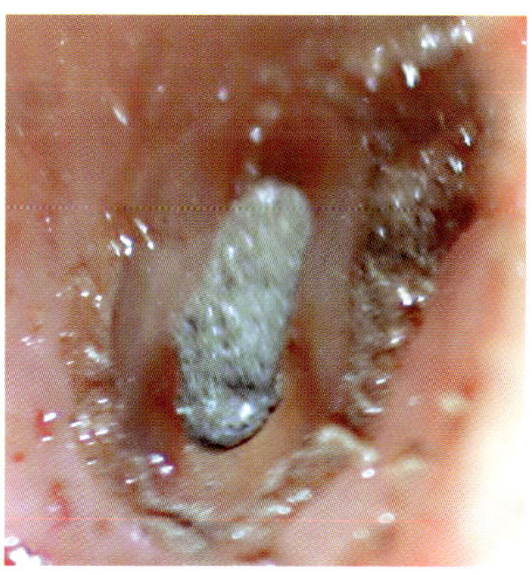

1-11b Retrograde obturation with ProRoot MTA (Dentsply). Note the outline of the cavity; the oval shape was created during the preparation stage of the initial treatment.

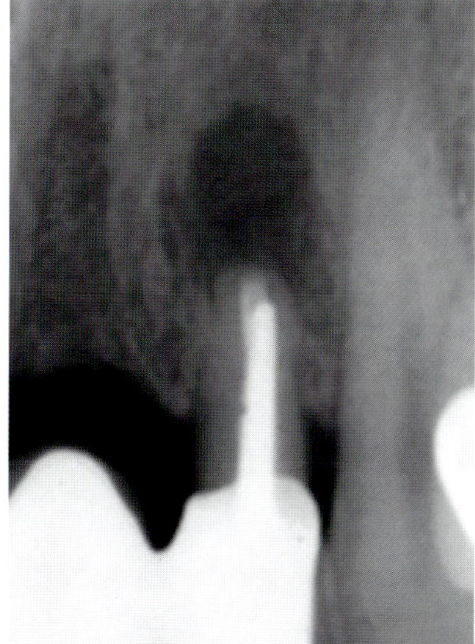

1-11c Immediate postoperative radiograph.

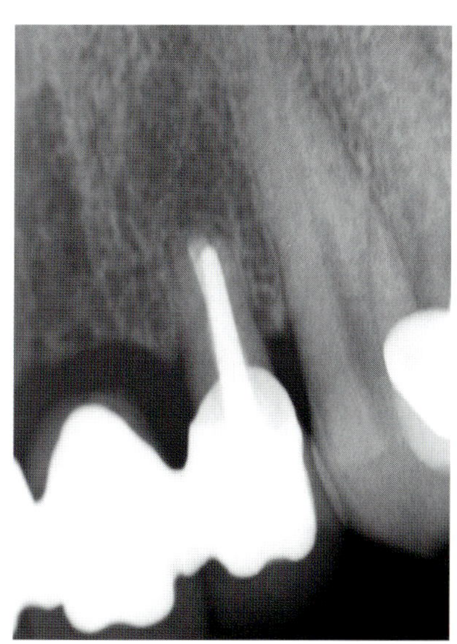

1-11d Radiograph taken 3 years postoperatively.

is associated with marked widening of the apical foramen. Treatment failures resulting from inadequate canal preparation and poor control of obturation material should be retreated first from a coronal approach (Figs 1-12a to 1-12c).

Nevertheless, surgical intervention may be necessary when material has been extruded in the following cases:

- When removal of the post and core is likely to result in root fracture or perforation
- Following failure of conventional retreatment and only when a period of monitoring has taken place over several months

Indications for surgical endodontic treatment are based on the technical limitations or failures of conventional retreatment. Thus, other than in exceptional cases, a conventional approach, though more time consuming, is preferred over surgical retreatment in the first instance.

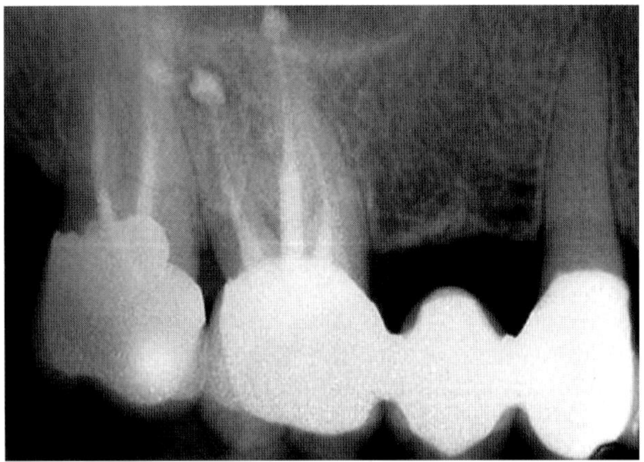

1-12a Preoperative periapical radiograph of first and second maxillary molars with periapical lesions and material extruded through the apex.

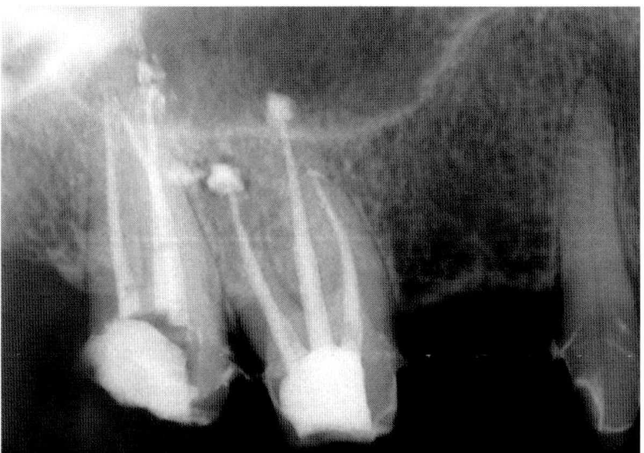

1-12b Postoperative radiograph following retreatment.

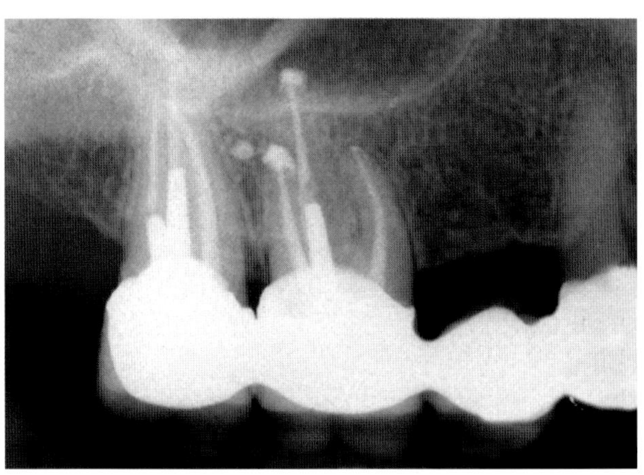

1-12c Periapical radiograph taken 2 years postoperatively. Good preparation, irrigation, and obturation of the canals has allowed healing despite the presence of the extruded material.

The goals of endodontic retreatment are to improve the existing situation and to transform a case that had been deemed a failure into one that can be described as a success. All the factors discussed in this chapter need to be considered when planning retreatment. The practitioner can then decide to undertake retreatment, choose an alternative treatment option, or refer the patient to a specialist.

Removal of Existing

2

Restorations

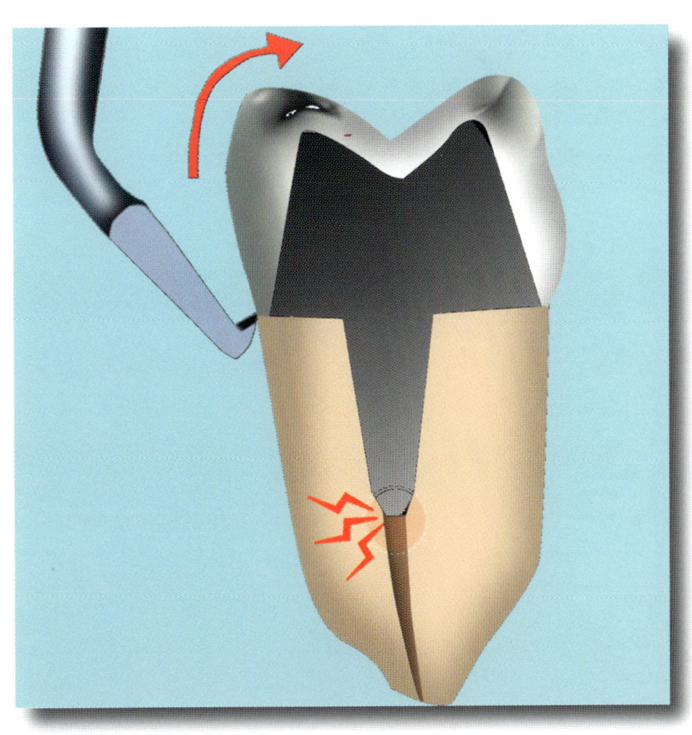

The first step in endodontic treatment is gaining access to the root canals. Gaining access in retreatment procedures might be complicated by a variety of factors:

- Presence of a direct or indirect coronal restoration
- Loss of the pulp chamber
- Complications created during the initial treatment (eg, poor access cavities, perforations)
- Presence of crowns or fixed partial dentures that, for esthetic or functional reasons, have been made to modify the occlusal morphology and/or the natural axis of the tooth
- Presence of a post

Overcoming or negotiating these obstacles is essential prior to any attempts to gain access to the root canal system. Preoperative radiographs and a thorough clinical examination can provide important information (Boxes 2-1 and 2-2). Additional information can be gathered from the patient notes and, if possible, from communication with the clinician who performed the previous treatment (Box 2-3). A treatment plan can then be drawn up.

Box 2-1	**Information derived from radiographs**
Long axis of the tooth	
Crown-root relationship	
Presence of and type of post (eg, passive, threaded, nonmetallic)	
Angulation, size, and shape of access cavity	
Type of obturation material	
Thickness of remaining pulpal floor	
Presence of perforations	
Number of canals treated	

Box 2-2	**Information derived from clinical examination**
Periodontal status	
Furcation involvement	
Type of coronal restoration (ie, crown, amalgam, composite)	
Relationship of adjacent teeth (passing floss interdentally helps determine if crowns are single units or attached to adjacent teeth)	
Restorative components used, the color of the material, and its toughness	

Box 2-3 Information obtained from the patient or previous clinician

Differentiation between an integrated post-retained crown and a tooth that has been restored with a separate post and crown. Only split pin posts are definitive evidence that the restoration is not a single unit.

Type of luting cement used.

Type of metal used for the post.

Nature of nonmetallic posts. Carbon fiber posts, glass fiber posts, and ceramic posts are often radiolucent, and it is very difficult to distinguish between them. Nevertheless, if possible, it is important to ascertain the post material, which determines the method of removal. Even after a thorough clinical examination, some things will remain unclear until the retreatment is actually begun. It is essential that the clinician has the necessary instruments and equipment available to deal with the different clinical scenarios that may arise as treatment progresses.

Should existing restorations be removed routinely?

It is strongly advisable to remove existing coronal restorations, since they may complicate access to the canal system and can cause errors to be made. The shape of the restored tooth often bears no resemblance to the original tooth morphology, and the coronal axis of the tooth also may have been masked by the restoration. When gaining access through a crown, it is very difficult to use the normal anatomic landmarks as a guide. Removing the crown before starting retreatment may reveal important information, such as the type of material used for the underlying core. All core material should be removed for proper assessment of the remaining tooth structure and detection of hidden cracks or fractures (Fig 2-1). Some argue that the crown should be kept and considered simply as a separate restoration placed prior to the endodontic treatment. It is nevertheless preferable to remove the existing crown while preserving as much tooth tissue as possible. After removing the existing crown and all the underlying core material, the practitioner can use this crown as a provisional restoration, lining it with either a luting cement or glass-ionomer cement. Thus, removing the crown not only reveals necessary information for proper assessment of the tooth, but also provides a good provisional restoration. In exceptional cases where access has to be gained through the crown, the coronal access cavity should be prepared larger than in natural teeth to allow better visualization.

To guarantee a good coronal seal and prevent recontamination of the root canals, a definitive restoration must be placed soon after treatment. The existing crown must not be used as the final restoration but, if necessary, should only be used as a provisional restoration during the monitoring period while waiting for healing to occur.

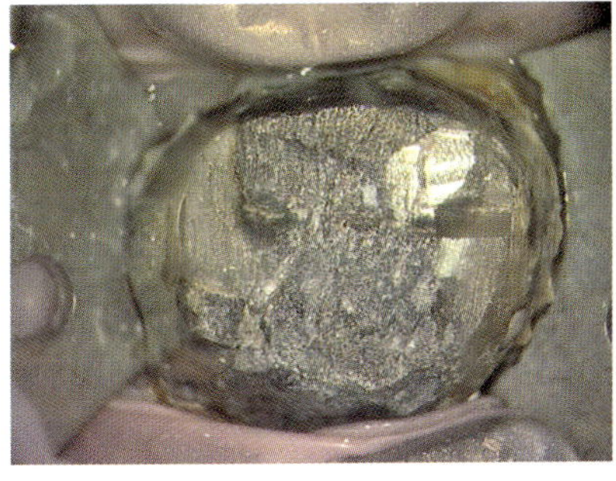
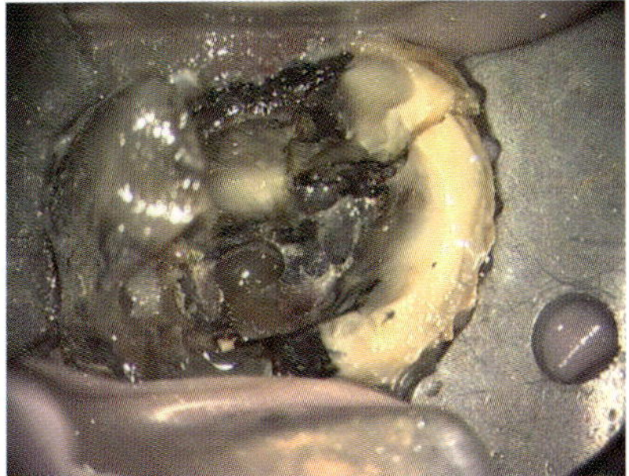

2-1 Removing the crown and underlying core material allowed a previously unseen fracture to be identified.

Removal of Coronal Restorations

Direct restorations

Direct restorations can easily be removed by cutting the material out. If an amalgam restoration is being removed, precautions must be taken to prevent fragments of amalgam from entering the root canals. A simple way of removing the restoration is to run a bur along the cavity wall, around the edge of the amalgam; using this technique, the restoration is often removed in one piece. Good irrigation and suction are essential. It is also advisable to place rubber dam to protect the patient from mercury vapor and aerosol droplets.
Composite restorations can be removed in a similar way with a high-speed handpiece and copious amounts of water. It can be difficult to distinguish between the restoration and the tooth if a good color match has been achieved. To preserve as much tooth tissue as possible, sonic or ultrasonic instruments can be used; these allow more precise movements and maintain a clear field of vision.

Intact crowns

Individual crowns can be removed intact by decementation, or they can be removed in sections.

To remove a crown intact or "decement" it, the cement seal between the crown and the underlying tooth or core material must be broken; the crown itself remains intact. While this technique is the method of choice for provisional crowns, it is rarely used for definitive restorations. Decementation occurs only when sufficient force is applied to break the cement seal. Fuhrer pliers are advised for the removal of provisional crowns; these specialized pliers with a diamond-coated surface provide extra grip. The use of conventional crown removers (Fig 2-2a) to take off definitive crowns is strongly discouraged because of the transmitted force to the crown along one side of the tooth. The force is delivered along the axis of the crown remover and produces a tipping motion that does not correspond to the crown's path of removal. Thus, there is a high risk of fracturing the underlying tooth (Fig 2-2b). If the tooth contains a post, this tipping motion will be transmitted to the root and could cause root fracture (Fig 2-2c).

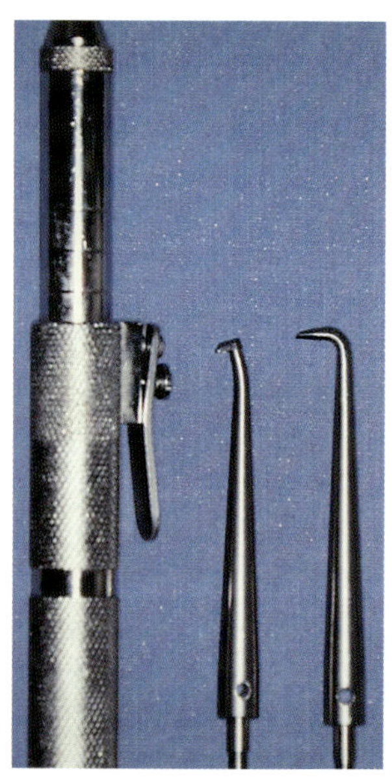

2-2a Crown remover and two different tips.

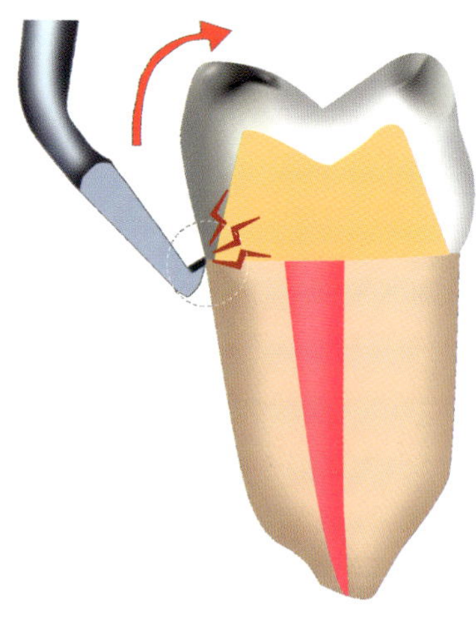

2-2b The force transmitted by the crown remover can damage or fracture the underlying tooth.

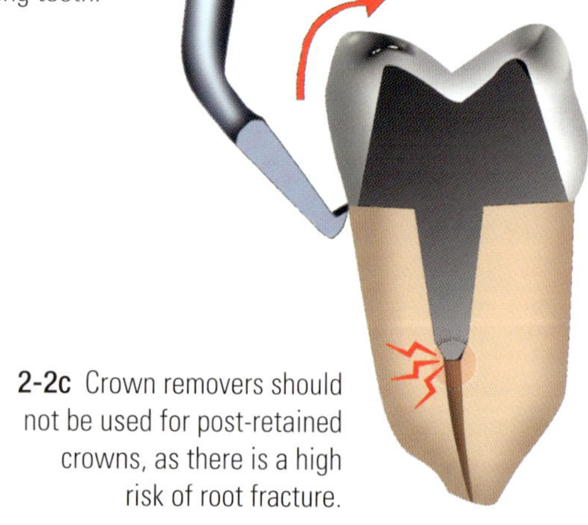

2-2c Crown removers should not be used for post-retained crowns, as there is a high risk of root fracture.

Crown removers powered by electric motors and compressed air are available (Fig 2-3). They deliver repetitive shockwaves (up to 20 per second) to attempt breaking the cement seal; the force and the frequency of these shockwaves are controlled by the operator. These devices, though effective, must be handled with care, especially when rigid tips are used. To remove fixed partial dentures, the parachute technique described below is far safer and less traumatic.

The Metalift (Metalift) crown removal system is a useful instrument based on the principle of a self-threading screw (Fig 2-4a). A small hole is created in the occlusal surface of the crown (Fig 2-4b) to expose the metal substructure in porcelain-fused-to-metal crowns. A drill that corresponds to the diameter of the Metalift is used to penetrate through the metal (Fig 2-4c). The Metalift crown remover is then placed into the prepared channel and screwed in, threading into the metal as it is turned. It comes to rest on the occlusal surface of the underlying tooth. With continued turning, the Metalift pushes against the dentin/core, exerting a force along the long axis of the tooth and eventually breaking the cement seal and decementing the crown (Fig 2-4d). For porcelain-fused-to-metal crowns it may be prudent to remove the porcelain first to prevent it from fragmenting. Crowns removed with the Metalift system tend to show only minimal damage, so they can be lined with a luting agent and used as provisional restorations.

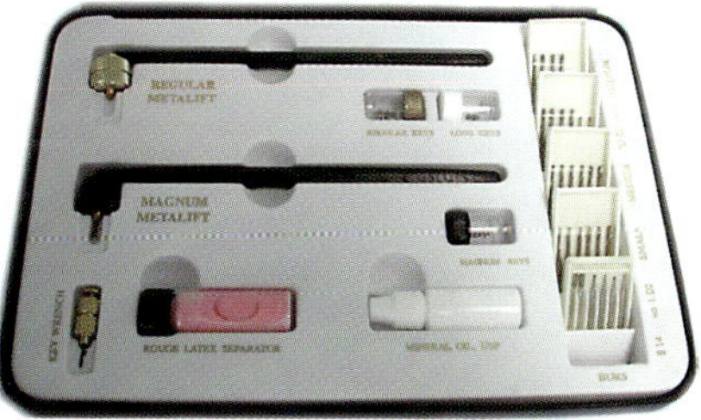

2-4a Metalift kit.

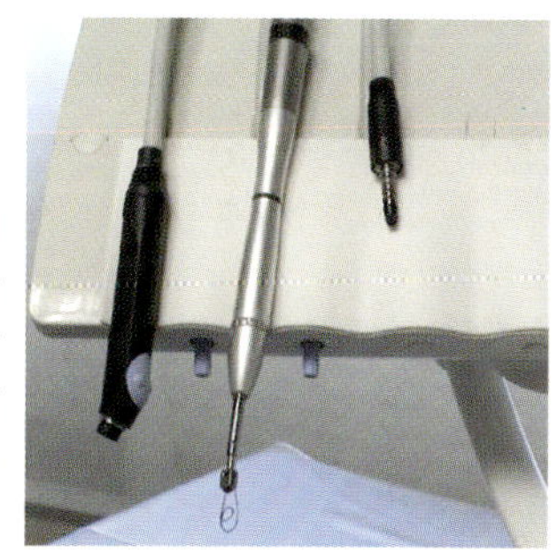

2-3 Safe Relax (Anthogyr) electric crown remover. The rigid tips must be used with caution to avoid fracturing the underlying tooth; the metal cables allow the crown remover to be used safely and efficiently in the parachute technique. The power and frequency of the shocks delivered by Safe Relax can be adjusted by the operator.

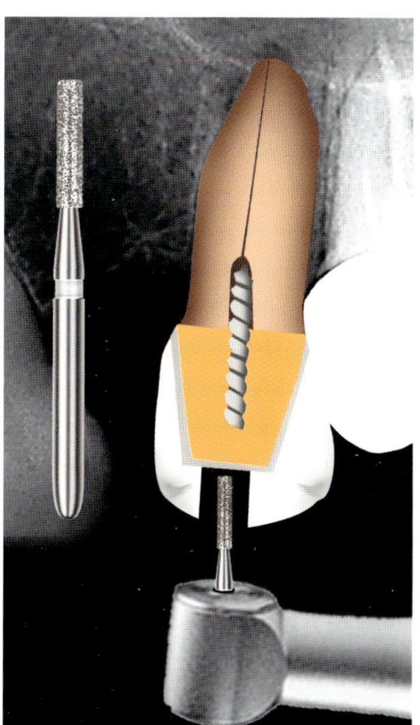

2-4b Porcelain on the occlusal surface of the crown is removed with a diamond bur.

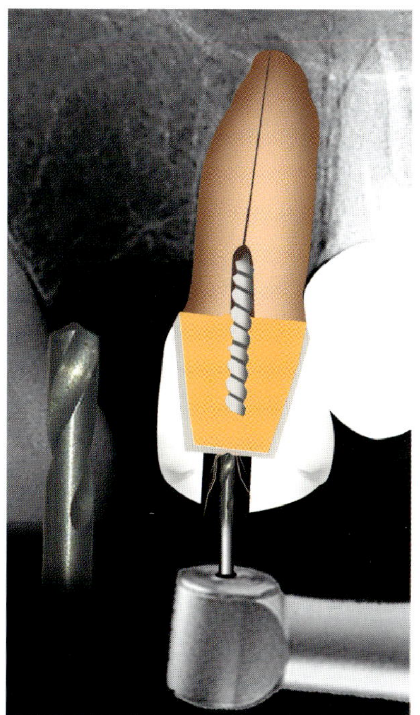

2-4c A tungsten carbide drill corresponding to the diameter of the Metalift is used to prepare a channel through the metal.

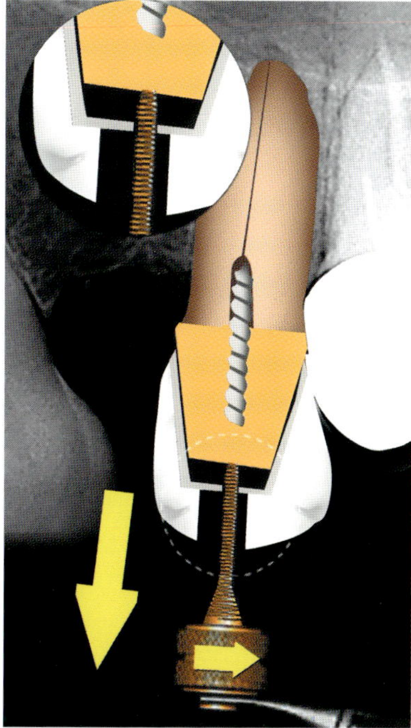

2-4d The Metalift is set in the prepared channel and screwed in; as it pushes against the underlying tooth, the cement seal breaks.

The use of a crown remover is, however, dependent on whether or not the channel through the crown has been prepared no deeper than the metal substructure. This can be difficult to gauge, as it is impossible to determine the thickness of the metal before starting the procedure.

The WAMkey (WAM) is currently the instrument of choice for removing crowns and even short-span fixed partial dentures intact (Figs 2-5a and 2-5b). Available in three sizes, the instrument is placed on the occlusal surface of the tooth and a rotating motion is used, allowing the crown to be lifted off. The design of the WAMkey tip prevents leverage forces from being applied when it is used. A window is prepared on the lateral aspect of the crown and the head of the WAMkey is inserted between the crown and the occlusal surface of the tooth; the instrument is then turned gently in a clockwise direction.

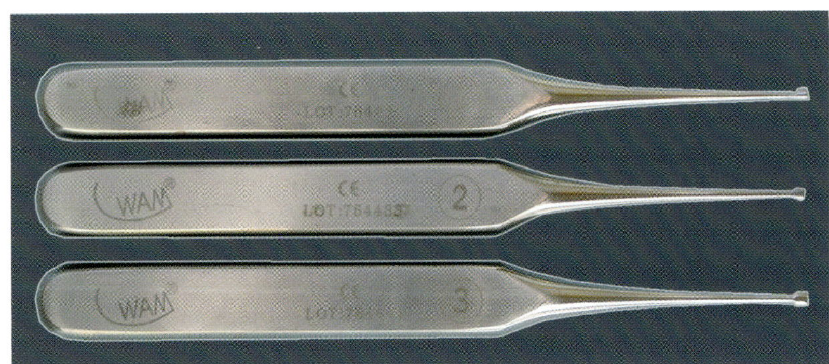

2-5a The WAMkey is available in three sizes.

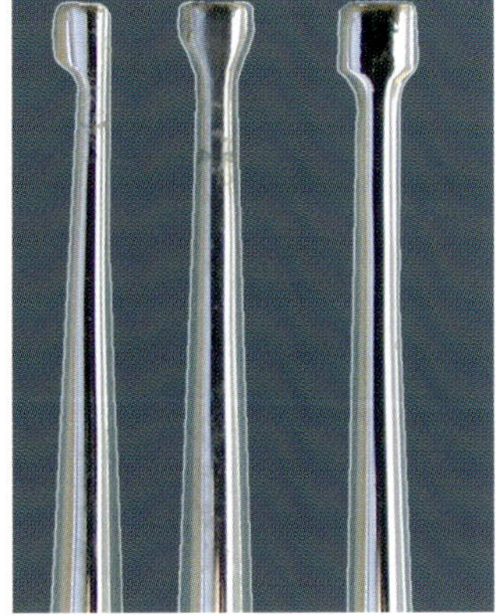

2-5b Each of the three WAmkeys features the distinctively shaped tip, characteristic of the product.

Use of the WAMkey on a porcelain-fused-to-metal crown

1. A round diamond 018 bur is used with plenty of water spray to remove porcelain from the buccal aspect of the crown (Fig 2-6a), creating a window in the porcelain. The window should be situated 2.0 mm to 2.5 mm below the buccal groove and extend depthwise until the metal substructure of the crown is just visible. It is important to use the buccal groove and not a buccal cusp as a reference point.
2. The window is then deepened and extended with a 012 transmetal bur to create a horizontal groove in the crown (Figs 2-6b and 2-6c).
3. The WAMkey #1 is inserted parallel to the occlusal surface and must penetrate through the full thickness of the crown (Fig 2-6d).
4. The instrument is rotated a quarter of a turn without forcing it and without applying any leverage. If WAMkey #1 spins with no effect, WAMkey #2 and then #3 are tried. Because of the instrument's shaped tip, rotation of the WAMkey gently lifts the crown and decementation is easily achieved (Fig 2-6e).

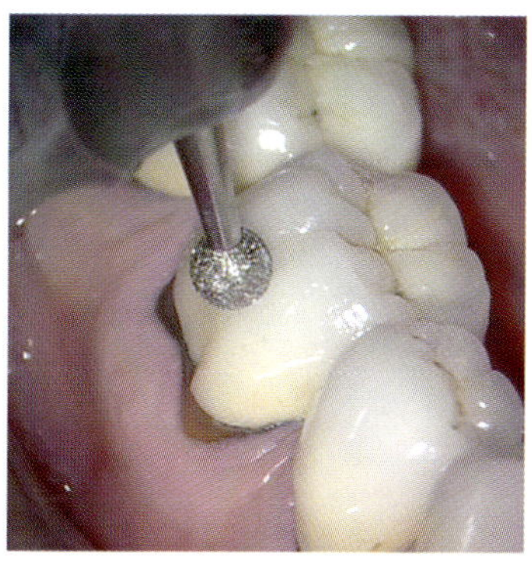

2-6a Porcelain is removed with a round diamond bur until the metal substructure of the crown is visible.

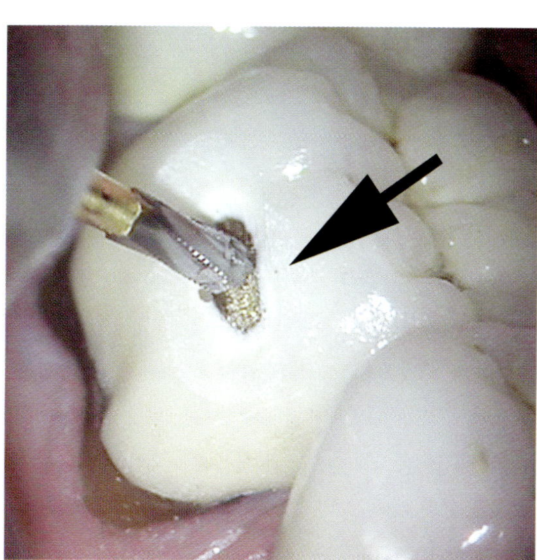

2-6b The margins of the cavity are bevelled (*black arrow*). The cavity is extended to create a horizontal groove in the crown that is parallel to the occlusal surface of the tooth. It is deepened to extend halfway into the tooth buccolingually.

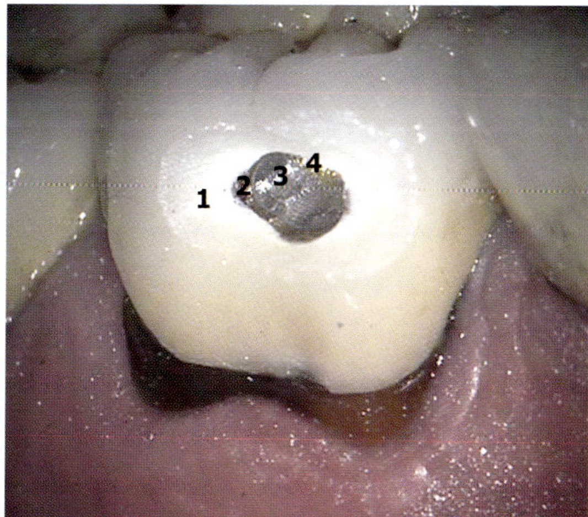

2-6c Note the following features: (1) porcelain; (2) metal substructure of the crown; (3) amalgam core; (4) gold post.

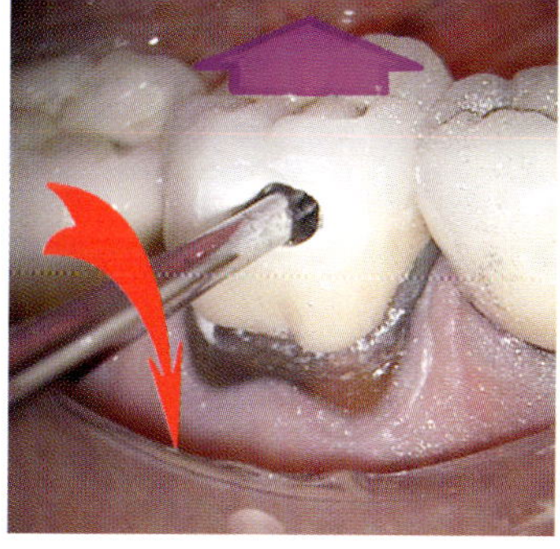

2-6d The WAMkey is inserted into the groove in the crown and positioned parallel to the occlusal surface of the tooth.

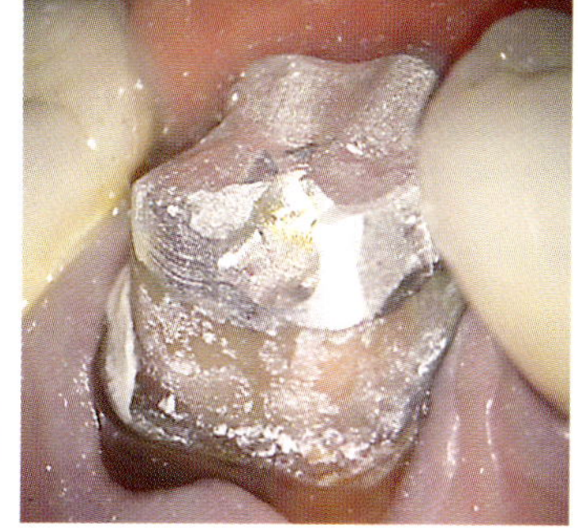

2-6e The instrument is gently rotated a quarter of a turn and the crown lifts off easily.

Use of the WAMkey on a metal crown

The technique for removal of metal crowns is the same as that for porcelain-fused-to-metal (PFM) crowns, but gaining access is slightly different. A metal crown is not as thick as a PFM crown, so the access groove in the metal crown is prepared just 1 mm below the buccal groove with a transmetal bur.

The WAMkey is suitable for removing posterior crowns in the majority of cases, where access can be gained from the palatal aspect, but it is not appropriate for use on anterior teeth.

One of the limitations of the WAMkey system is that it cannot be used for resin-bonded crowns that demonstrate good retention; these must be cut off. It is impossible to determine clinically if a crown has been cemented or bonded into place. If the crown proves impossible to remove with a gentle turn of the WAMkey, it should then be removed by sectioning. Persisting with the WAMkey in such cases may result in fracture of the instrument. The WAMkey is simple, quick, and easy to use. Since little damage is done to the crown during removal, it can be reused as a provisional restoration during endodontic treatment. Although other systems for crown removal are described in the literature (eg, modified enamel chisel, large burs), these techniques rely on a rocking movement and create leverage forces, which may fracture the tooth. The distinctively shaped tip of the WAMkey allows crowns to be removed atraumatically along the long axis of the tooth.

Sectioning crowns

Sectioning a crown involves sacrificing the crown to preserve as much of the underlying tooth structure as possible.

1. Using an appropriate bur (capable of cutting through both metal and ceramic, if necessary), the clinician makes a vertical cut in the buccal wall of the crown and extends it to the occlusal surface. This groove must go through the full thickness of the crown so that the cement layer is visible (Fig 2-7a).
2. A flat-edged instrument is inserted into the groove in the crown so that the two parts of the crown are separated; it is essential that no leverage forces are applied (Fig 2-7b).
3. An ultrasonic instrument placed between the crown and the underlying tooth breaks up the cement layer.
4. With an excavator placed at the margin, the crown is delicately removed.

If mechanical retention features have been used (slots, grooves), sectioning the crown in this way will not be sufficient. The additional retention features will determine the path of removal of the crown. In cases where little movement can be gained, it is better to section the crown into multiple pieces rather than to continue putting force on the tooth.

Regardless of the technique used, the clinician should never attempt to remove a crown by applying leverage forces, especially when the crown is post-retained. Removal must always be done gently and should be along the path of insertion. Use of excessive force risks fracture of the underlying tooth.

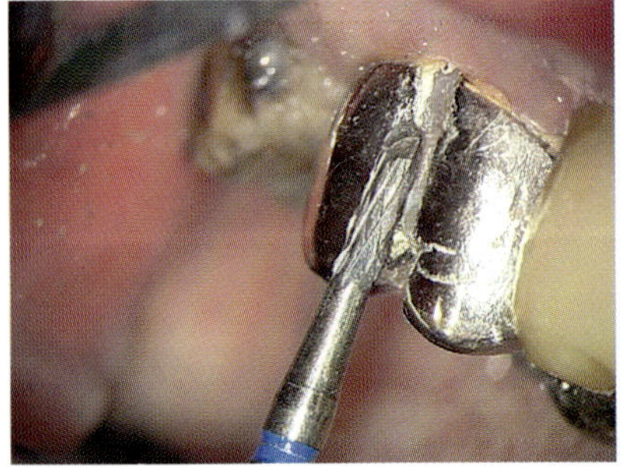

2-7a The crown is sectioned on the buccal and occlusal surfaces.

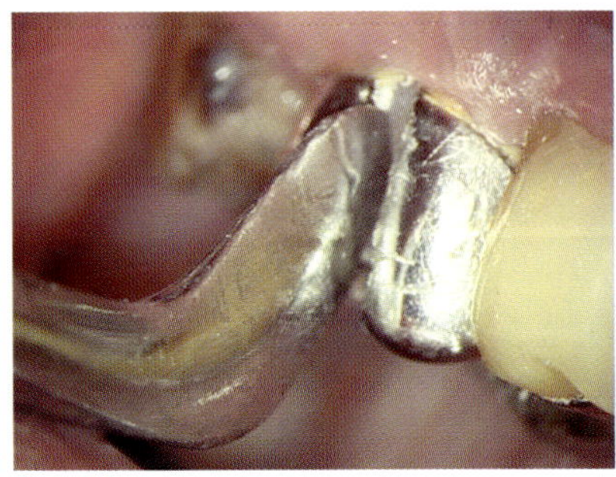

2-7b A flat-edged instrument is used to separate the two parts of the crown.

Fixed partial dentures

Removing a fixed partial denture (FPD) is more complicated than removing an individual crown because of the multiple abutment teeth. The path of removal can be difficult to identify, particularly in terms of buccolingual angulation. Only short-span FPDs (3 or 4 units) can be safely removed intact.

Use of a crown remover with the parachute technique

In the parachute technique, the cable is passed under the FPD and crossed back the other way to wrap around the pontic (Fig 2-8a). Once the electric crown remover is activated and the flexible cable aligns itself along the path of removal of the FPD, the device can be used to safely remove the FPD intact (Fig 2-8b). This technique is uncomfortable for the patient, particularly when used in the maxillary posterior region; this may be due to resonance in the maxillary sinus.

Use of the WAMkey

Each FPD retainer is treated as an individual crown. A horizontal groove is cut in the buccal aspect of each retainer, and the WAMkey is used on each in turn, breaking the cement seal and loosening the FPD. Once each of the retainers has been decemented, the FPD can then be lifted off in one piece (Figs 2-9a and 2-9b).

Long-span fixed partial dentures

Long-span FPDs should be sectioned between the abutment teeth, and each part should be removed as though it were a short-span FPD or an individual crown.

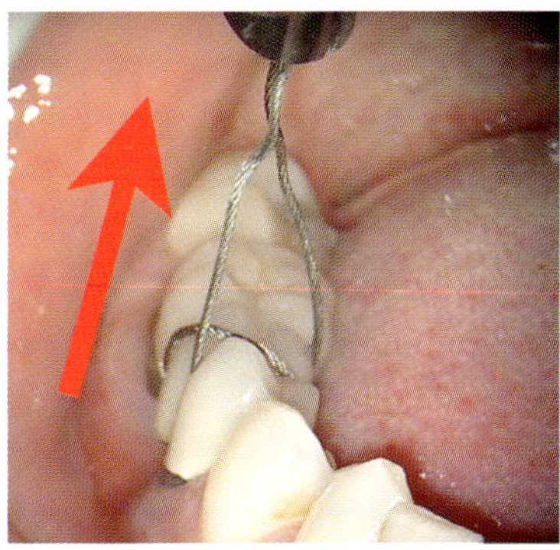

2-8a The parachute technique is the only method of FPD removal that ensures that forces are transmitted down the long axis of the teeth.

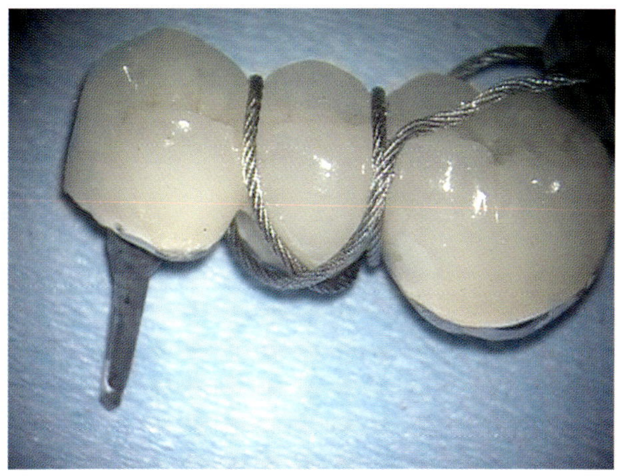

2-8b Passing the cable around the pontic allows short-span FPDs to be safely removed.

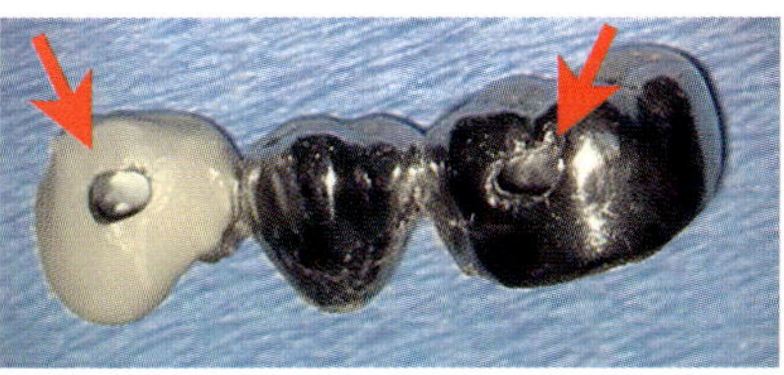

2-9a Short-span FPDs can be removed with the WAMkey. Each retainer is treated as an individual crown.

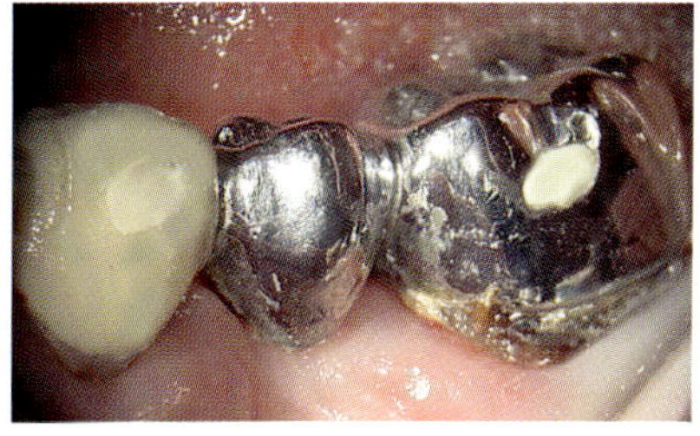

2-9b Since it is removed intact, the FPD can be used as a provisional restoration until a definitive restoration is placed.

The decision of which crown/FPD removal technique to use for a particular case must be made with the aim of preserving as much of the underlying tooth structure as possible. If there is any doubt about the type of restoration or the nature of the underlying core, the crown/FPD should be sectioned and removed in pieces; attempts to remove it intact may harm the remaining tooth structure. Regardless of the removal method, the old restoration should never be refitted as a definitive restoration. If it is removed intact, it may be used temporarily as a provisional restoration.

Removal of Restorative Material and Posts

A tooth that has been restored with a post-retained crown must have the post removed before conventional root canal retreatment can be undertaken. Posts are not visible on clinical examination; only a preoperative radiograph will provide the necessary information about the type and shape of post used. Specific techniques for removal of each of the following will be discussed: passive posts, threaded posts, indirect posts, split pin posts, carbon fiber posts, glass fiber posts, and ceramic posts.

Passive posts

Passive posts are sometimes known as *smooth-sided posts*. In reality, they are rarely totally smooth and tend to have slight irregularities, which the luting agent flows into, thus improving the retention. Although generally made of stainless steel, they can also be made from titanium. The posts can be parallel, tapered, or a combination of both. Because of the parallelism of the tooth's walls, a parallel post is harder to remove than a tapered one.

Once the crown has been removed, the post must be gently loosened with ultrasonic vibration. Post removal relies on breaking the cement seal; the easiest and quickest way of doing this is with ultrasonic instruments. A large ultrasonic tip (Insert ETPR, Acteon) or a ball-ended tip (ProUltra no.1, Dentsply) should be used at maximum power and placed on the coronal aspect of the post. The vibrations are transmitted down the length of the post and cause the cement seal to break. The instrument is used without water spray and directed up and down the visible part of the post. It must not remain stationary on the post.

When the post loosens, it is carefully removed with tweezers. With passive posts, even slight movement of the post indicates that the cement seal has been broken and that there is no need for further ultrasonic instrumentation. Because ultrasonic vibrations create heat and the instrument is used without water spray, it is important to check the handpiece regularly during the procedure to ensure it is not heating up. Instruments that overheat can induce bony necrosis and periodontal complications.

Threaded posts

These can usually be easily identified on radiographs. The most common type is the Screw Post (Henry Schein), but other brands such as Flexi-Post (Essential Dental Systems) are also widely used. Posts are rarely screwed or threaded into dentin because of the risk of microcrack formation. The thread of the post offers a form of secondary retention: the luting agent locks into the threads and provides good mechanical retention.

Before a threaded post is removed, it is impossible to determine whether it has been screwed into the canal or simply cemented in; the technique for removal is the same in both cases. These posts must be unscrewed to be removed. A simple elevation force risks fracturing the post or the root. The cement should be carefully cleared away to reveal the coronal part of the post (Figs 2-10a to 2-10c). The ultrasonic instrument (ProUltra no.1) is set to maximum power and placed against the top of the post. Keeping the instrument in contact with the post, the operator moves the ultrasonic tip in a counterclockwise direction to unscrew the post (Fig 2-10d).

Manual screwdrivers for removing threaded posts are also available (Fig 2-11). Screwdrivers can be difficult to use if the post is damaged, and great care must be taken when clearing around the coronal part of the post. A trephine with a known diameter can be used to modify the diameter of the post. A calibrated tubular tap can then be threaded onto the post in a counterclockwise direction, thus unscrewing the post.

If a post fractures during removal, the ProUltra no. 2 and no. 3 ultrasonic tips can be used to create a trench around the fractured post (Figs 2-12a and 2-12b). A ball-ended ultrasonic tip is then inserted in this trough and used at maximum power in a counterclockwise direction to unscrew the fragment (Figs 2-12c and 2-12d). This technique aims to preserve as much tooth tissue as possible.

2-10a and 2-10b The coronal part of the post is carefully revealed.

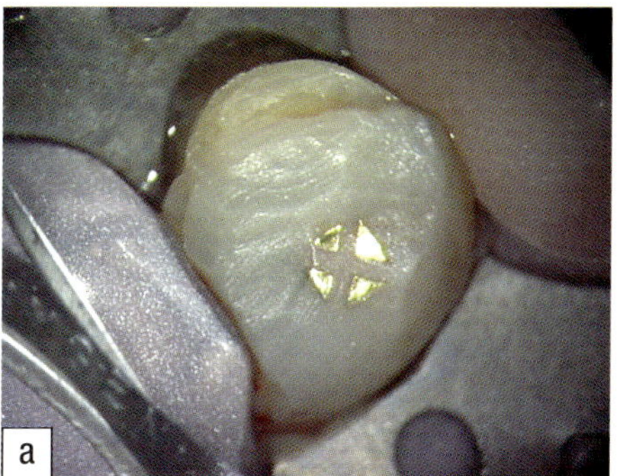

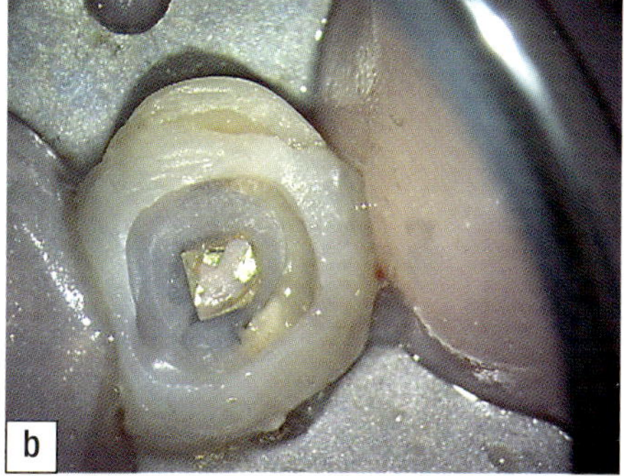

2-10c An ultrasonic instrument (ProUltra no. 2 or no. 3) is carefully used to completely free the top of the post without damaging it.

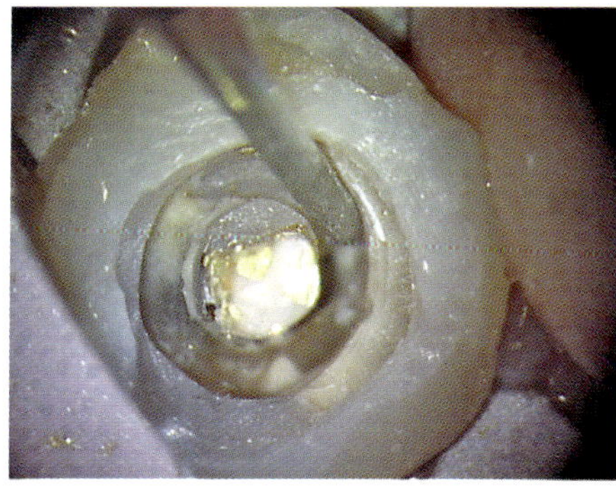

2-10d The ProUltra no. 1 ultrasonic tip is used at maximum power and rotated in a counterclockwise direction around the post to unscrew it.

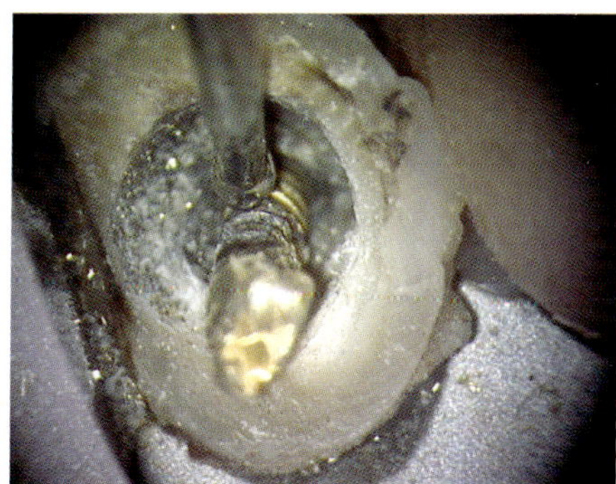

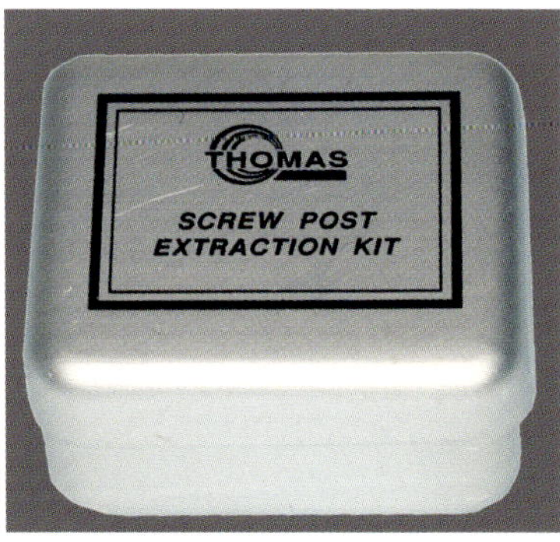

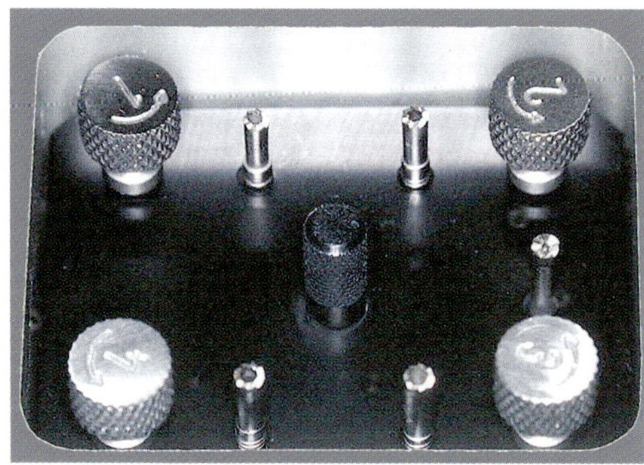

2-11 This screw post extraction kit (FFDM-Pneumat) offers four screwdrivers of different sizes.

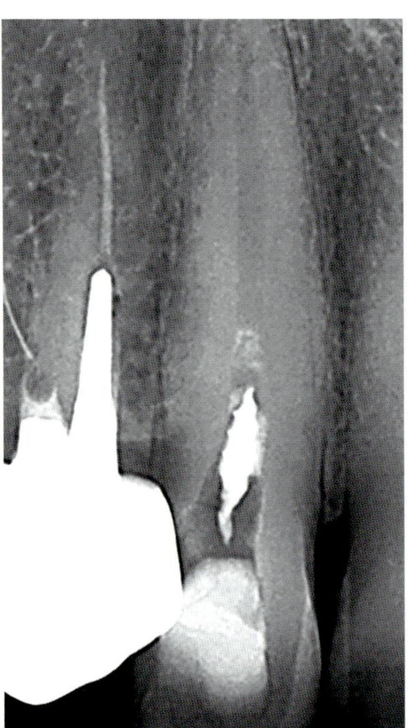

2-12a Preoperative radiograph of a maxillary canine with a fractured post.

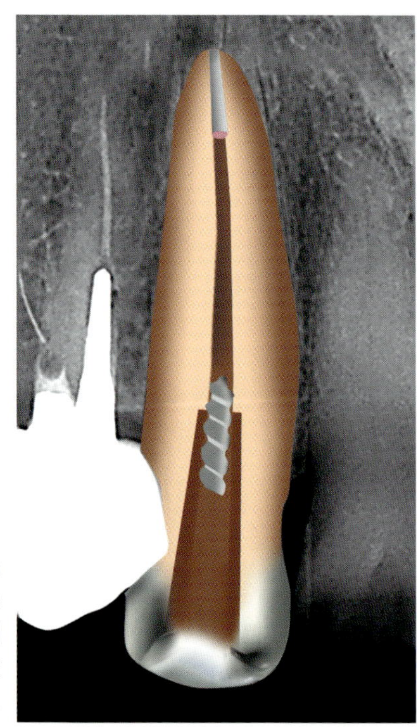

2-12b An ultrasonic tip is used to create a trough around the fractured post (ProUltra no. 2 or no. 3).

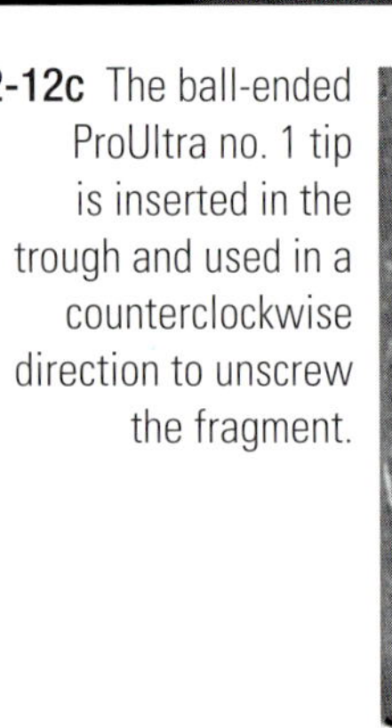

2-12c The ball-ended ProUltra no. 1 tip is inserted in the trough and used in a counterclockwise direction to unscrew the fragment.

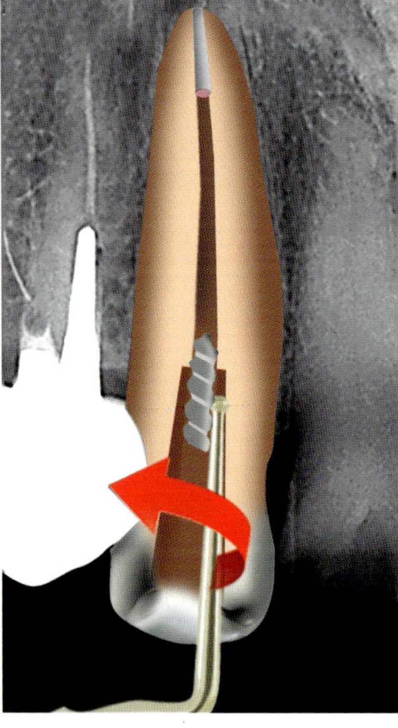

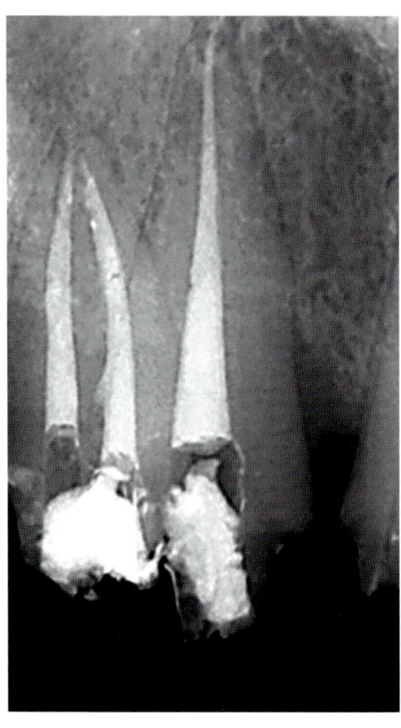

2-12d Once the fractured post is removed, the retreatment can be completed.

Indirect casted posts

Indirect posts are cast to fit the root canal perfectly. They are highly retentive and therefore can prove difficult to remove. The greater the length and the diameter of the post, the greater the surface area for cementation. An endodontically prepared tooth with only thin residual walls is particularly fragile. A long, wide, parallel post will be more difficult to remove than a short, narrow, tapered post. Casted posts are often placed for a post-retained crown or as part of a split pin post restoration. Removal of casted posts is similar to removal of direct posts: the first step is to free the coronal part of the post. The difficulty and speed with which this is done depends on the type of coronal restoration in place. *This stage is done using a water-cooled high-speed handpiece. Several bur changes may be necessary to replace burs blunted by the metal.* This action transforms the post-retained crown into a simple post. The vibrations of the ultrasonic instruments should then be sufficient to dislodge the remaining restoration; no attempts should be made to remove the post by applying lateral force, as the risk of root fracture is high.

Universal Post Remover

The Gonon post remover was introduced more than 40 years ago. It was recently modified to include four stainless steel tubular taps that work in a counterclockwise direction, which means the system can now also be used for the removal of active threaded posts. A color-coded system has been incorporated to facilitate the use of the Universal Post Remover (Fig 2-13).

The device exerts traction on the post while applying a downward force on the tooth itself. The design of the extractor with its metal and rubber washers ensures that the extraction force is always applied along the path of insertion (Machtou, 1993). When used correctly, the universal post remover is very successful: 99.4% of passive posts can be removed without the risk of root fracture (Abbott, 2002).

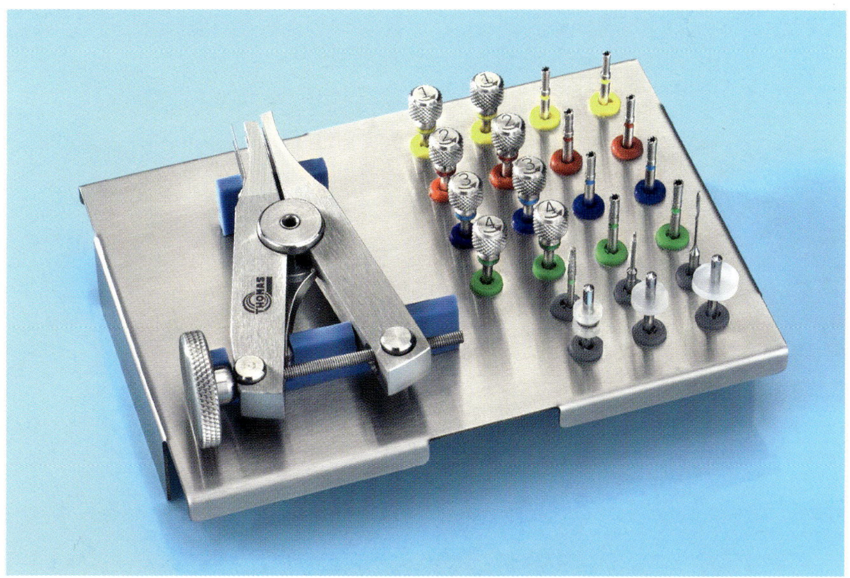

2-13 There are fewer instruments in this updated version of the universal post remover kit (FFDM-Pneumat). The new tubular taps are used in a counterclockwise direction, contrary to the original version.

Technique

1. The post and core or post-retained crown must be transformed into a simple post and modified to match the cylinder shape of the tubular tap (Figs 2-14a to 2-14c).
2. The top of the post is rounded off with a diamond bur.
3. The diameter of the post is gauged, and the appropriate tubular tap with the same diameter is selected.
4. The post is modified and its diameter calibrated (Fig 2-14d) using the trephine that corresponds to the selected tubular tap.
5. The tubular tap includes a brass washer, a convex steel washer (if the edges of the root are irregular), and a rubber washer that lies against the tooth.
6. The tubular tap is then gently screwed onto the post in a counterclockwise direction; in this way the device threads into the metal of the post (Figs 2-14e and 2-14f).
7. An ultrasonic tip is placed on the tubular tap to vibrate the post.
8. The universal extractor is positioned and the wheel is turned slowly and evenly in a clockwise direction. The rotation of the wheel causes the jaws of the extractor to open; the lower jaw rests on the tooth while the upper jaw exerts traction on the tubular tap and therefore indirectly on the post along its long axis (Fig 2-14g).
9. The post is removed easily, and the endodontic treatment can begin (Figs 2-14h and 2-14i).

Necessary precautions

- The axis of the post must not be modified during the preparation stages; if the angle were to be altered, the traction force would not be exerted correctly along the long axis of the post.
- The largest possible tubular tap should be selected.
- A drop of oil can be placed on the inside of the tubular tap to make it easier to thread it onto the post.

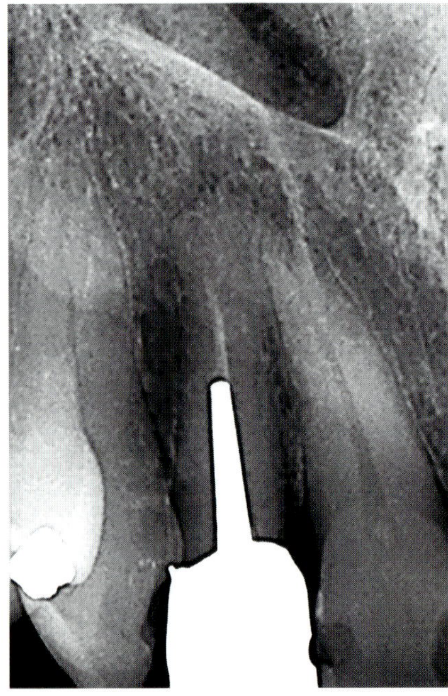

2-14a Preoperative radiograph of a maxillary lateral incisor restored with a post and core.

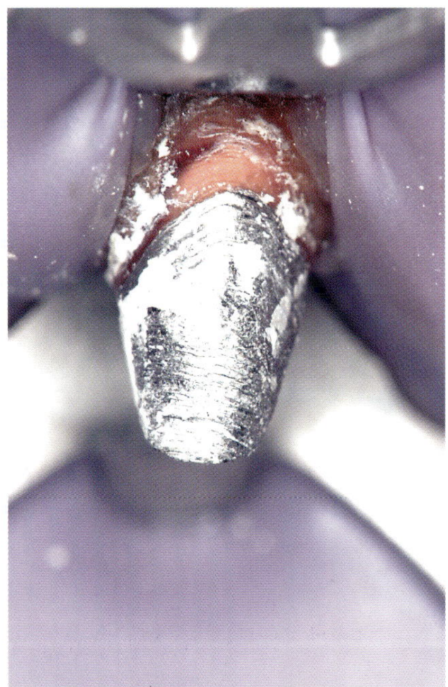

2-14b The crown is removed first.

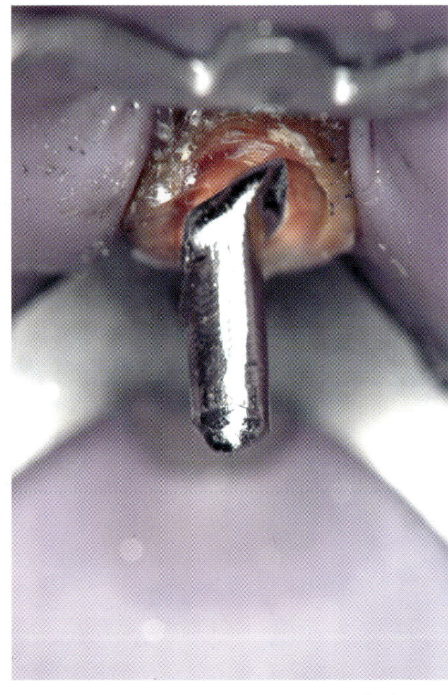

2-14c The post is modified to match the cylinder shape of the tubular tap. The top of the post is rounded off with a diamond bur.

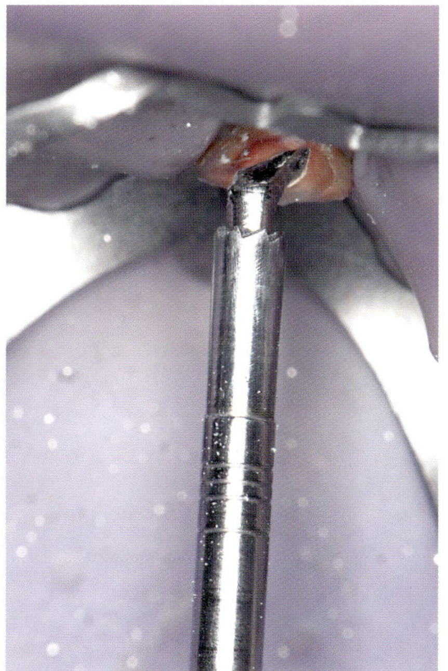

2-14d The stump is calibrated with a size 4 trephine.

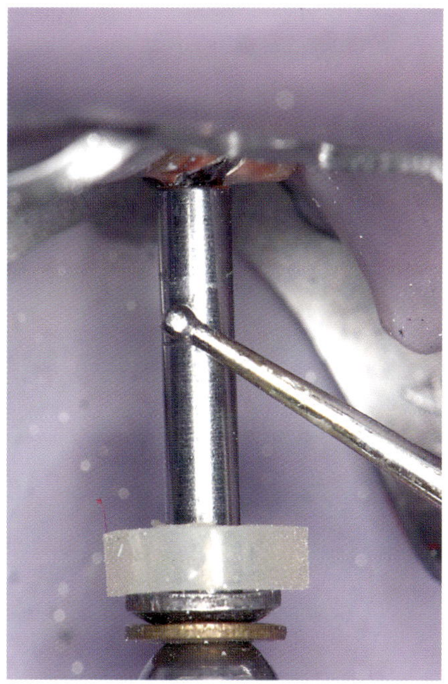

2-14e The size 4 tubular tap is screwed onto the post in a clockwise direction and the ensemble is vibrated with an ultrasonic tip.

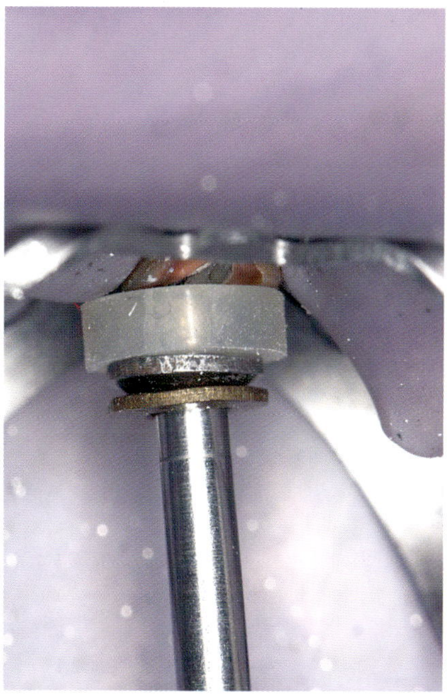

2-14f The washers are placed on the tubular tap in the following order: rubber washer, convex steel washer, brass washer.

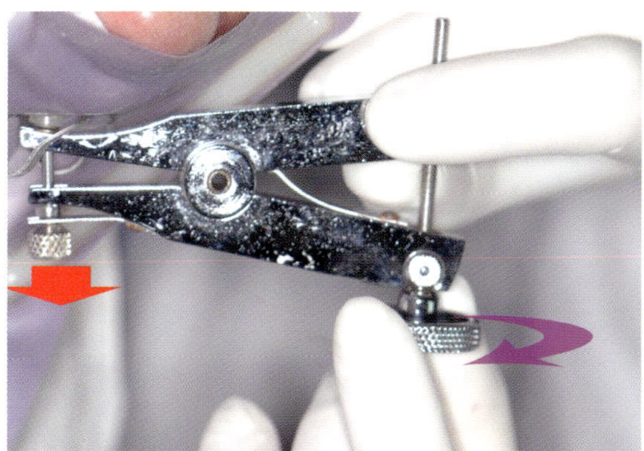

2-14g The jaws of the extractor are positioned. The rotation of the wheel allows the extractor to open; the lower jaw rests on the washers and the tooth, and the upper jaw exerts traction on the tubular tap.

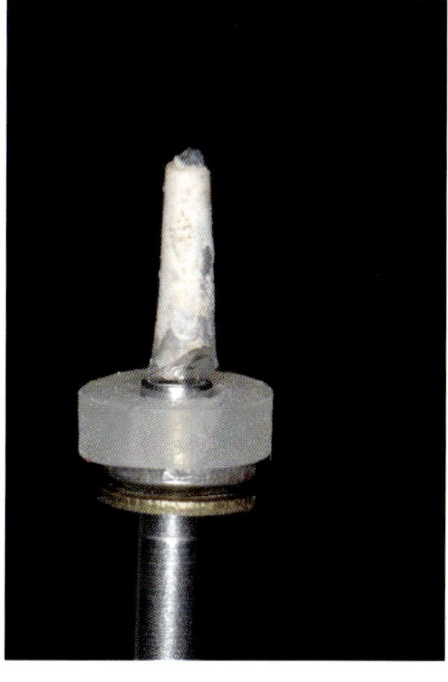

2-14h The post is removed along the path of insertion without harming the root.

2-14i The canal is now accessible and ready for retreatment.

WAM X

The WAM X (WAM) is a post removal system consisting of a set of forceps and three pairs of pronged attachments. The attachments can be mounted on the forceps and freely rotated in any direction on their axis (Figs 2-15a to 2-15c). The clinician cuts horizontal grooves mesially and distally through the full thickness of the crown, allowing the forceps with its prongs to be positioned. The force produced by the forceps is enough to break the cement seal. The rotation of the attachments directs the force along the correct axis and thus limits the risk of root fracture.
Although attractive in principle and effective in practice, the WAM X is difficult to operate. The WAM X system is most commonly used for removing post-retained crowns, as it avoids the laborious preparation stage needed to use the universal device. The grooves that are cut into the sides of the crown expose the root face on which one of the attachments will rest (Figs 2-15d to 2-15h). However, as post-retained crowns tend to have a ledge at the gingival or just subgingival level, this maneuver can be risky for both the tooth and the interproximal gingiva.

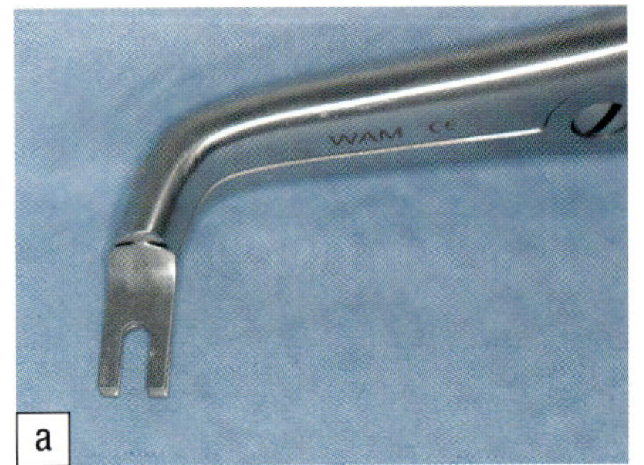

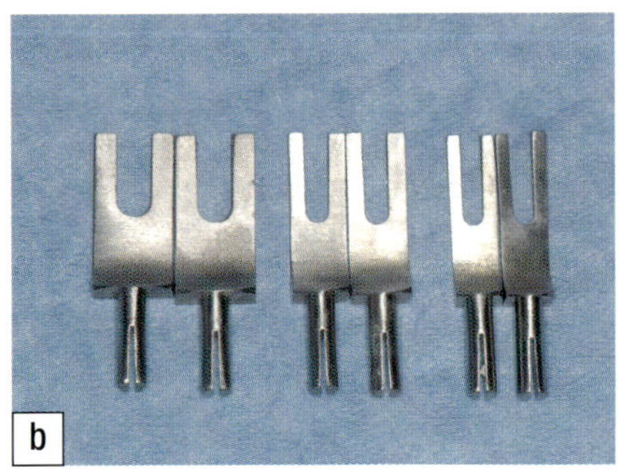

2-15a and 2-15b The WAM X system consists of a set of forceps and three pairs of pronged attachments.

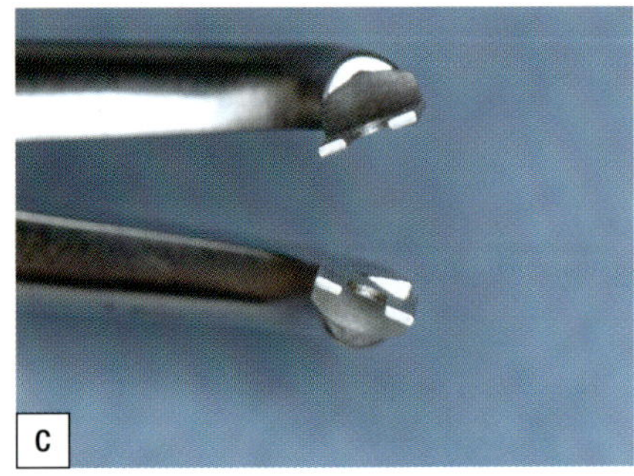

2-15c The free rotation of the prongs directs the force along the correct axis without risking any harm to the root.

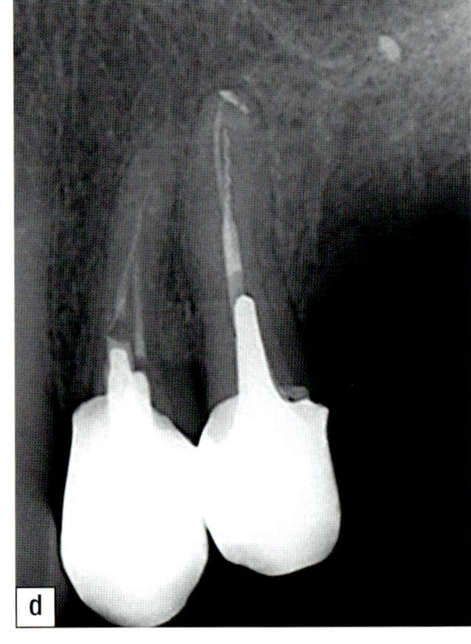

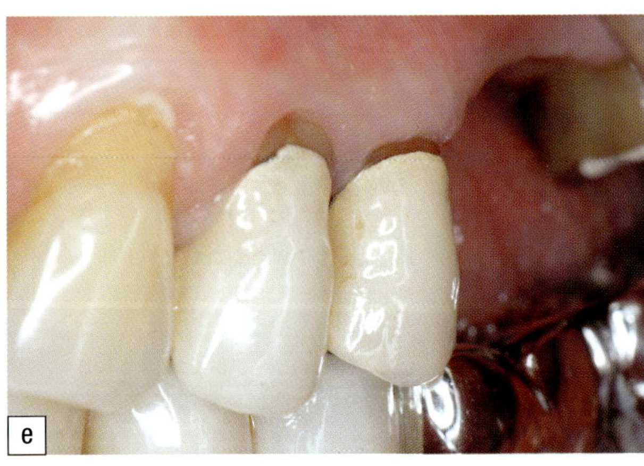

2-15d and 2-15e The post-retained crown on the maxillary left second premolar needs to be removed so endodontic retreatment can be performed.

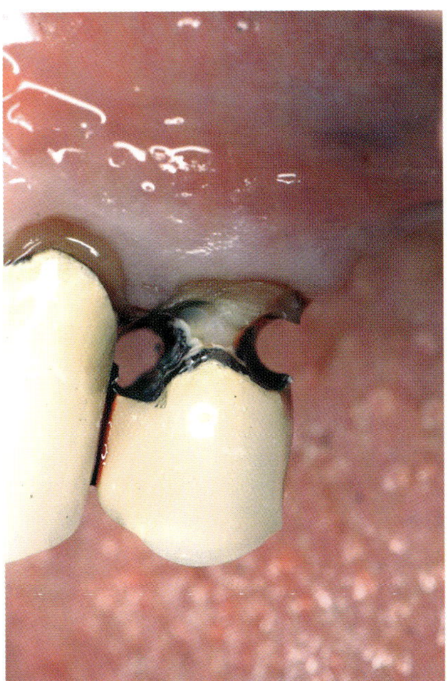

2-15f Horizontal grooves are cut in the sides of the crown and should extend the full depth of the crown. The root face must be laid bare so the attachments can be positioned on the surface.

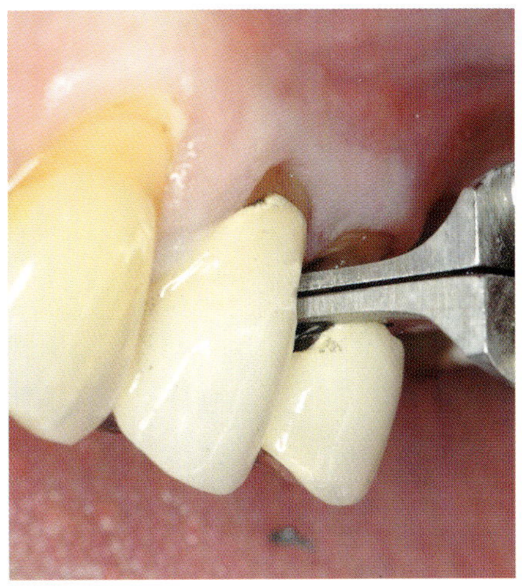

2-15g The grooves must be large enough to allow two of the pronged attachments to be positioned on top of each other.

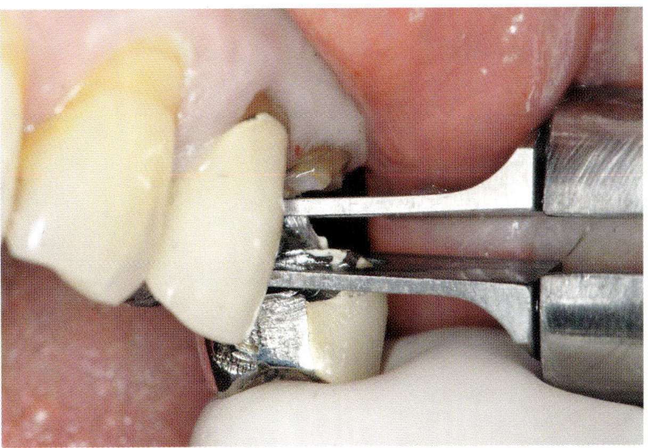

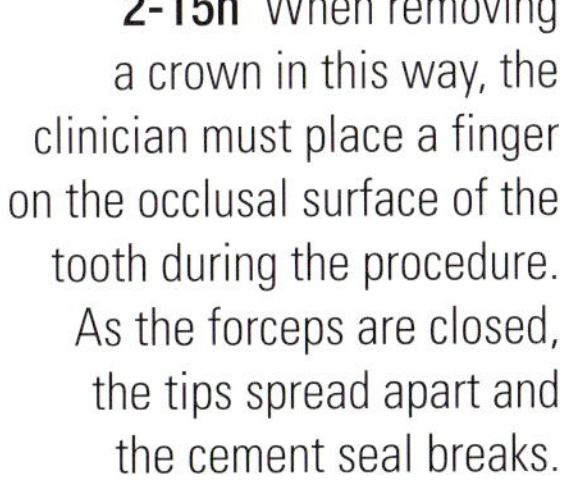

2-15h When removing a crown in this way, the clinician must place a finger on the occlusal surface of the tooth during the procedure. As the forceps are closed, the tips spread apart and the cement seal breaks.

Split pin posts

Split pin posts must be sectioned into as many fragments as there are posts in order to be removed (Figs 2-16a to 2-16h). The difficulty lies in sectioning the coronal aspect. A transmetal bur should be used in a high-speed handpiece; a low-speed handpiece is not suitable. Great care must be taken when sectioning a split pin post to ensure the pulp chamber floor is not damaged or perforated.

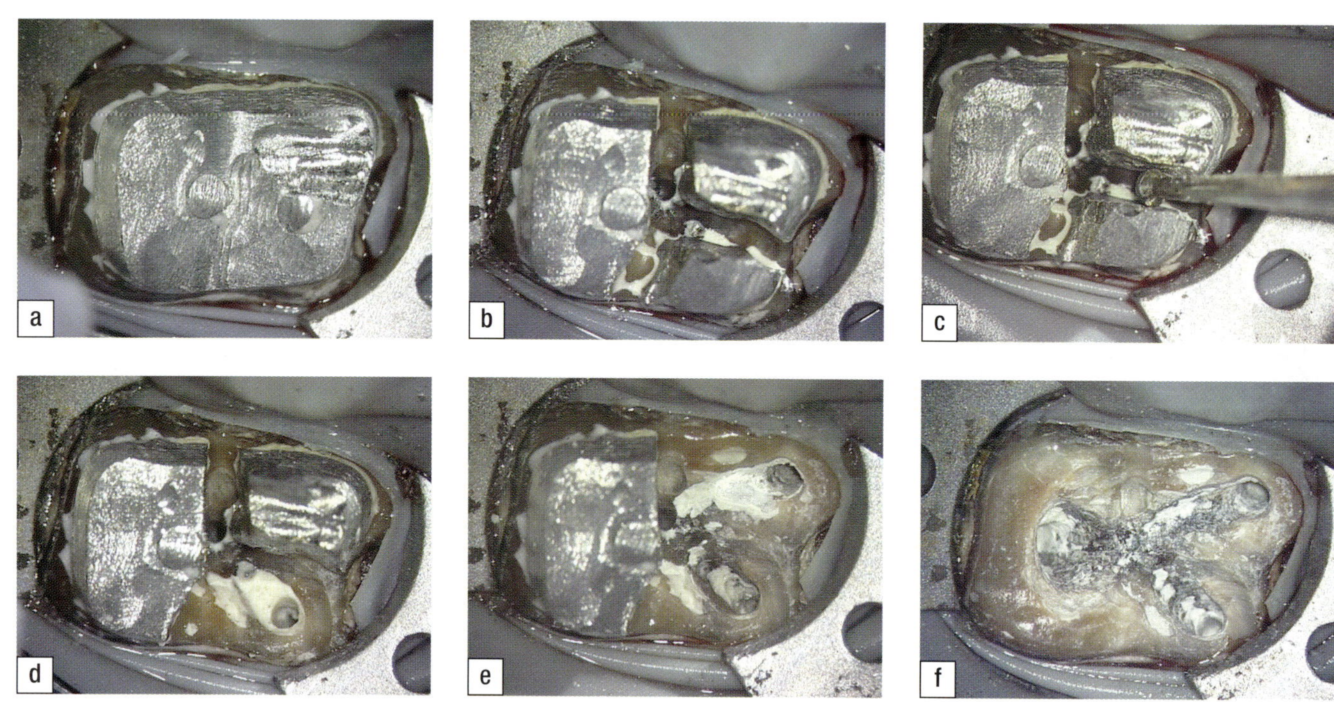

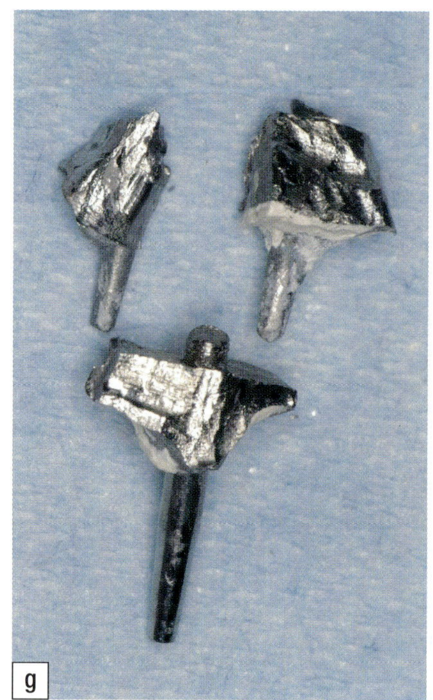

2-16 *(a)* This molar was reconstructed with the use of a split pin post. *(b)* To be removed, the split pin post had to be sectioned into three pieces with a transmetal bur. *(c to e)* Each section is removed with the use of an ultrasonic tip at maximum power. *(f and g)* With the split pin post removed, *(h)* retreatment can be undertaken.

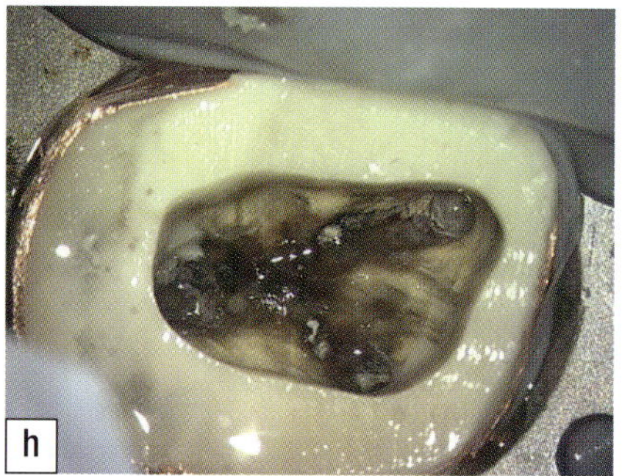

Bitewing radiographs can be a useful guide as to the thickness of the remaining material (Figs 2-17a to 2-17c). Once separated, each section is then treated as a simple post and ultrasonic vibration is used to break the cement seal.

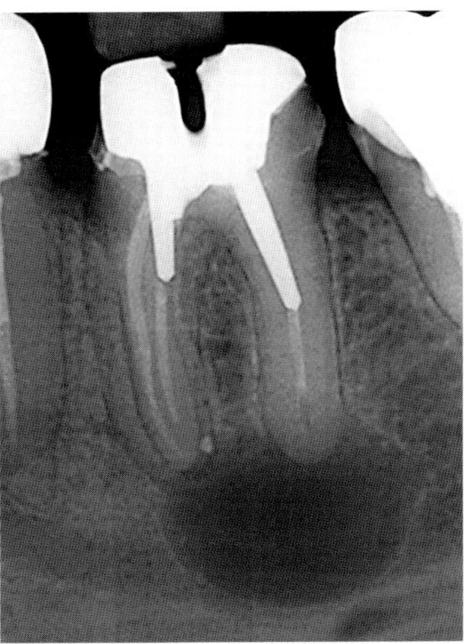
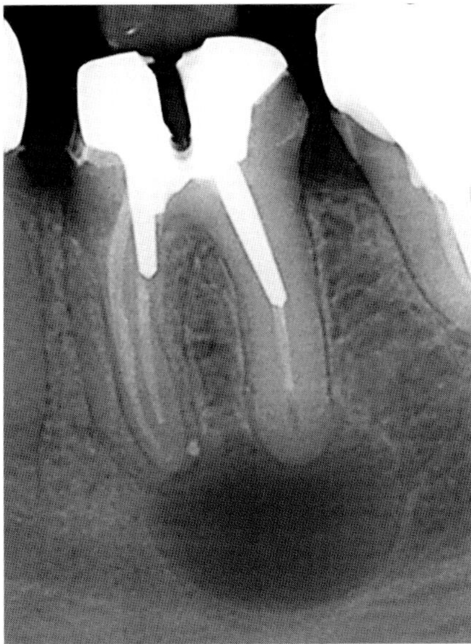
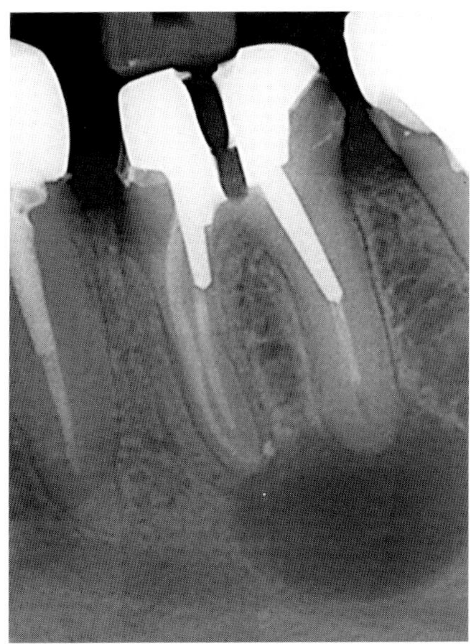

2-17a, 2-17b and 2-17c Periapical radiographs taken during the removal of a split pin post allow the procedure to be assessed midtreatment. They also help ensure the pulpal floor is not damaged. This technique is not applicable to the maxillary molars.

Fiber posts

In recent years nonmetallic posts have been used more and more frequently to restore teeth with bonded post-retained crowns. These posts are made up of carbon fibers (black posts) or glass fibers (white posts) embedded in a resin matrix. Because these posts are not radiopaque, the canal appears empty on radiographic examination. After they are bonded into the prepared canals, these posts cannot be simply dislodged but must be drilled out (Figs 2-18a and 2-18b).

Technique for removal

1. The coronal restoration is removed and the pulp chamber is thoroughly cleaned. Contrary to metal posts, fiber posts are sectioned at the orifice of the canal, and the top of the post is removed (Fig 2-18c).
2. A small hole is made in the center of the fiber post with a small round diamond bur (Fig 2-18d).
3. The length of the post is assessed from preoperative radiographs and is marked with a rubber stop on a size 1 Gates Glidden drill (Dentsply-Maillefer).
4. The tip of the drill is placed in the prepared hole, and it is rotated at 800 rpm (Fig 2-18e).
5. The pathway is then enlarged with Gates Glidden drills size 2, 3, and 4 (Fig 2-18f), and the remainder of the post is removed (Figs 2-18g and 2-18h).

Some authors recommend the use of ultrasonic instruments to remove fiber posts. However, this is a time-consuming process and, if used for carbon fiber posts, generates a cloud of black dust.

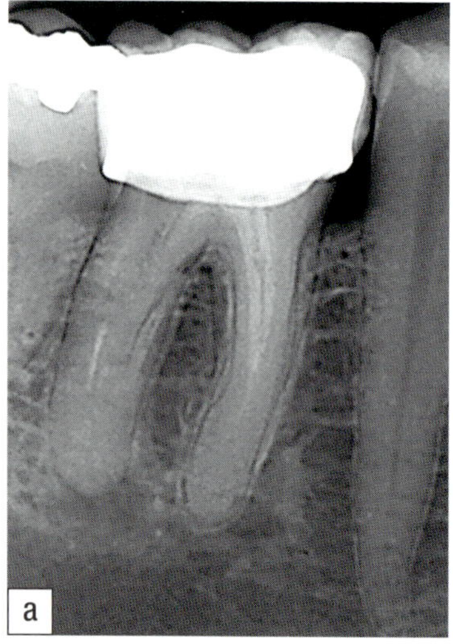

b

2-18a and 2-18b The carbon fiber post in the distal root of this mandibular molar could not be detected radiographically.

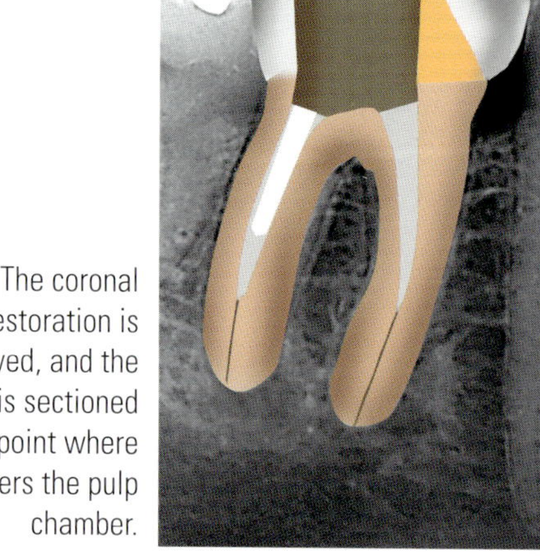

2-18c The coronal restoration is removed, and the post is sectioned at the point where it enters the pulp chamber.

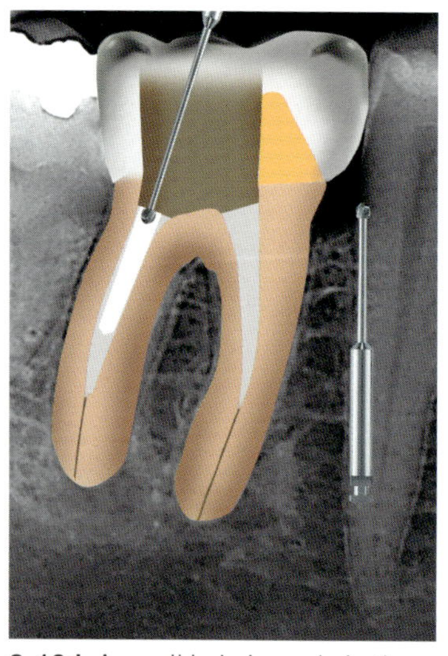

2-18d A small hole is made in the post with a round diamond bur.

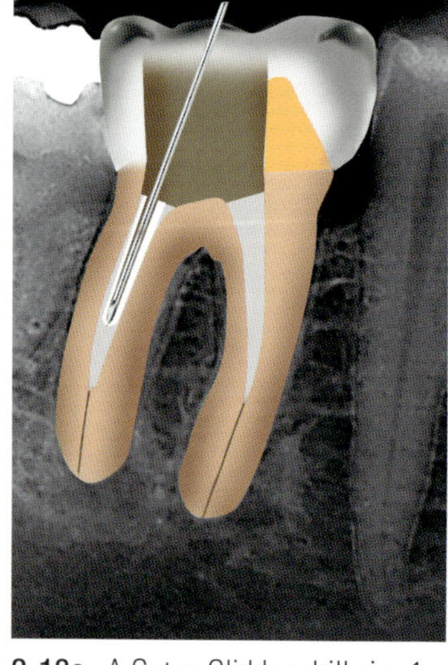

2-18e A Gates Glidden drill size 1 is used at 800 rpm to penetrate between the fibers of the post.

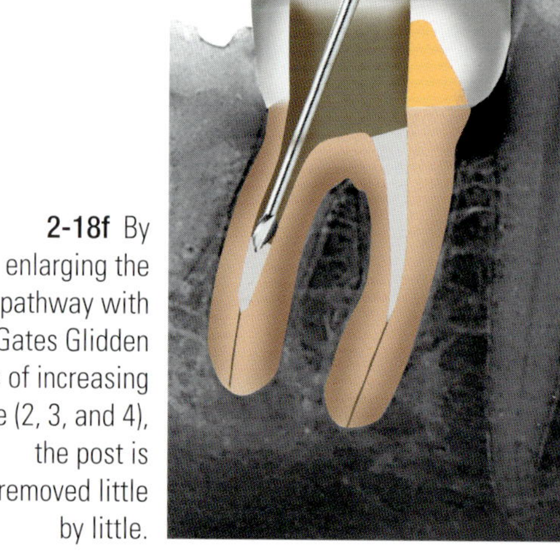

2-18f By enlarging the pathway with Gates Glidden drills of increasing size (2, 3, and 4), the post is removed little by little.

2-18g Once the post has been removed, a file can be used to negotiate the canal to the apex.

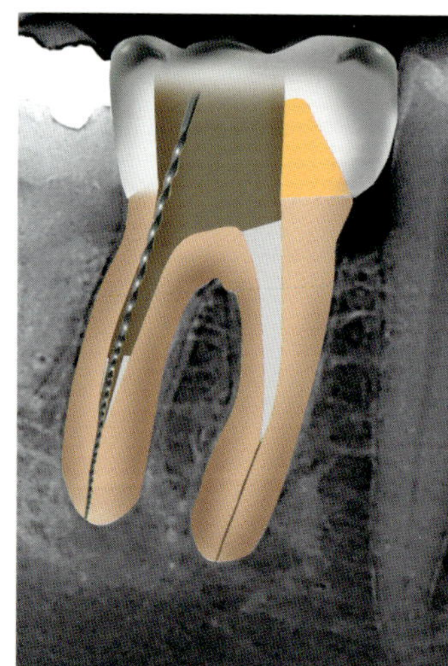

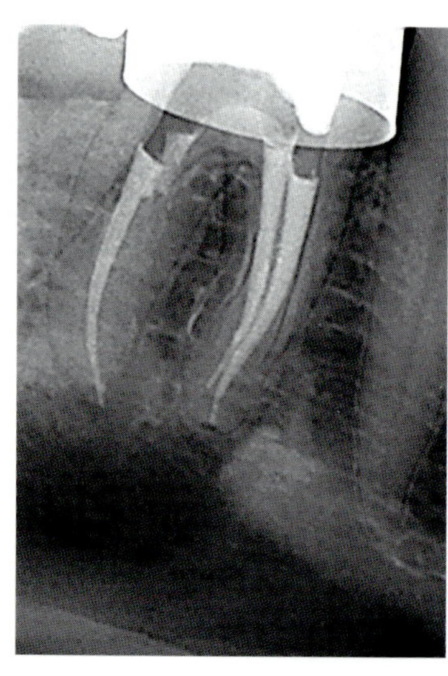

2-18h Endodontic retreatment can now be completed.

Ceramic posts

Ceramic posts are bonded into the root canal, and removing them is difficult. They cannot be merely "debonded." The strength of the material makes it impossible to vibrate them out with ultrasonics, simply grip them, or thread a post remover onto them. The only way to remove them is to drill them out (Figs 2-19a to 2-19f). This is a delicate procedure that must be done under magnification—ideally a microscope. Perforations can be prevented by studying the preoperative radiographs to determine the angulation of the post. Diamond or tungsten carbide burs can be used but will need to be replaced regularly. The procedure must be performed with copious water spray to avoid overheating the ceramic and endangering the periodontal tissues.

2-19a and 2-19b Preoperative clinical and radiographic views of a lateral incisor with a fractured ceramic post.

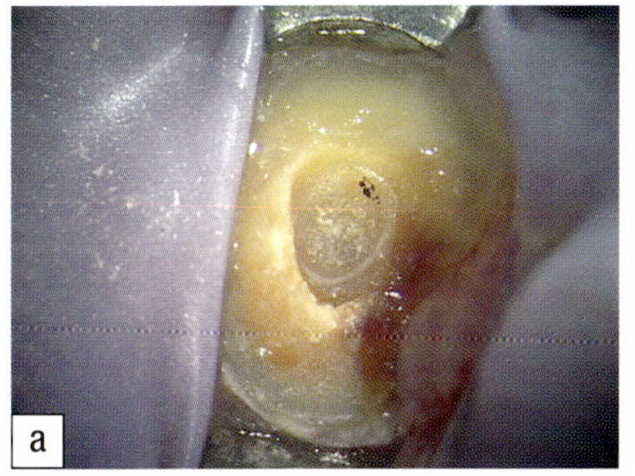

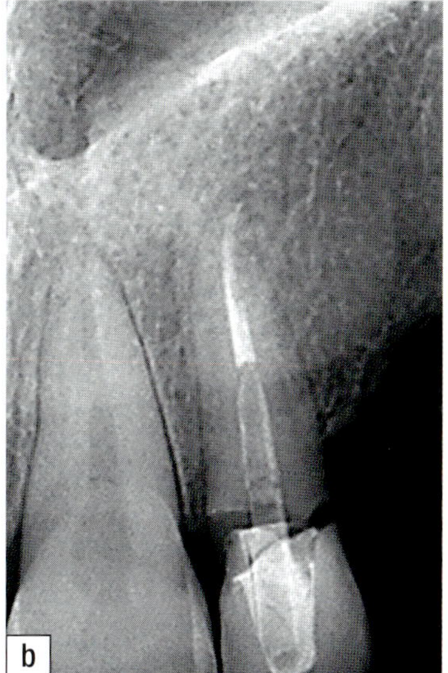

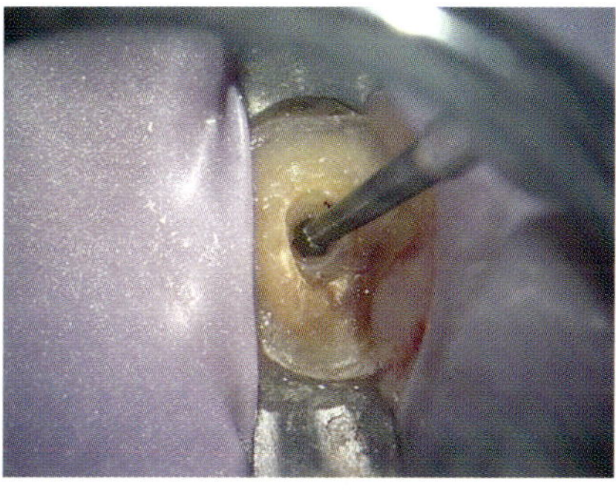

2-19c The post is carefully drilled away. A tungsten carbide bur is used in a high-speed handpiece, with lots of water spray.

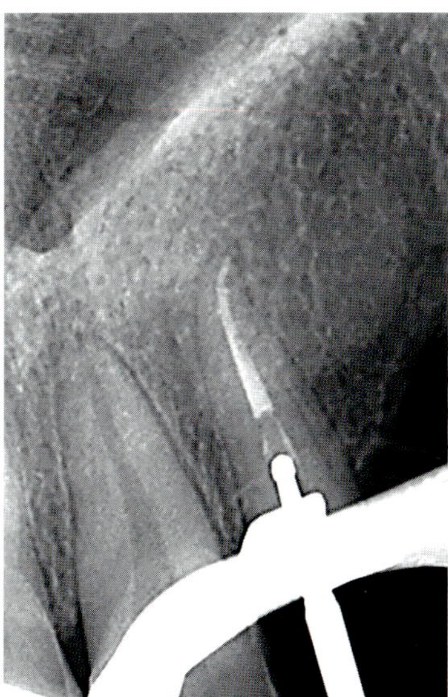

2-19d Radiographs can be taken at regular intervals to verify the angulation of the drill.

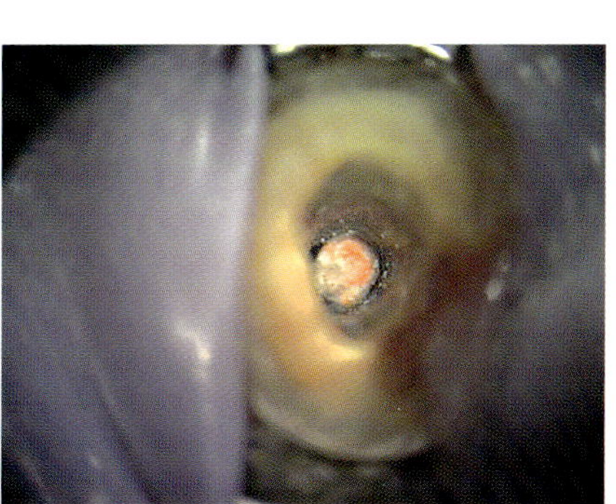

2-19e Little by little, the post is completely removed, and the obturation material in the apical part of the canal becomes visible.

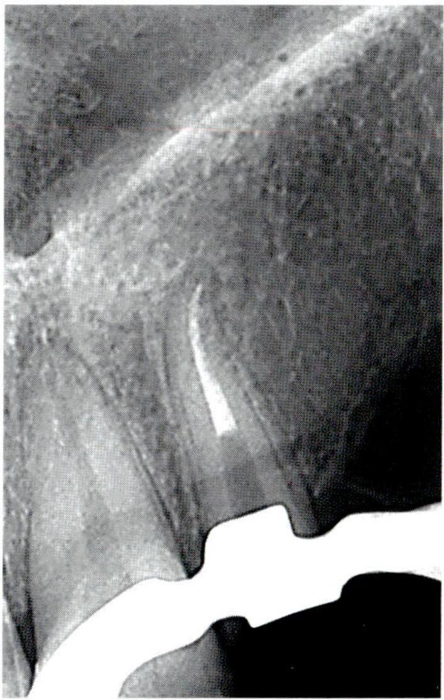

2-19f Postoperative radiograph.

Once the crown and the root filling have been removed, the tooth is restored. The missing walls are replaced so that a rubber dam clamp can be positioned and a stable four-walled access cavity can be prepared.

Access, Removal of Obturation Materials,

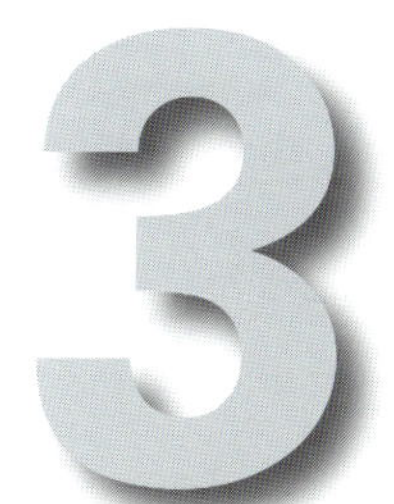

and Negotiation of Canals

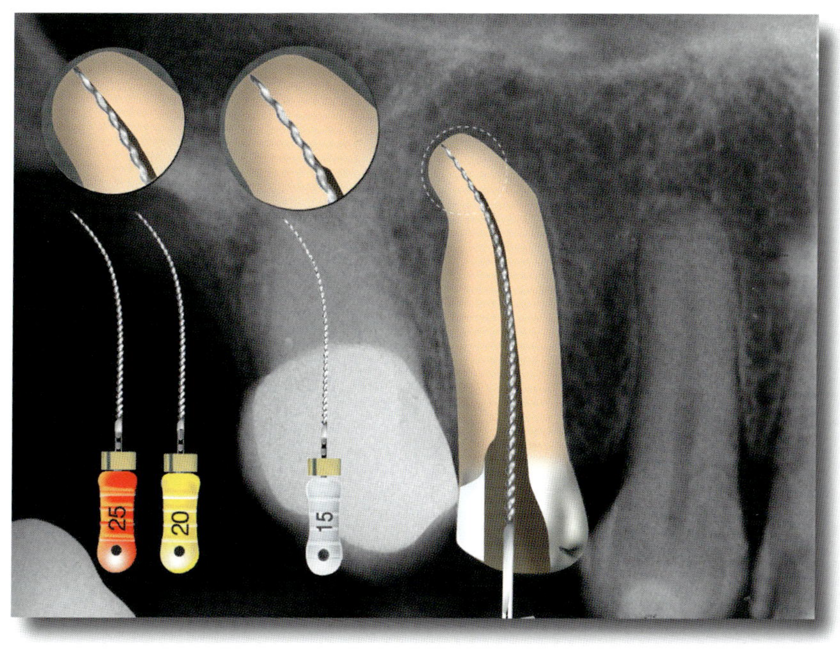

After both the crown and the post have been removed, the next step in retreatment is to improve the coronal access, identify untreated canals, and remove any blockages (eg, obturation material, fractured instruments). Once all the canals have been located and previously uninstrumented areas have been negotiated (often the most difficult stage), the root canals are prepared, cleaned, and obturated in the same way as for initial treatment. Failure of initial endodontic treatment is commonly associated with the following:

- Lack of knowledge of tooth anatomy and morphology (coronal and radicular)
- The impossibility of producing an accurate image of the three-dimensional pulp chamber on a radiograph
- Restricted vision
- The complex root canal anatomy of posterior teeth, along with the restricted access in this area
- Poor access cavity design

Access cavities should allow the identification and preparation of canals. Inadequate access hampers this process and makes optimal preparation of the root canal system impossible. Poorly designed access cavities can also prevent the establishment of straight-line access. This, in turn, leads to a loss of control over instruments in the apical third; uncontrolled dentin removal can result in overpreparation, blockages, and fractured instruments.

Improving Access

After removing both the crown and the post, the clinician must reassess and modify the access cavity before attempting the removal of root filling material. Modifications to the access cavity should include the following:

- Clearing any caries lesions or unsupported enamel.
- Thorough debridement of the access cavity and pulp chamber.
- Provision of a coronal restoration. This creates a four-walled access cavity to act as a reservoir for the irrigant. It also facilitates the placement of a rubber dam clamp and enables a stable temporary dressing to be placed that is capable of resisting occlusal forces and preventing bacterial leakage.
- Extending the access cavity as necessary, often in a buccolingual direction.
- Identifying extra canals.

A detailed description of the anatomic landmarks to locate, the clinical stages to follow, and the materials to use is found elsewhere (Pertot and Simon, 2003). Here, the basic stages are presented and some important points are highlighted.

Canal Anatomy and Clinical Implications

In the maxilla

- *Incisors*
  Incisors usually have single roots containing just one canal; occasionally a second canal is present (Figs 3-1a to 3-1c). The most common mistake is to prepare the access cavity too far buccally because of a failure to appreciate the palatal inclination of the tooth. This can result in coronal blockages during the preparation stage, or even a perforation.

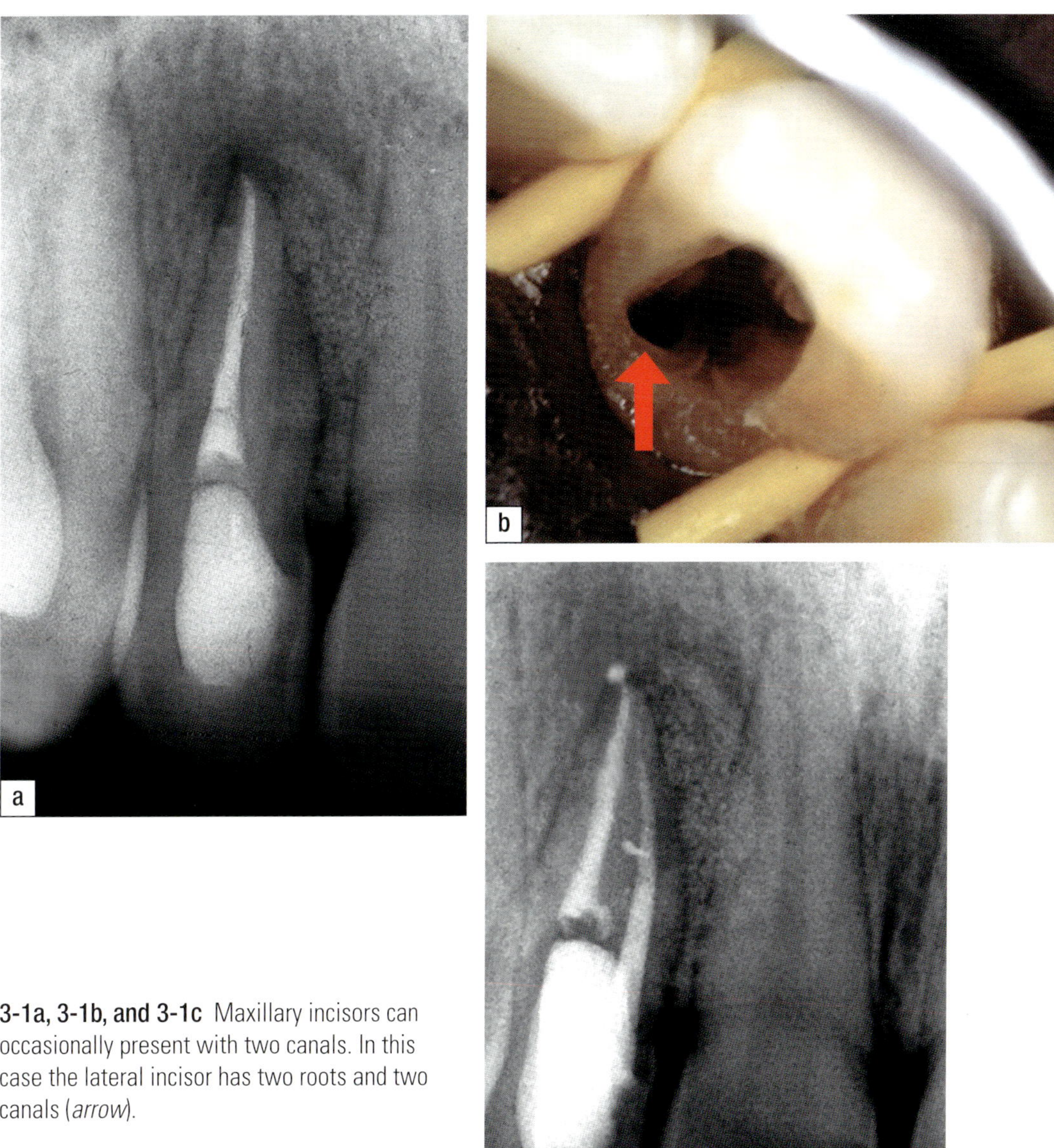

3-1a, 3-1b, and 3-1c Maxillary incisors can occasionally present with two canals. In this case the lateral incisor has two roots and two canals (*arrow*).

- *Premolars*
  Premolars can present with the following: an oval root with a canal that is widened buccopalatally, an oval root with two canals that may be connected by an isthmus, or two roots with a single round canal for each. Thus, when retreating a premolar, if the clinician discovers a small access cavity and a single round canal slightly displaced from the center, it suggests that the original access cavity is inadequate and there is likely to be an untreated canal.

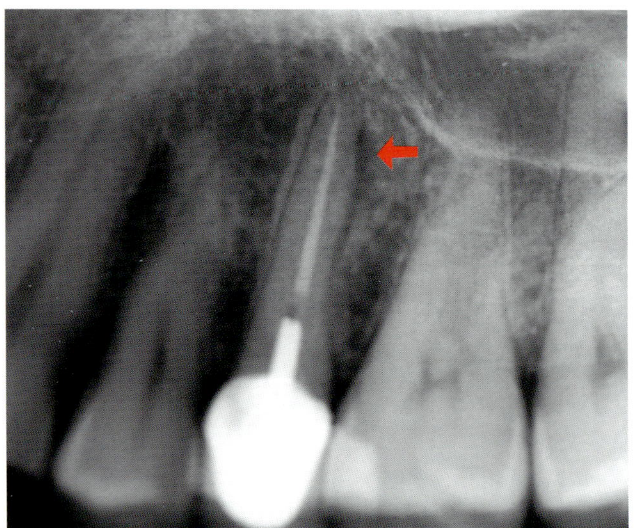

3-2a Preoperative radiograph of a maxillary second premolar with a lateral radiolucency (*arrow*).

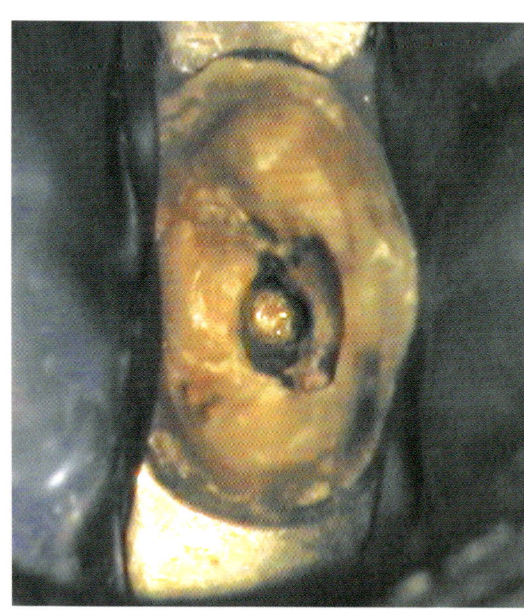

3-2b Midtreatment photograph (after removal of the post and crown) displaying the inadequate access cavity.

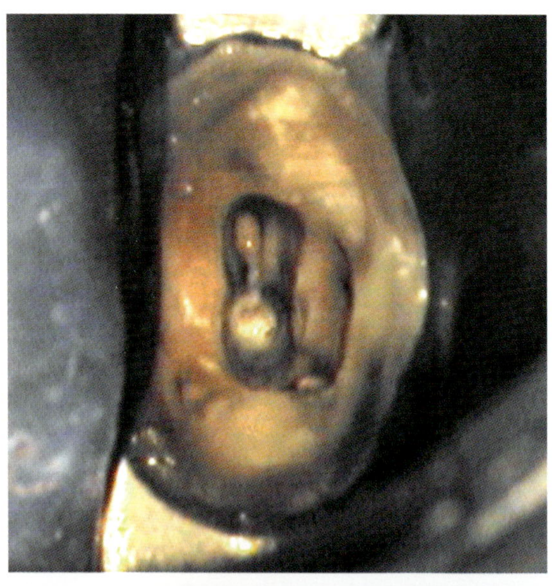

3-2c Extending the access cavity lingually reveals the oval canal.

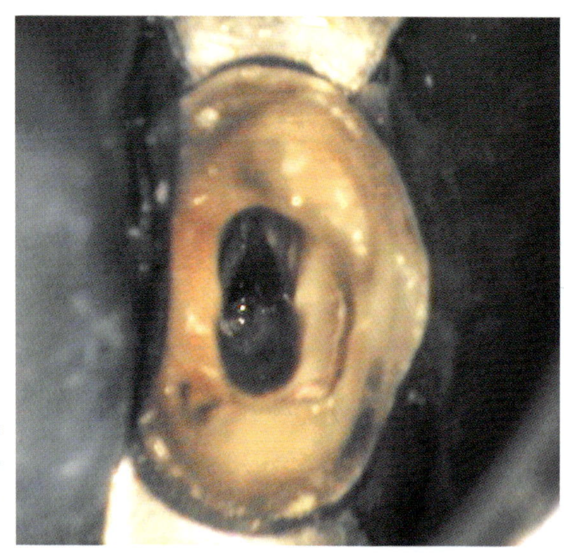

3-2d View of the canal after the preparation stage.

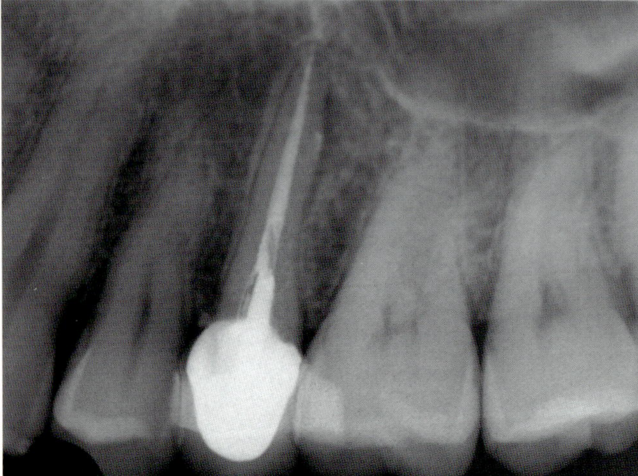

3-2e Postoperative radiograph demonstrates the presence of a lateral canal.

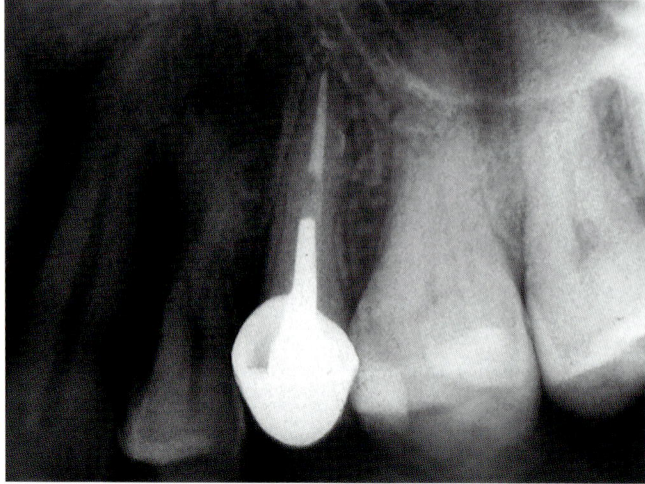

3-2f Radiograph taken 1 year postoperatively shows healing of the lateral lesion. Unfortunately, the post hole was overprepared in this case.

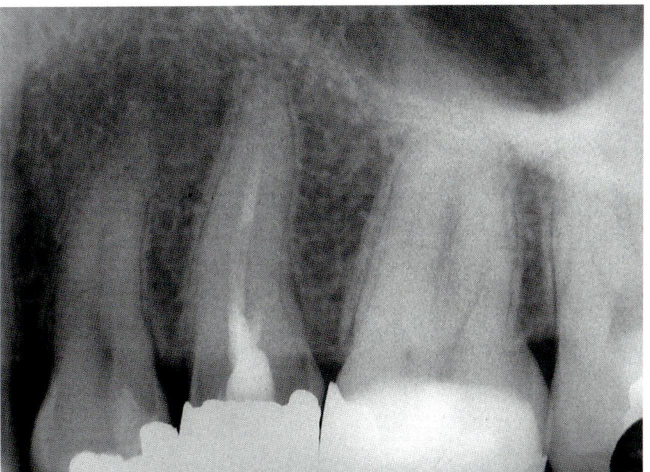

3-3a Preoperative radiograph of a maxillary second premolar that has an inadequate root filling in place.

3-3b Clinical photograph of the extended access cavity and the two prepared canals.

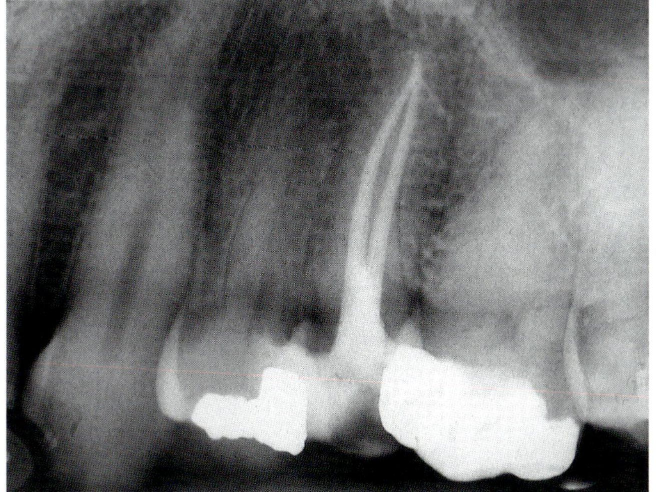

3-3c Angled postoperative radiograph shows the two canals.

Traditionally, in premolar retreatment cases, the access cavity prepared during the initial treatment is found to be underprepared in a buccolingual direction (Figs 3-2a and 3-2b). Before attempting to regain access to the canals, the operator must extend the coronal access cavity bucco-lingual so any untreated canals can be located (Fig 3-2c). In cases with flattened oval roots, a conventional periapical radiograph is not sufficient, since the majority of the endodontic work is performed in a buccolingual direction and will not appear on the radiograph (Figs 3-2d to 3-2f).

Maxillary first premolars sometimes present with three canals (two buccal and one palatal). In this situation, the access cavity should be prepared in a T shape with the horizontal branch extending mesiodistally, parallel to the buccal wall, and the vertical branch extending toward the palatal aspect.

- *Molars*

  A molar access cavity that is insufficiently extended often causes difficulty with preparation of the mesiobuccal canal. Moreover, a second mesiobuccal canal is found in 90% of maxillary first molars and in almost 50% of maxillary second molars. This second canal is frequently not identified and not treated (Figs 3-4a to 3-4e). Occasionally the palatal root of a maxillary molar has two canals.

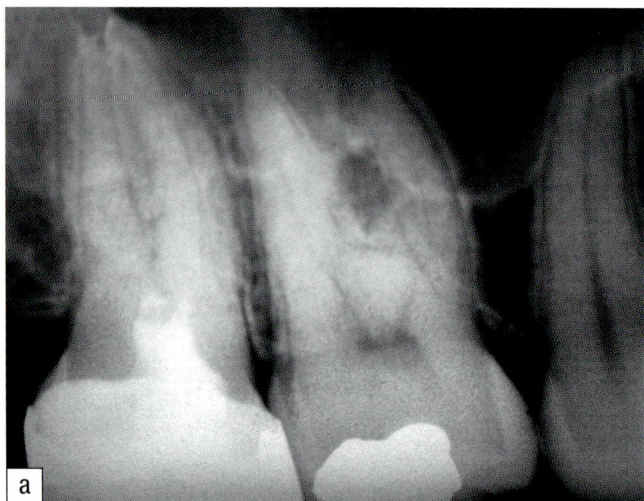

3-4a Preoperative radiograph of a maxillary second molar with an inadequate root filling in place.

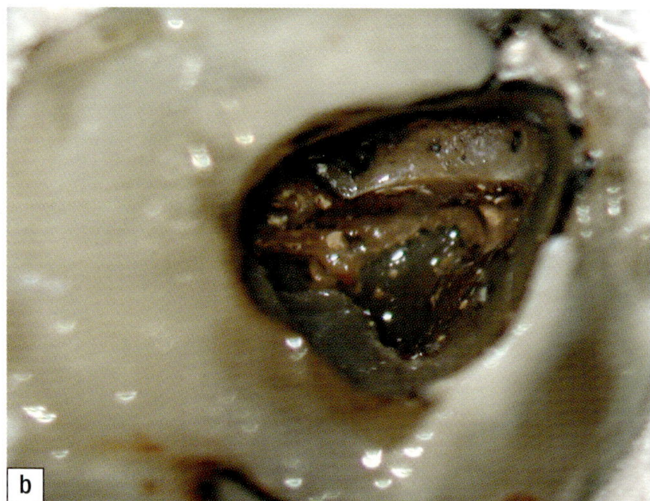

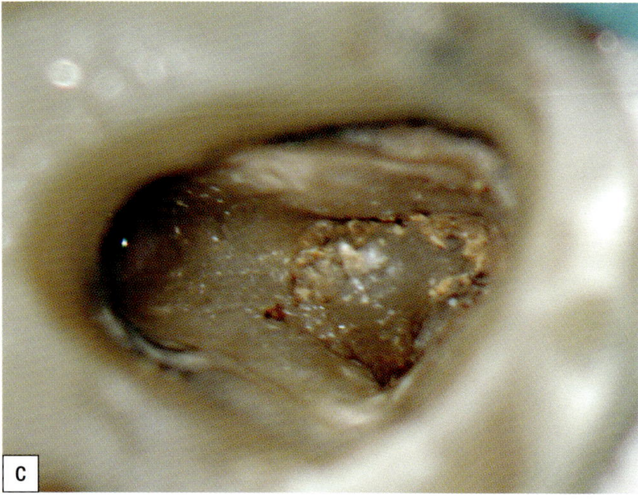

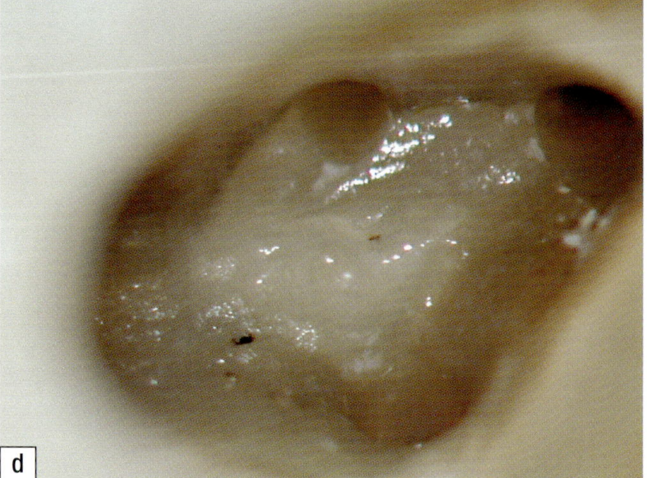

3-4b, 3-4c, and 3-4d Views of the access cavity after removal of the crown, debridement of the pulp chamber, and identification of the second mesiobuccal canal.

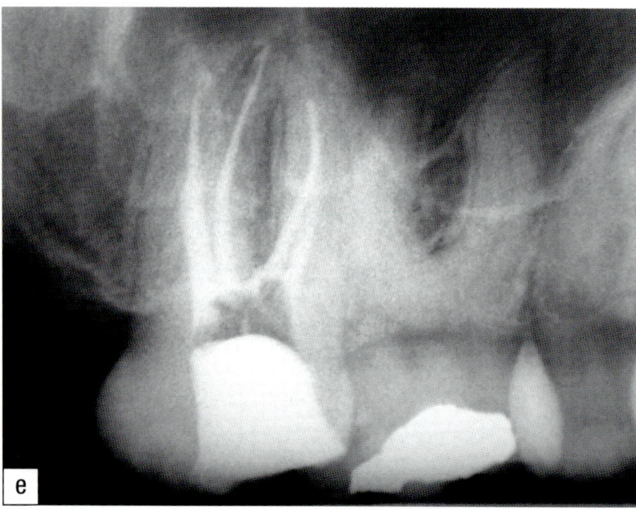

3-4e Angled postoperative radiograph displaying the four canals.

In the mandible

- *Incisors and canines*
  Mandibular incisors and canines have a flattened root with either a single canal or, in 45% of cases, two canals. The access cavity must therefore be oval in shape. For retreatment procedures, the access cavity should be extended buccolingually to allow the clinician to look for a second canal and to ensure the root canals can be properly cleaned and prepared (Figs 3-5a and 3-5b).

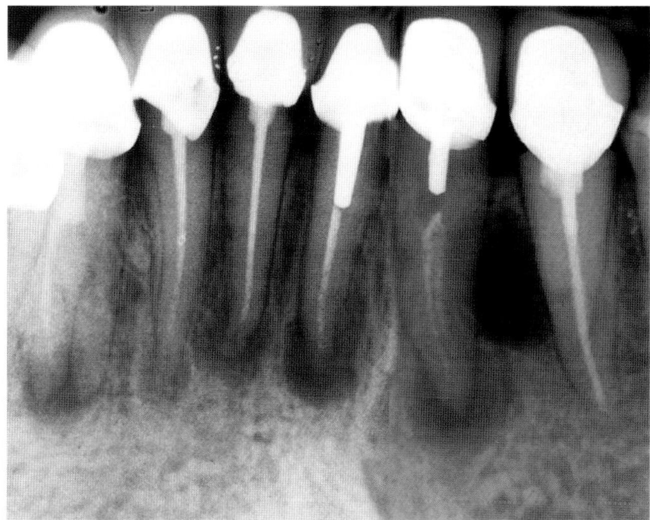

3-5a Preoperative radiograph of mandibular incisors and canines, each of which has an associated radiolucency.

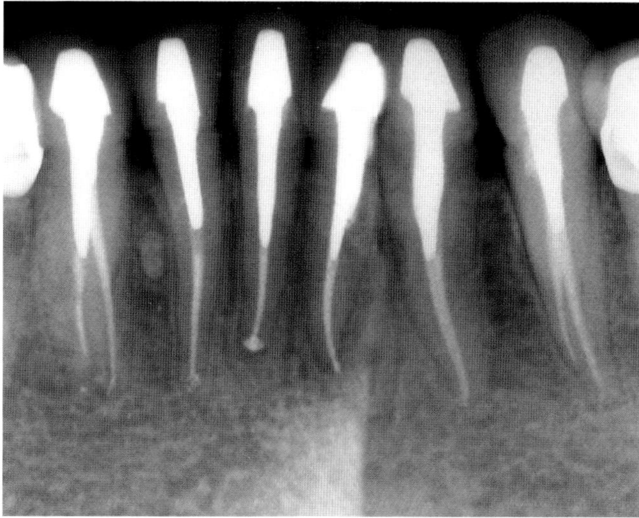

3-5b Radiograph taken 7 years postoperatively demonstrating the healing that has occurred. Note the double-rooted canine.

- *Premolars*
  The anatomy of mandibular premolars is highly variable, and configurations include a single root with a single oval canal, a single root with two canals (Figs 3-6a and 3-6b), and two roots each with one or more canals (Figs 3-7a and 3-7b). Very rarely there may be three roots. The same rules listed earlier for extending the access cavity in maxillary premolars apply, but in the mandibular premolars the access cavity should be extended slightly more buccally because of the lingual inclination of these teeth.

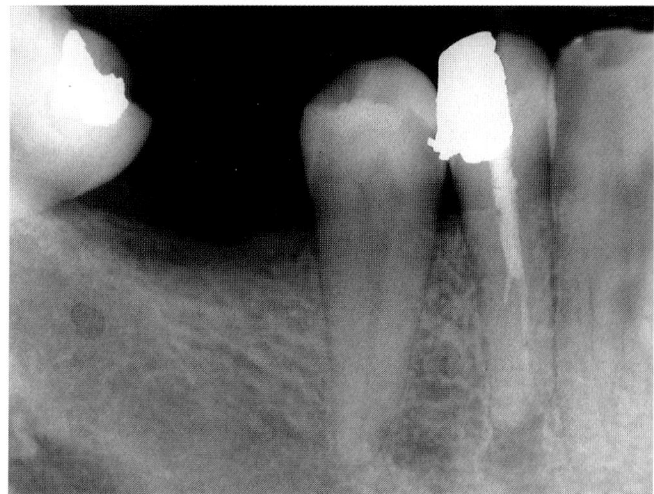

3-6a Preoperative radiograph of a mandibular first premolar; the endodontic treatment failure is a result of poor access cavity design.

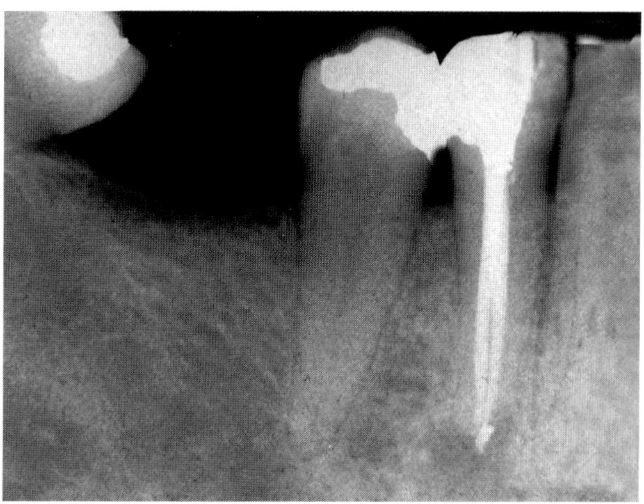

3-6b Postoperative radiograph after retreatment. The modified access cavity allowed both canals to be treated.

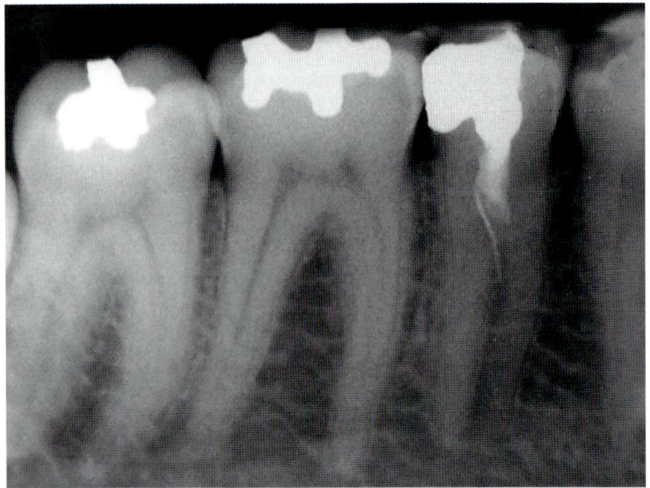

3-7a Preoperative radiograph of a mandibular second premolar displaying an inadequate root filling and a fractured instrument.

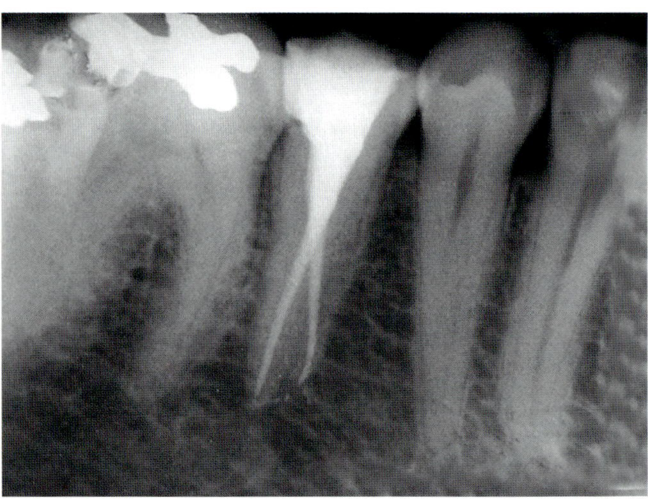

3-7b Postoperative radiograph showing the two treated canals.

- *Molars*

  The mesiobuccal canal in mandibular first and second molars is often underprepared because the access cavity is not extended far enough buccally. The canal orifice is situated below the mesiobuccal cusp, so it is essential that the access cavity is extended in this direction. The space between the two mesial canals should be explored and the possibility of a third canal investigated. A third canal is present in 4% of cases (Figs 3-8a to 3-8d).

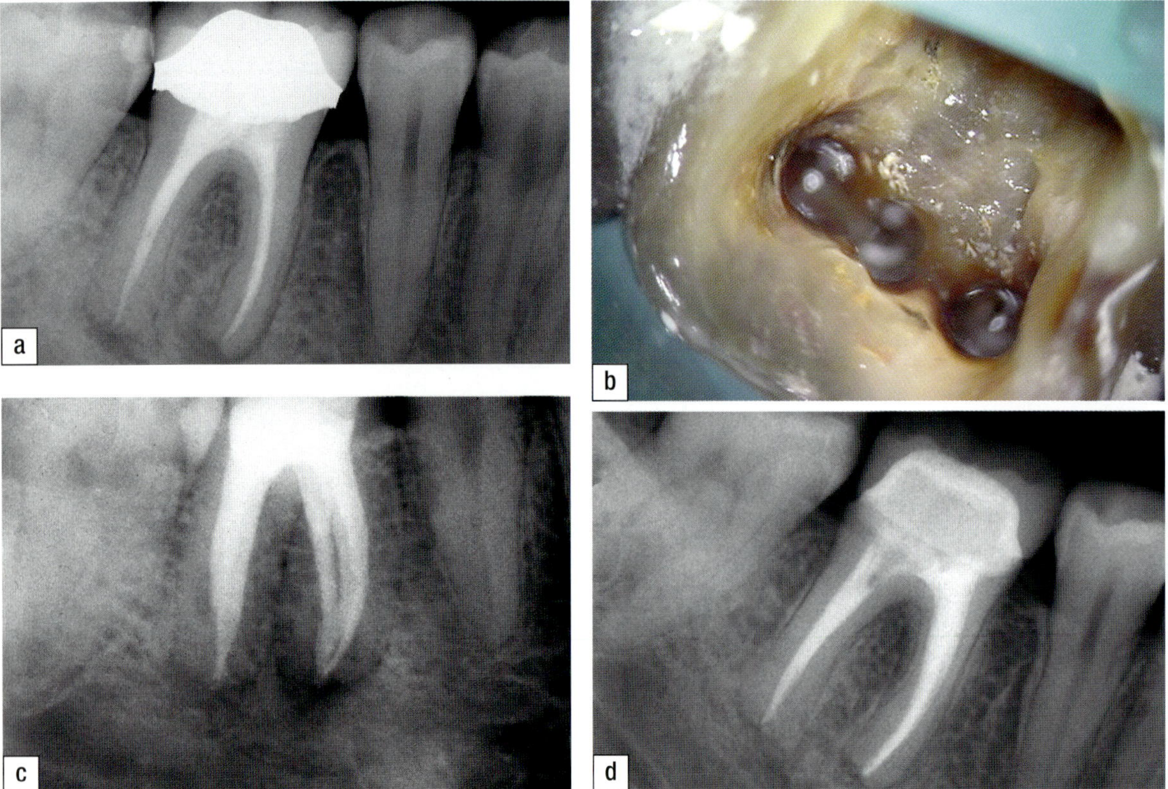

3-8a, 3-8b, 3-8c, and 3-8d *(a)* The mesial root of mandibular molars has three canals in almost 4% of cases. *(b)* Here the third (central) canal can be seen from the access cavity and *(c)* on the angled postoperative radiograph. *(d)* Identification and treatment of all of the canals resulted in healing by 24 months postoperatively.

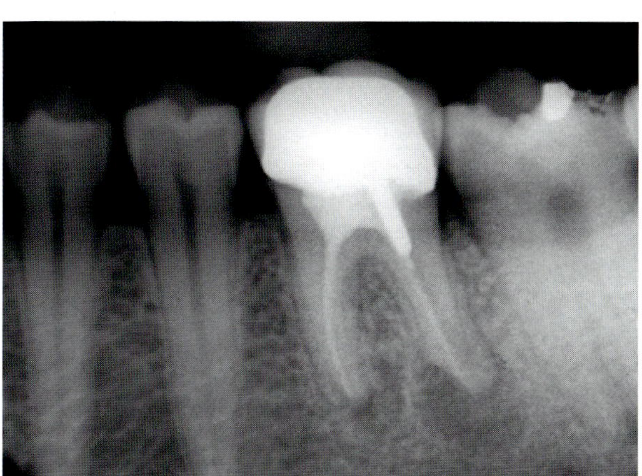

3-9a Preoperative radiograph of a mandibular first molar revealing inadequate endodontic treatment and periapical radiolucencies associated with both the mesial and distal roots.

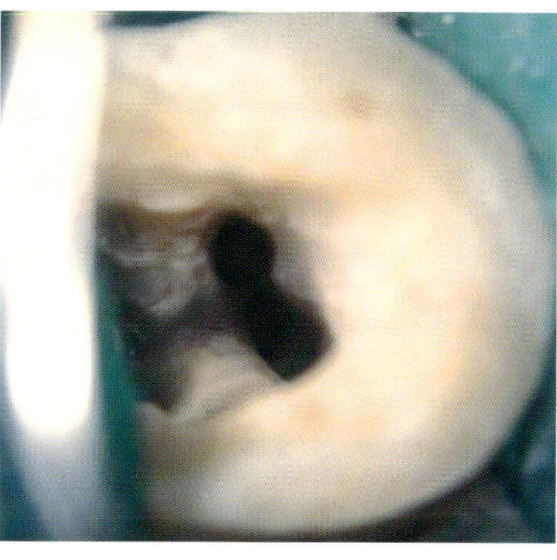

3-9b Midtreatment view of two distal canals.

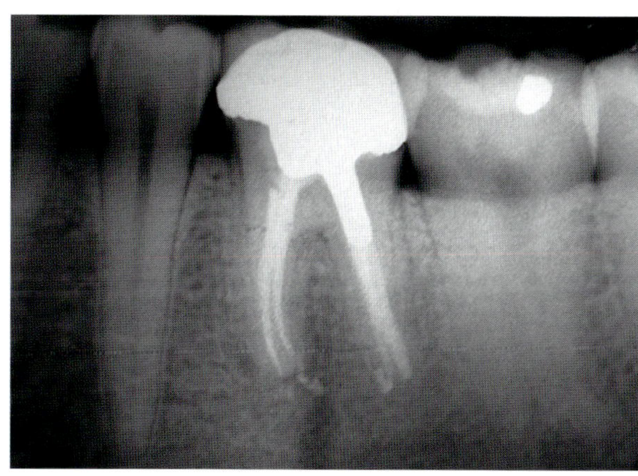

3-9c Radiograph taken 3 years postoperatively showing the four canals and demonstrating that healing has occurred.

The distal root of mandibular molars has a second canal in almost 50% of cases. Where there is only a single canal, it tends to be oval in shape and relatively large buccolingually. If a single round canal is discovered slightly displaced from the center, the likelihood of a second canal should be investigated (Figs 3-9a to 3-9c). Some mandibular molars exhibit C-shaped canals that join the mesial and distal canals.

Materials and equipment

- *Radiographs*

Preoperative radiographs, both conventional periapical views and angled views, in conjunction with a comprehensive understanding of root canal anatomy, allow for the identification of extra canals.

- *Magnification tools*

Tools to improve vision such as loupes, microscopes, and enhanced lighting are invaluable in endodontics. The use of magnification and an additional light source vastly improves operating conditions and gives the clinician greater control; it is especially useful in root canal retreatment, as it allows accessory canals to be detected while minimizing the risk of perforation. The most frequent and the most damaging perforations are the result of using rotary instruments in an uncontrolled manner by clinicians searching blindly for accessory canals.

- *Long-shank burs*

Once the access cavity has been extended, the use of long-shank low-speed burs without water spray is advised (LN Burs 012 and 014 diameter, Dentsply-Maillefer). The long shank ensures that the head of the handpiece does not restrict vision, therefore enabling the preparation to be done under direct vision (Fig 3-10).

- *Ultrasonic tips*

Dedicated endodontic ultrasonic tips are available to remove dentin safely and assist with the identification of accessory canals (ProUltra Endo no. 2, Dentsply-Maillefer; ETBD and ET18D, Satelec). These are used without water spray so the operator's vision is not impaired.

- *Dye*

Dyes such as methylene blue (Canal Blue, Dentsply) can prove helpful in locating root canals. A drop is placed in the access cavity and left for a minute before being washed off. The dye is absorbed by the canal orifices and isthmuses (and cracks) and makes the anatomy visible.

After preparation of the root canals, the access cavity should be filled with sodium hypochlorite and examined for bubbles. This "champagne effect" is a result of the reaction of hypochlorite on organic residue and indicates either that there is organic debris remaining or an accessory canal has been identified.

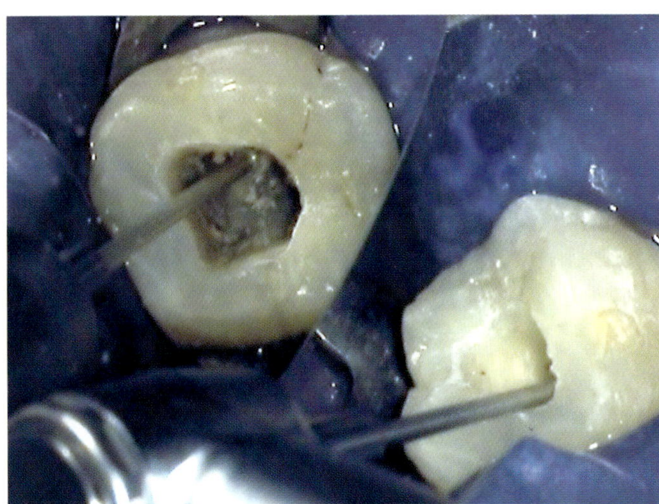

3-10 Long-shank tungsten carbide burs (LN Bur, Dentsply) used without water spray at low speed (below 1,000 rpm) in a micro-handpiece allow direct vision of the operating field and therefore minimize the risk of perforation.

Once located, any untreated accessory canals can be prepared, cleaned, and filled in the normal way as if it were the initial treatment (Figs 3-11a to 3-11c). Retreatment of canals, however, is far less predictable and may be complicated by many factors. Each case must be managed on an individual basis.

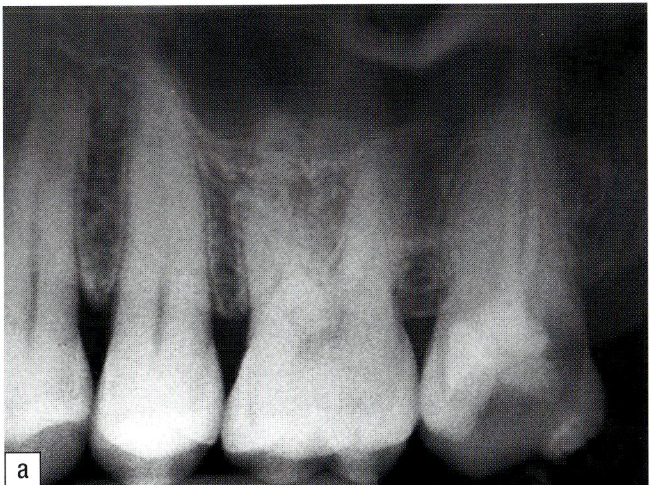

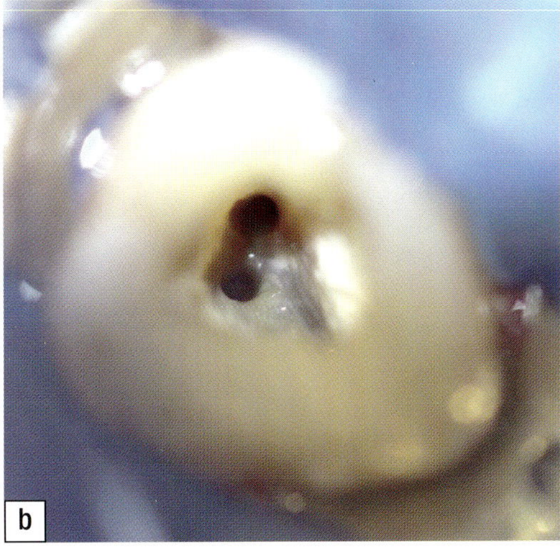

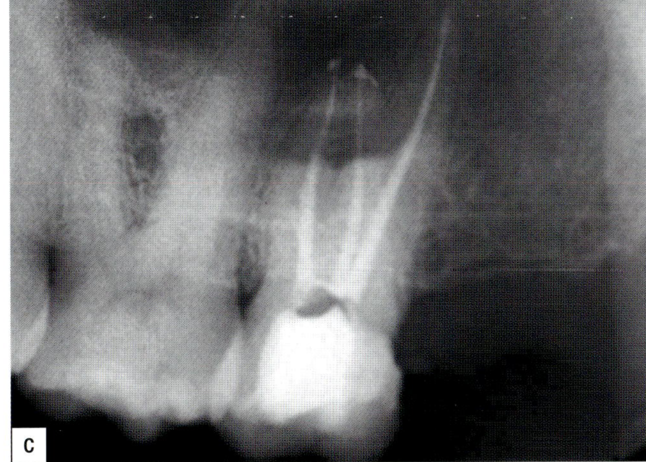

3-11a, 3-11b, and 3-11c Treatment of the mesiobuccal canal in this maxillary second molar is conducted according to conventional guidelines for primary endodontic treatment. Retreatment of the previously treated canals could prove less predictable.

Removal of Obturation Material

General guidelines

Regardless of the technique adopted for removing obturation material, some simple rules must be followed to avoid further complications.

1. After penetrating just a few millimeters into the canal, the clinician must reassess the angulation of the preparation and modify it as necessary to allow straight-line access and ensure good control of the instruments (Figs 3-12a and 3-12b). Failure to gain straight-line access may lead to coronal blockages, make further instrumentation of the canal difficult, and increase the chances of creating a perforation or obstruction.
   This first stage in refining the access preparation should be completed with a Gates Glidden bur (Dentsply-Maillefer) or with dedicated nickel-titanium instruments designed for this purpose. The instruments must never be forced apically but should be carefully introduced a few millimeters into the canal and then withdrawn, removing dentin on the upstroke.

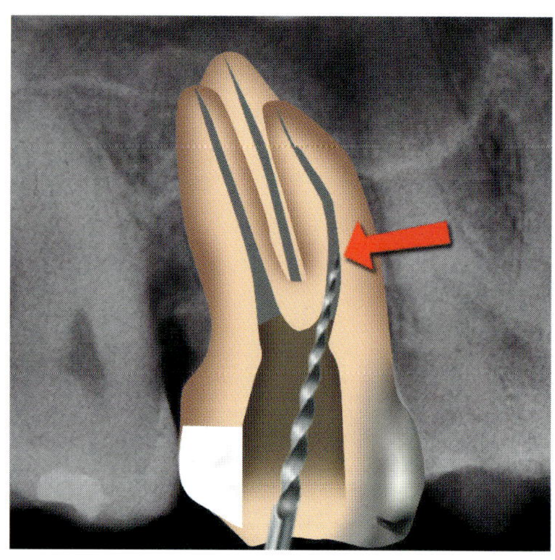

3-12a If coronal access is not modified at the beginning of the procedure, it will be difficult to advance instruments further down the canal. The risk of blockages and perforations is high (*arrow*).

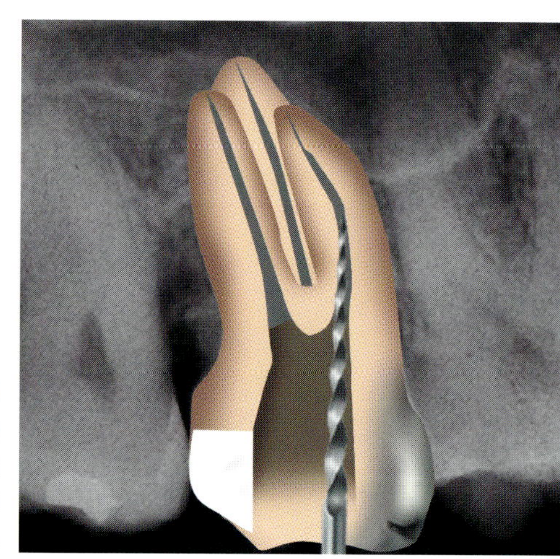

3-12b Eliminating the coronal shoulder of dentin opens up the access preparation, thus ensuring straight-line access for instrumentation.

2. The obturation material should be removed progressively as the instruments are advanced further down the canal; this prevents material extrusion through the apex.
3. All files and instruments should be regularly wiped clean on damp gauze so the clinician can assess them for any signs of damage or loss of threading that could lead to instrument fracture.
4. If excessive resistance is encountered, instruments should not be forced. A radiograph may reveal the cause of the obstruction. *Forcing instruments apically into a ledge is the chief cause of iatrogenic perforations during retreatment procedures.* There are two possible causes for resistance: *(1)* there is obturation material remaining in the canal, but the instrument being used has too large a diameter; and *(2)* the obturation material has been removed and the resistance is due to a ledge or calcification of the canal. In both these situations, a fine, precurved file should be used to help negotiate the canal further; careful use of the instrument will either allow the remaining obturation material to be removed or enable the ledge to be bypassed.

Identifying the obturation material

The obturation material may be visible at the level of the canal orifice, but this is not the case in teeth that have been restored with a post-retained crown.

If the material is not visible at the canal orifice

After the removal of a post, any residual cement in the base of the preparation (eg, zinc phosphate, zinc polycarboxylate, glass ionomer) hinders access to the canal and interferes with the action of solvents (Fig 3-13a). The most effective way of removing this material is with the use of ultrasonic instruments (ProUltra Endo 6 to 8, Dentsply-Maillefer; or ET20 and ET25, Acteon) or wide-diameter ultrasonic files (diameter 35/100, Acteon). These instruments should be used only under direct vision in order to avoid perforations or transportation of the canal. The ultrasonic tip is placed in the canal, resting on the plug of material (Fig 3-13b), and activated for a few seconds. The canal is then irrigated and dried, and a drop of solvent is placed. A stainless steel hand file is used to check whether the cement has been removed; if the plug of material remains in place, the same procedure can be repeated. Once the residual cement has been eliminated, removal of the obturation material further down the canal can be attempted (Figs 3-13c to 3-13e).

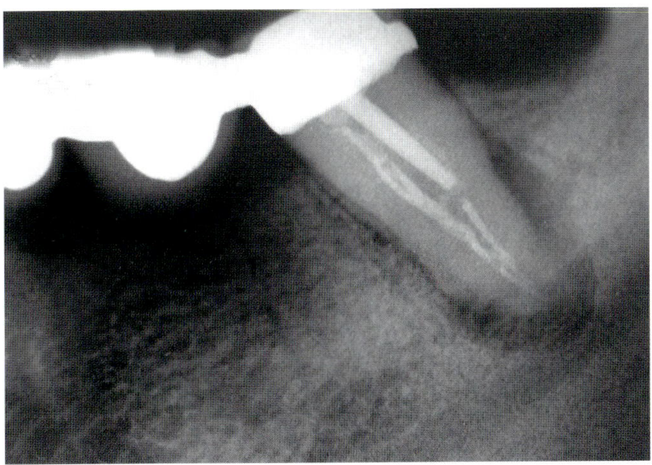

3-13a Preoperative radiograph of a mandibular second molar (fixed partial denture abutment) with a periapical radiolucency.

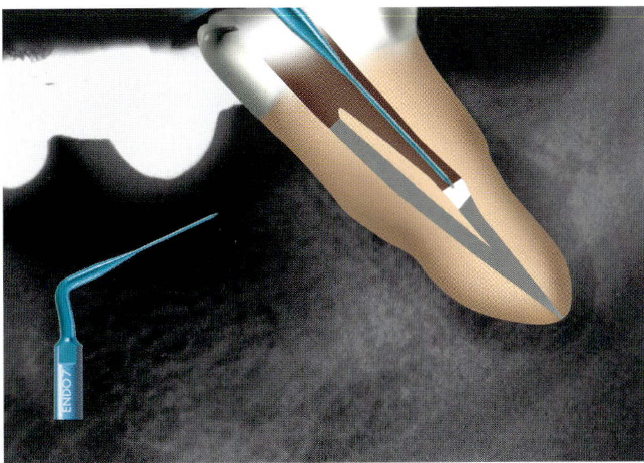

3-13b To remove the residual plug of luting agent, an ultrasonic tip is placed on the material and activated for several seconds.

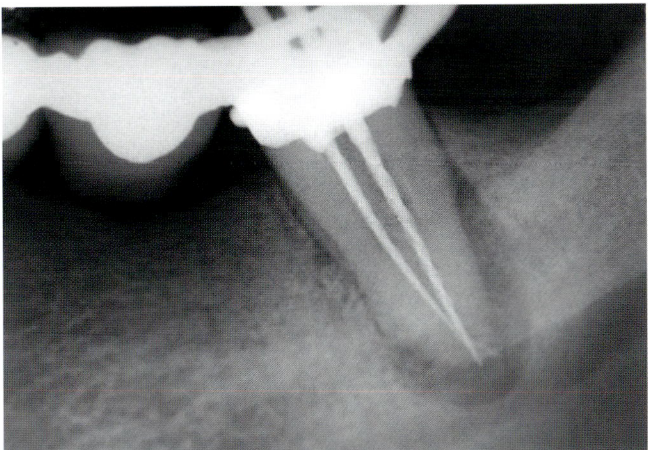

3-13c With the plug of material removed, solvents can be used to dissolve the obturation material.

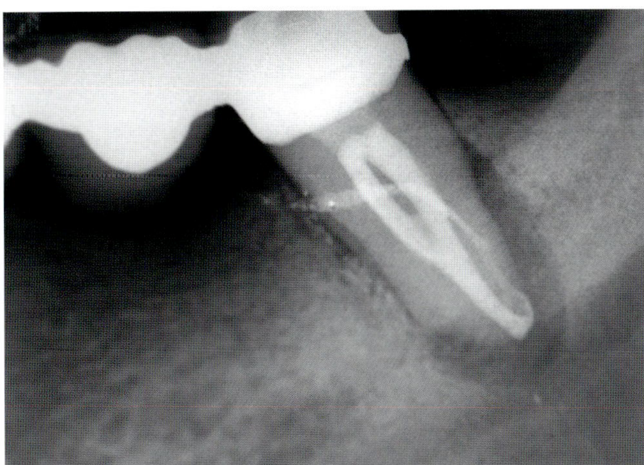

3-13d Immediate postoperative radiograph. Note the extrusion of the sealant along the sinus tract.

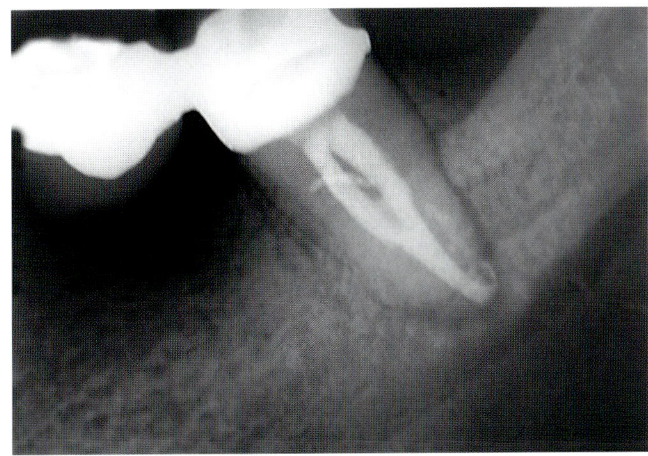

3-13e Radiograph taken 2 years postoperatively demonstrates healing of the lesion.

If the material is visible at the canal orifice

The ease with which the obturation material is removed depends on the nature of the obturation material, the amount of canal preparation done for the initial treatment, the curvature of the canal, and the length of the root filling. The majority of inadequate root canal fillings are unsatisfactory because of insufficient preparation and obturation of the entire root canal system. If the obturation material is soluble, the iatrogenic complications (eg, obstructions, sclerosis, curvature) are the clinician's main concern; removal of the material should not be difficult.

Techniques for removal of obturation material

Removal of pastes

Once the access cavity has been modified, the pulp chamber debrided, and additional canals located, a DG-16 probe (Hu-Friedy) is used to test the hardness of the obturation material. A drop of solvent is then placed in the pulp chamber to assess its effect on the obturation material. Although some canals are still obturated with hard pastes, the majority of obturation pastes are zinc oxide–eugenol based and are largely dissolvable. Some examples include ethyl acetate solvents (DPC7, Dentsply; DMS IV, Dentsply), tetrachloroethylene solvents (Endosolv E, Septodont; Désocclusol, Pierre Rolland), orange essence (Dentsply), and xylene.

Hard pastes

If the obturation material proves insoluble (phenoplastic resin or Bakelite) and the solvents are ineffective, the material must be drilled out or chipped out using a combination of endodontic tips (ProUltra Endo 4 and 5, Dentsply-Maillefer; ET20 and ET25, Satelec) and ultrasonic files (diameter 20/100 or 25/100, Satelec); the ends of these instruments can be sectioned to give them greater cutting ability in the coronal part of the canal. The endodontic tips break up the first few millimeters of obturation material, and the ultrasonic files are then used to progress further down the canal. *Ultrasonic instruments should be used only under direct vision in straight portions of the canal.* Once the first few millimeters of material have been removed, precurved stainless steel hand files are used to advance further apically.

As these obturation pastes are often harder than dentin, it is impossible to use tactile feedback to help guide the direction of the instruments. Removal of hard pastes can be time consuming and difficult, especially in curved canals. Frequent radiographs, both conventional and angled views, should be taken to check progress and angulation, ensuring there is no danger of transporting the canal or creating a perforation (Figs 3-14a to 3-14d). Resin-based root fillings tend to be denser coronally because of the obturation technique that is employed; once this coronal portion has been removed, progression further down the canal might not prove difficult. Poor access and inadequate preparation often results in the obturation of only the central part of oval canals (premolars, mandibular incisors and canines, distal roots of mandibular molars, and palatal roots of maxillary molars). In such cases, once access has been modified, hand files should be introduced down the lateral aspect of the canal, alongside the obturation material, into the untreated region of the canal.

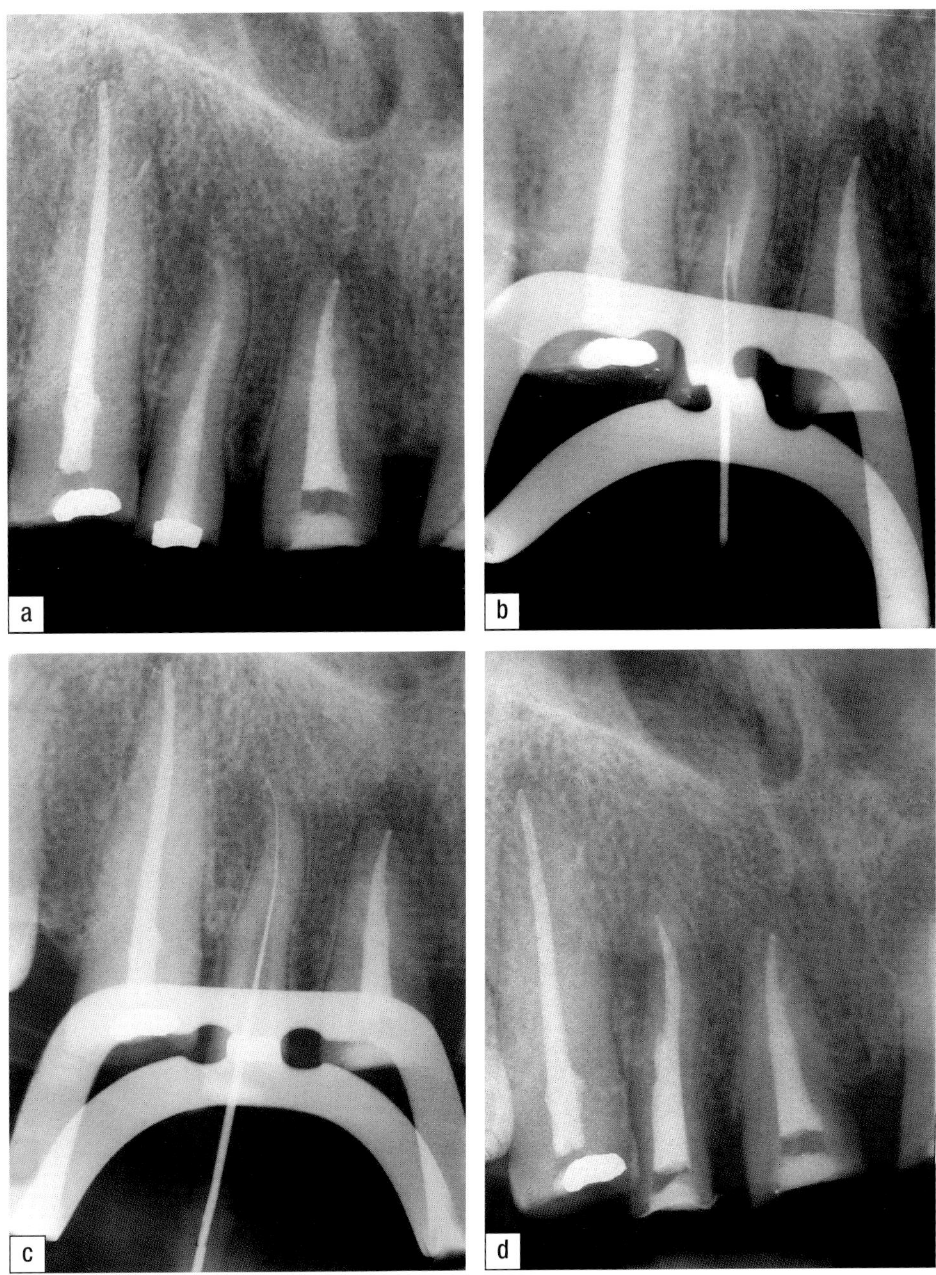

3-14a to 3-14d Removal of Bakelite obturation material can prove time consuming and risky even in cases that appear straightforward. Frequent midtreatment radiographs allow the angle of the instruments to be checked and adjusted as necessary, thereby avoiding perforations.

Soft pastes
This procedure relies on the use of instruments of sufficient rigidity and solvents. The dimensions of the canal should be gauged and an instrument of appropriate diameter chosen. Large-diameter instruments should be used first to clear the coronal part of the canal, allowing finer instruments to penetrate further apically. Soft pastes can be removed effectively with either stainless steel hand files or nickel-titanium rotary instruments; removal with rotary instruments is likely to be quicker. The amount of solvent needed depends on the nature and the hardness of the obturation material. If excessive amounts are used, the material will develop a liquid consistency, making its removal more difficult. The material should

be softened enough to allow instruments to "bite" into it but at the same time should be solid enough to allow it to be chipped away, which is particularly important when rotary instruments are being used.

If a canal has been obturated to its full length, removal of the obturation material is relatively easy and should not pose many problems. Nevertheless, care should be taken to ensure material is not extruded through the apex.

If a canal has been obturated short of the apex, there are two possible scenarios. *(1)* The apical portion of the canal is not calcified or blocked; it needs to be explored and negotiated with small-diameter stainless steel hand files. *(2)* A ledge may have been created apically during the initial treatment and this section of the canal has eventually calcified; such situations can be complicated further by curvature of the canal that may or may not be detected radiographically. *Rotary nickel-titanium instruments should never be used to negotiate the canal in such cases.*

Instrumentation

Stainless steel hand files

For practitioners not equipped with rotary instruments, the hand file of choice is an H-file; this has a relatively aggressive point that allows the paste to be removed as the file is worked in and out of the canal while being advanced apically. A Gates Glidden drill is used initially to clear the first 2 to 3 mm of obturation material from the canal orifices and to modify the access preparation, always working away from the furcation (Figs 3-15a and 3-15b). This enables the operator to achieve straight-line access and also creates a reservoir coronally. A drop of solvent is placed in the canal orifices and an H-file that is 21 mm long (file diameter should be appropriate for canal dimensions) is used to progress down the canal (Fig 3-15c). The lateral walls of the canal are cleaned as the file is advanced and the canal is irrigated with sodium hypochlorite. The canal is then dried, more solvent is introduced, and instrumentation of the canal is continued. When this large-diameter file begins to bend and cannot be taken any further apically, it is replaced with a file of smaller diameter (Figs 3-15d and 3-15e). When two successive files refuse to progress, a radiograph should be taken. If the canal is blocked, a small-diameter C+-file is used to negotiate the canal and establish the working length (Figs 3-15f and 3-15g). The apical portion of the canal can then be prepared, cleaned, and obturated (Fig 3-15h).

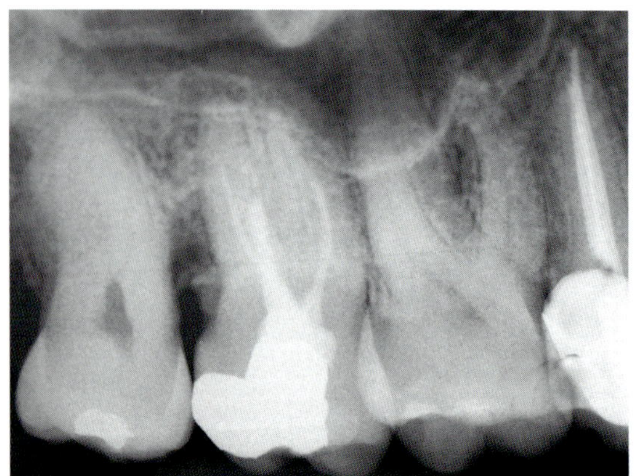

3-15a Preoperative radiograph of a maxillary first molar with an inadequate root filling.

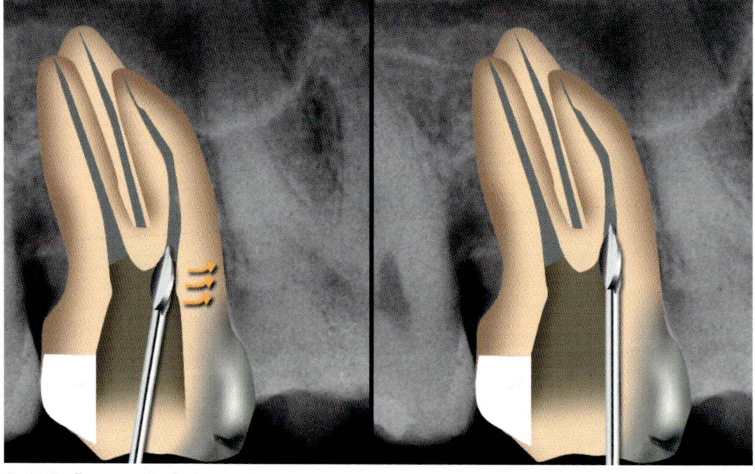

3-15b Removal of obturation material always begins with modification of the access preparation to ensure straight-line access.

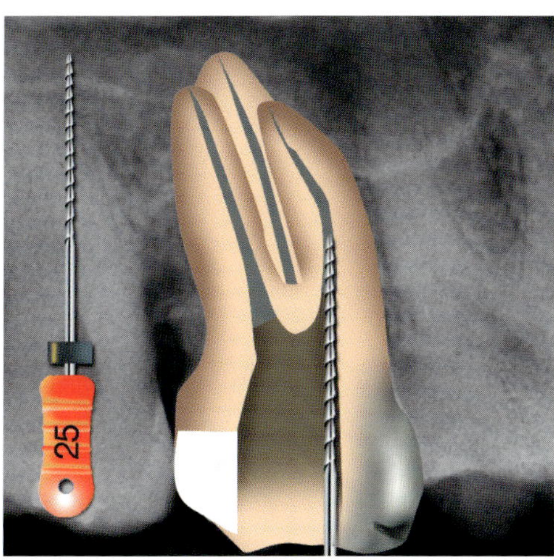

3-15c Once the solvent has been introduced into the canal orifices, a size 25 H-file is used; the obturation material is removed as the file advances down the canal.

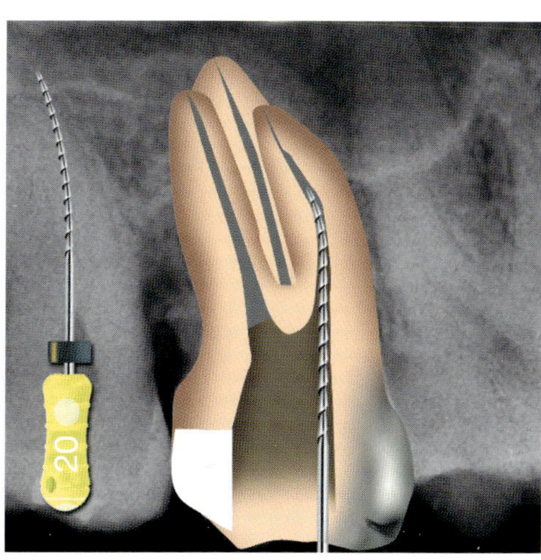

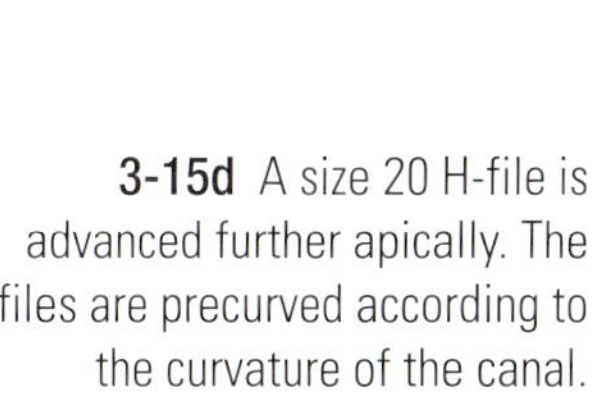
3-15d A size 20 H-file is advanced further apically. The files are precurved according to the curvature of the canal.

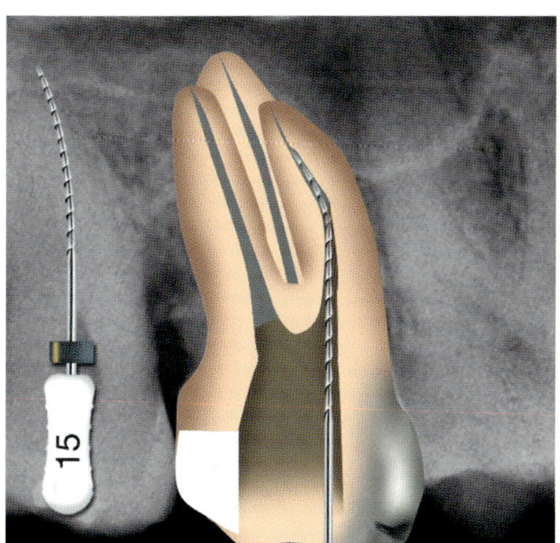

3-15e A size 15 H-file continues the apical progression. Instruments are never forced if a blockage is encountered.

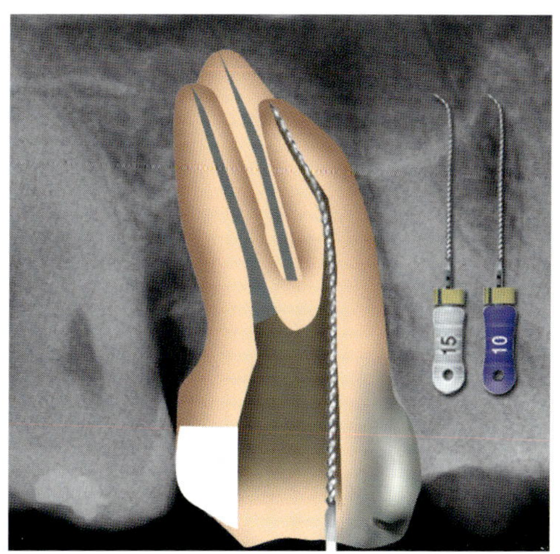

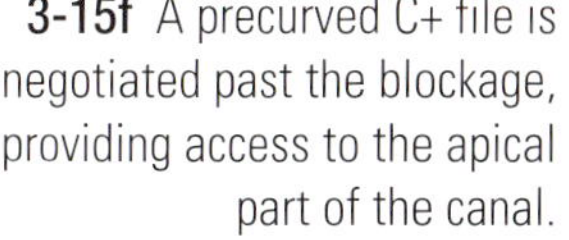
3-15f A precurved C+ file is negotiated past the blockage, providing access to the apical part of the canal.

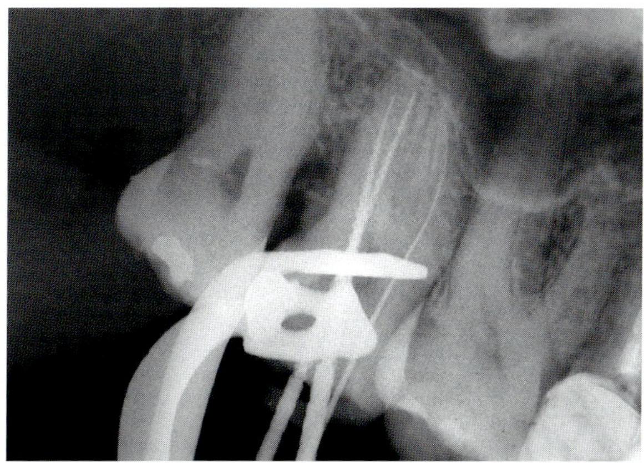

3-15g Working length radiograph. The canals can be prepared, cleaned, and obturated.

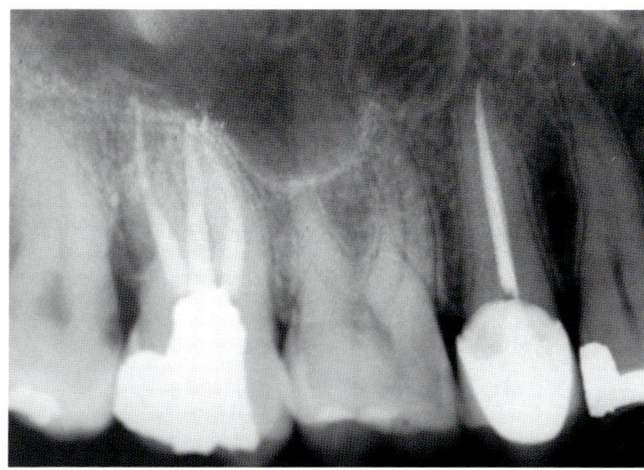

3-15h Postoperative radiograph.

Rotary nickel-titanium instruments

Although rotary instruments specifically designed to remove obturation material are now available (R-Endo System, Micro-Mega; ProTaper Universal retreatment files, Dentsply), most of the existing systems (eg, Hero 642, Micro-Mega; Hero Shaper, Micro-Mega; FlexMaster, VDW Endodontic Synergy; Mtwo, VDW Endodontic Synergy; ProFile, Tulsa Dental; K3, SybronEndo) can be used in a crown-down technique to remove soluble obturation materials.

The R-Endo System is composed of an Rm hand file (length 17 mm, diameter 25/100, taper 4%), which is designed to pierce the surface of the obturation material, and five rotary instruments (Fig 3-16): *(1)* a 15-mm Re file with a tip size of 25/100 and a taper of 12%, *(2)* a 15-mm R1 file with a tip size of 25/100 and a taper of 8%, *(3)* a 19-mm R2 file with a tip size of 25/100 and a taper of 6%, *(4)* a 23-mm R3 file with a tip size of 25/100 and a taper of 4%, and *(5)* a 25-mm Rs file to finish with a tip size of 30/100 and a taper of 4%. These instruments are used sequentially in order of decreasing taper. They form part of the InGeT system (Micro-Mega) (Fig 3-16) and are used in a specially designed high-speed handpiece with a small head, allowing greater visibility and improved access. These instruments can be used only in the specially adapted handpieces, but another version for use with conventional handpieces is available.

The ProTaper Universal Retreatment system includes three retreatment instruments of varying taper and diameter (Fig 3-17): *(1)* a 16-mm D1 with a cutting tip size of 30/100 and a taper varying from 9% for the first 3 mm to 7% for the remainder of its length; *(2)* an 18-mm D2 with a non-cutting tip of 25/100 and a taper of 8% for the first 3 mm and 6% for the remainder of the instrument; and *(3)* a 22-mm D3 with a non-cutting tip of 20/100 and a taper of 7% for the first 3 mm and 6% for the remainder of the instrument. The decreasing taper allows each instrument to be active while avoiding a "screwing" effect and a potential coronal blockage. These rotary instruments feature a standard handle and can be used in conventional nickel-titanium high-speed handpieces.

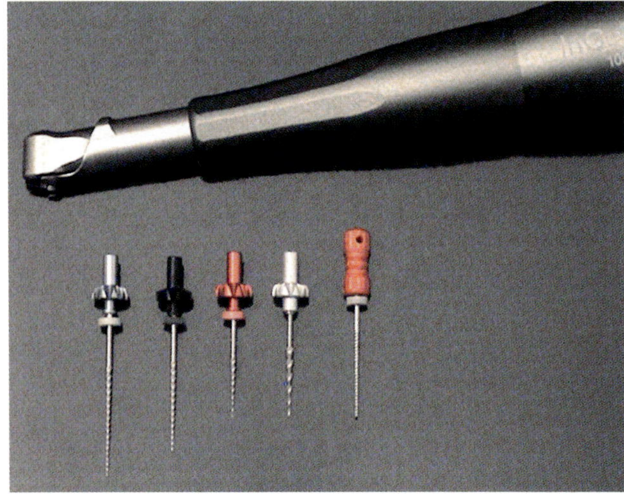

3-16 R-Endo System includes the InGeT high-speed handpiece and rotary instruments for removal of obturation material. *(right to left)* The Rm file and the instruments Re, R1, R2, and R3.

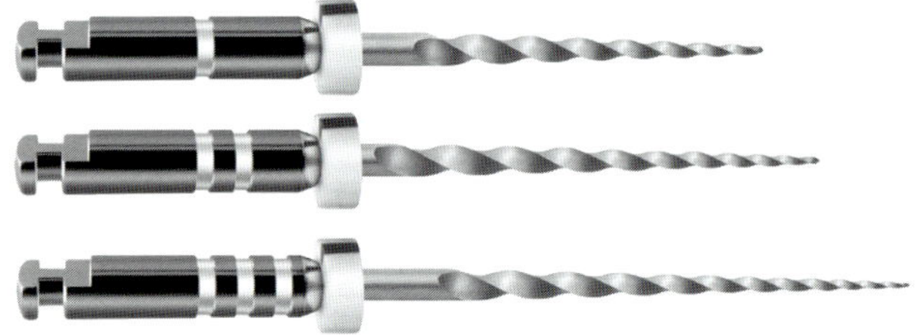

3-17 ProTaper Universal system is designed specifically for removal of obturation material. *Top* to *bottom*: the instruments D1, D2, and D3, with varying taper.

Whichever system is used, instruments of wider diameter and greater taper are used initially to remove obturation material from the coronal part of the canal; instruments with smaller diameter and smaller taper can then be used to progress further apically (Figs 3-18a and 3-18b). The material is removed by slowly advancing the instruments down the canal, moving them in and out with controlled apical pressure but not excessive force. The instruments must be cleaned regularly during use. Solvent is added and the next file is used to progress further down the canal (Figs 3-18c and 3-18d). As soon as an obstruction is encountered, a radiograph is taken; if a ledge is identified, a precurved stainless steel hand file is used to negotiate further (Figs 3-18e and 3-18f). The ledge is then eliminated, and the apical part of the canal is prepared, cleaned, and obturated (Fig 3-18g and 3-18h).

Rotary instruments facilitate this stage of the retreatment process and save invaluable time for the operator.

Nevertheless, rotary instruments can *only* be used to remove obturation material that has already been softened by a solvent; they should never be used in an attempt to bypass a ledge or an apical obstruction. Ledges are frequently encountered during endodontic retreatment and must be addressed by using precurved stainless steel hand files.

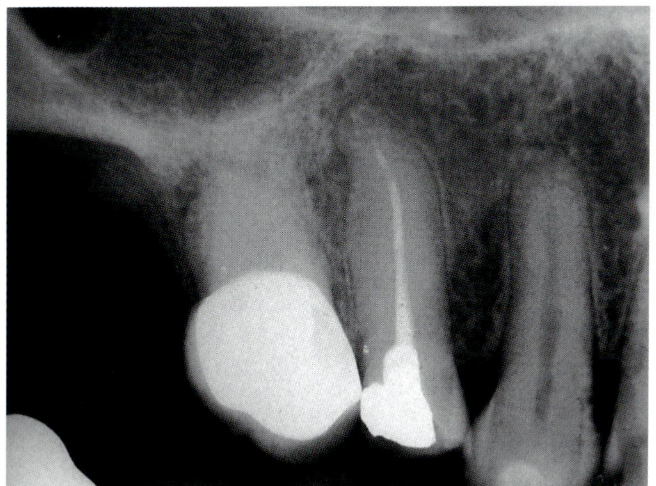

3-18a Preoperative radiograph of a maxillary premolar with an inadequate root filling.

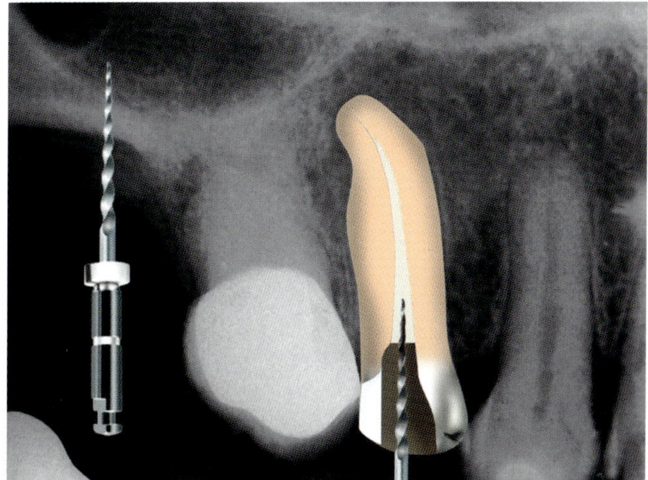

3-18b Removal of obturation material with ProTaper D1.

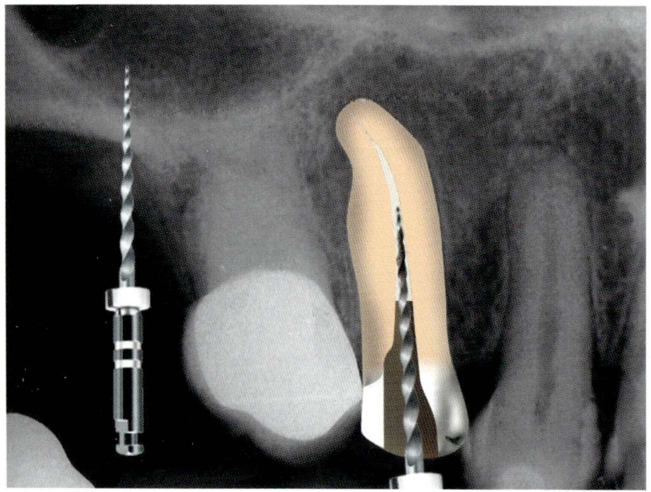

3-18c Removal of obturation material with ProTaper D2.

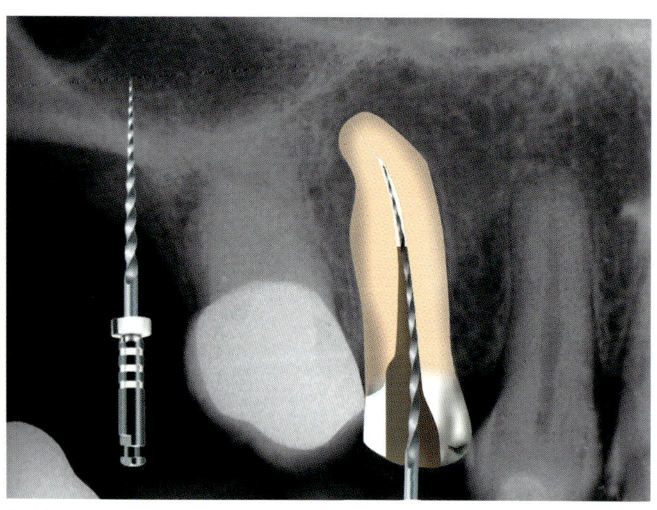

3-18d Removal of obturation material with ProTaper D3.

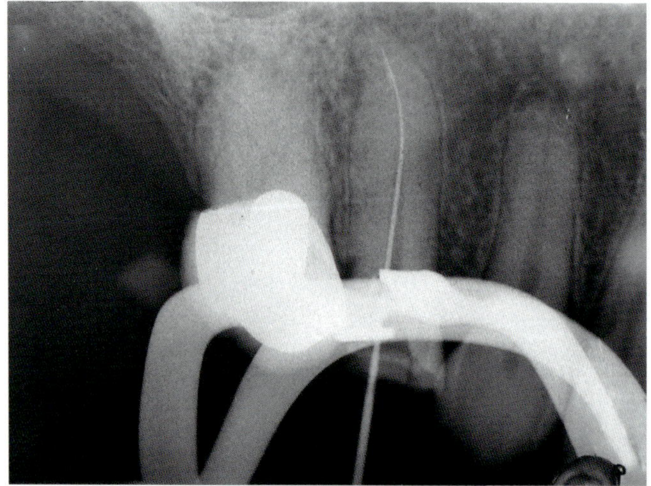

3-18e If an obstruction is encountered, the instruments must not be forced apically. A radiograph is taken to verify the cause of the blockage.

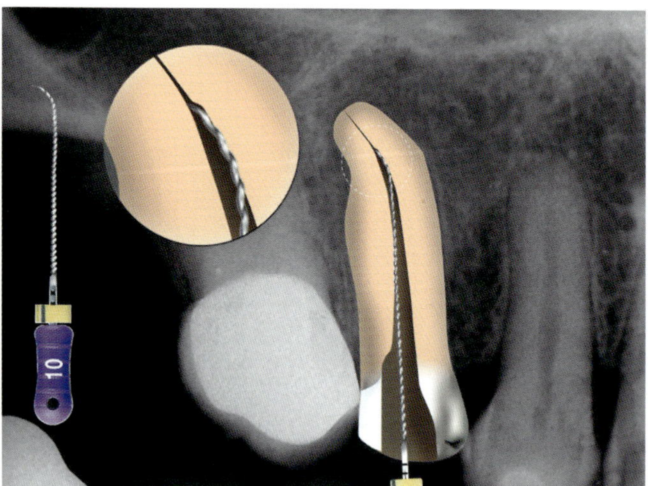

3-18f The apical part of the canal is negotiated with precurved stainless steel hand files, and the working length is established.

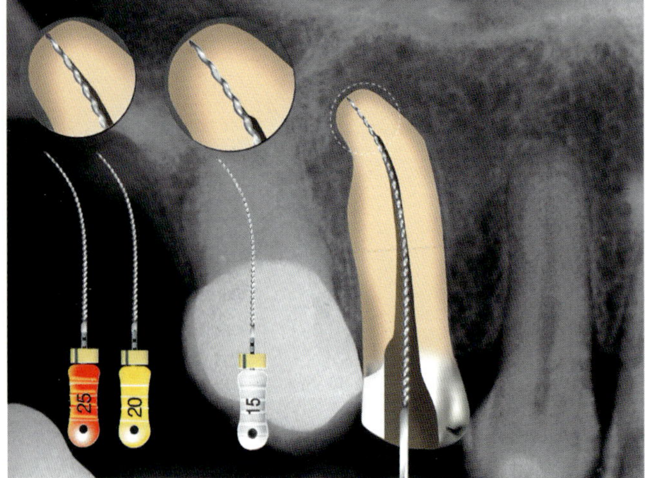

3-18g The apical part of the canal is prepared and cleaned.

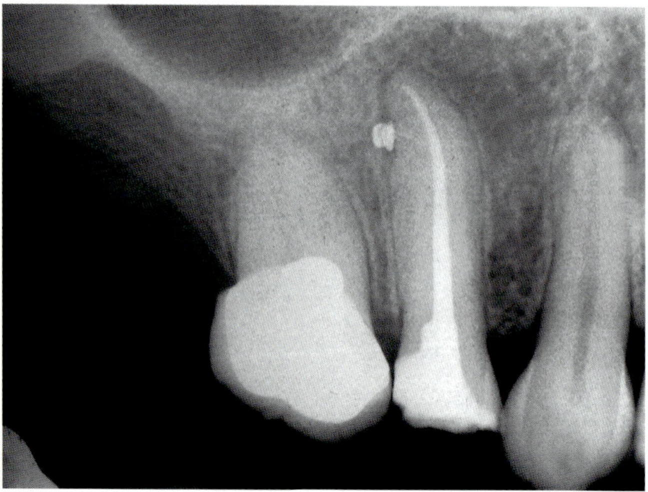

3-18h Postoperative radiograph.

Removal of gutta-percha

Removal of gutta-percha generally poses no problems; it is usually more easily removed than other obturation materials unless a thermocompaction technique has been used for obturation.

If *cold lateral condensation* or a *single-cone technique* has been used for obturation, it is not advisable to apply a solvent; use of a solvent would cause the gutta-percha and the sealer to form a sticky paste that is difficult to remove. If the coronal gutta-percha appears as a compact mass, a Gates Glidden drill is used without solvent to open up the canal orifice and clear the first few millimeters of the canal (Fig 3-19a). Following this, the preferred technique is to use an appropriately sized H-file to slowly advance down the canal along the length of the gutta-percha in an attempt to remove all the gutta-percha in one piece (Fig 3-19b). Once the gutta-percha is removed, the canals are cleaned, prepared, and obturated (Figs 3-19c and 3-19d).

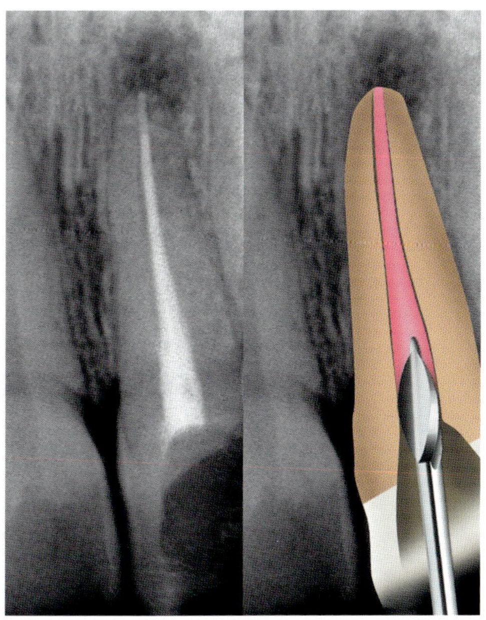

3-19a If it is radiographically evident that gutta-percha has been used for obturation, a Gates Glidden drill is used to remove the coronal portion of obturation material.

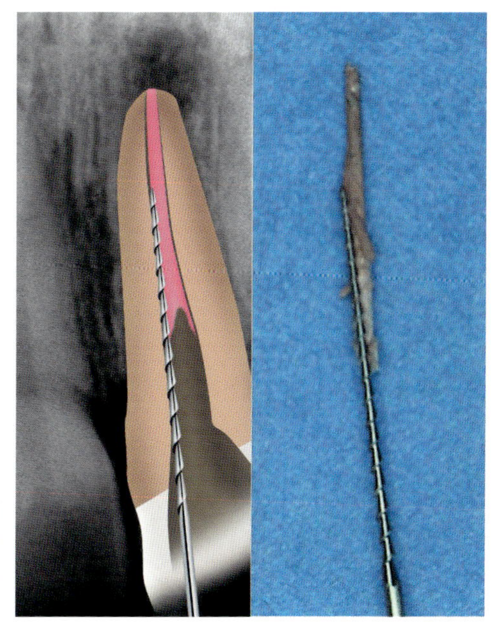

3-19b A large-diameter H-file is then advanced slowly down the canal and rotated in an attempt to retrieve the gutta-percha cones intact.

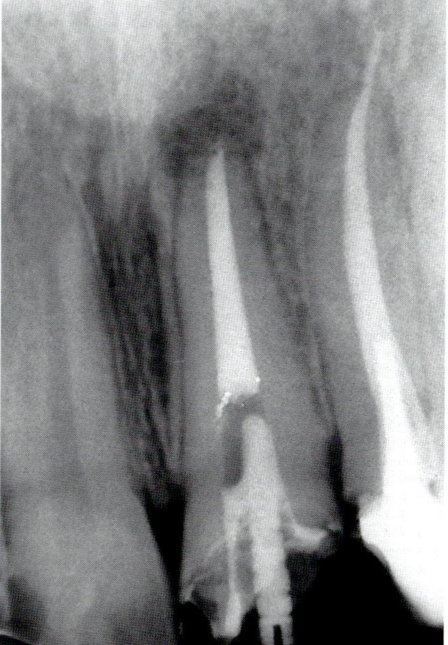

3-19c Postoperative radiograph.

3-19d Radiograph taken 3 years postoperatively. In certain cases rotary nickel-titanium instruments can be used to retrieve gutta-percha cones using the same technique.

In cases where the gutta-percha appears as a compact mass, hand files and rotary instruments can be used as described earlier for the removal of pastes; this allows effective removal of the obturation material without difficulty.
To remove gutta-percha, some authors suggest the use of rotary nickel-titanium instruments, without solvent, at speeds of 700 to 1,200 rpm. When used at these speeds without any form of coolant, the instruments heat the gutta-percha, thereby softening it; owing to the design of the instruments, the softened obturation material is propelled coronally. This technique should be used only in straight canals and might be dangerous because of the increased risk of the instrument screwing into the canal or fracturing; this technique offers no major advantage over more controlled methods.

Whichever technique is used (rotary instruments or hand files) it is very important to remember the following rule: *When an instrument cannot be advanced further down the canal, it must not be forced.*

When an instrument cannot be advanced further, the operator must first check that there is still obturation material remaining within the canal and there is no other cause for the obstruction. A drop of solvent is then added and a smaller-diameter instrument is advanced apically. Attempting to force an instrument apically in a blocked canal risks fracturing the instrument and increasing the ledge or even creating a perforation.

Removal of silver points

Immediate retrieval of silver points should never be attempted. Even if a silver point appears to be poorly adapted to the coronal two-thirds of the canal, it may fit well in the apical third. Silver points will often be affected by corrosion and can be quite fragile. Grasping the coronal aspect of a silver point, without any prior preparation to loosen it, risks fracturing the silver point (Machtou, 1993).

The procedure to remove silver points is as follows:

1. The coronal restoration is removed with a high-speed handpiece and ultrasonic instruments; this step must be performed with care to ensure the coronal tip of the silver point is not removed (Figs 3-20a and 3-20b). The pulp chamber is then debrided with ultrasonic instruments.
2. Solvent is placed in the pulp chamber and hand files are used down the canal along the length of the silver point to remove the sealer (Fig 3-20c).
3. After the sealer is eliminated, an ultrasonic file with a diameter of 15/100 is introduced, with copious irrigation, along the length of the silver point (Fig 3-20d). The ultrasonic vibrations are sometimes sufficient to free the silver point and remove it.
4. When the silver point has been loosened, the coronal aspect can be grasped gently with Steiglitz forceps, an Instruments Removal System (IRS, Dentsply), or a Masserann extractor (Micro-Mega) (Figs 3-20e and 3-20f).
5. If the silver point resists removal, it must not be forced; ultrasonic vibration can be applied directly to the forceps holding the silver point in an attempt to loosen it.

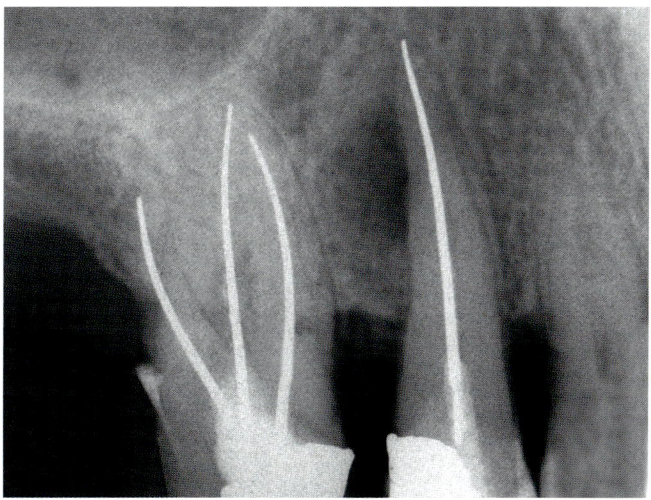

3-20a Preoperative radiograph of a maxillary molar and premolar obturated with silver points. Note the lateral lesion associated with the premolar and the periodontal problems affecting the molar, which necessitated the sectioning of the distal root.

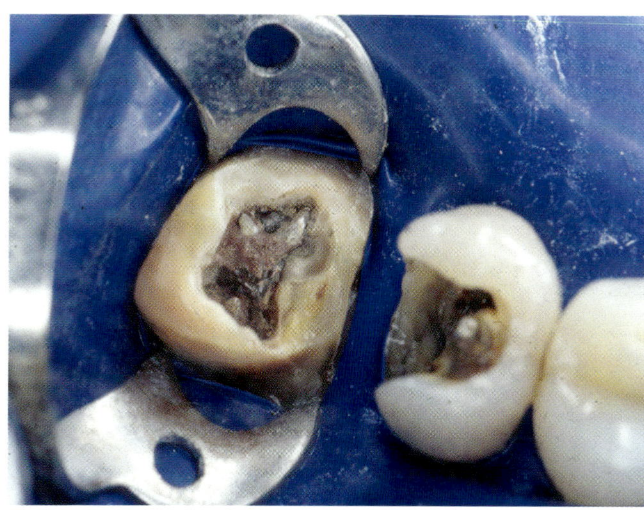

3-20b The tips of the silver points have been carefully uncovered without being damaged.

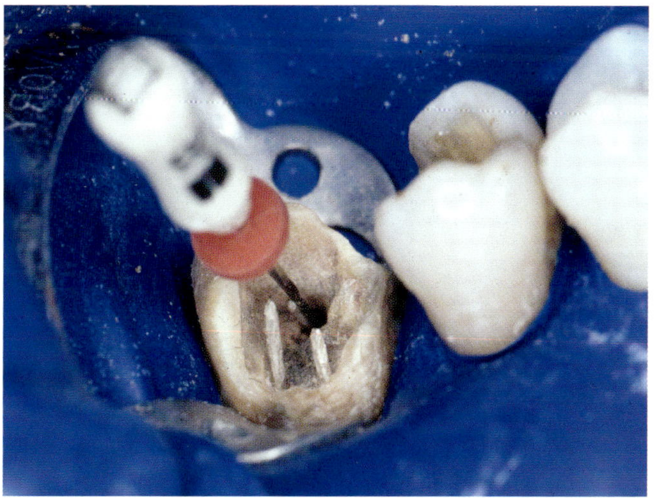

3-20c A drop of solvent is placed and hand files are used to remove the sealer from around the silver points.

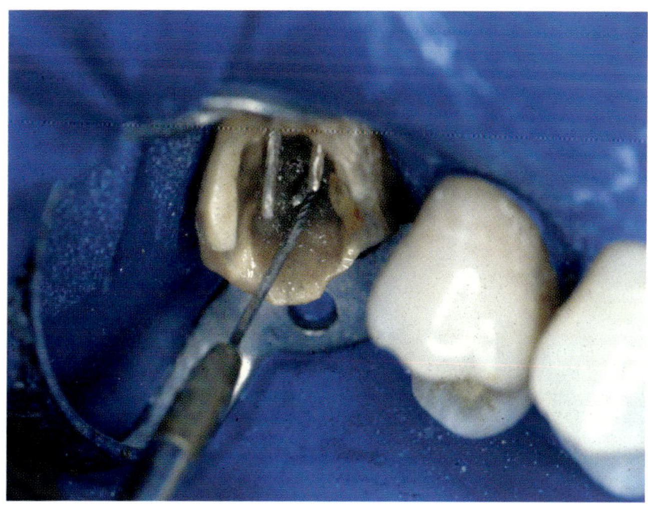

3-20d The silver points are then vibrated with ultrasonic files, under copious irrigation. It is only at this stage that the silver points can be retrieved.

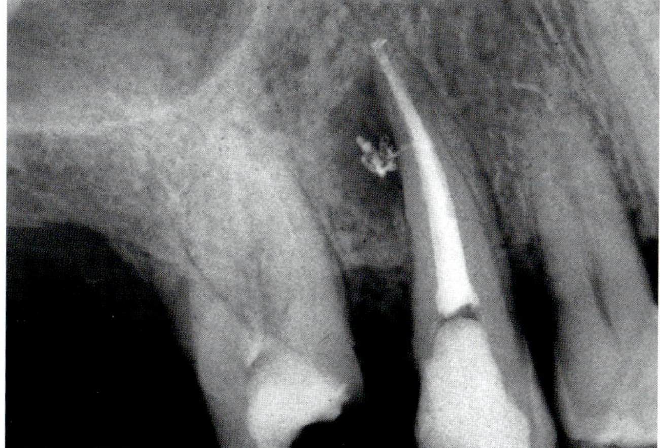

3-20e Postoperative radiograph of the premolar.

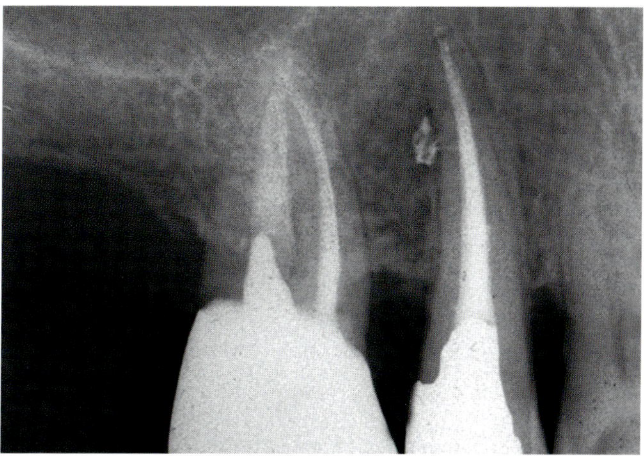

3-20f Radiograph taken 3 years postoperatively.

The techniques used to remove carrier-based obturation material (Thermafil Plus, Dentsply; Soft-Core, Axis Dental) resemble the techniques used to remove gutta-percha. In large or oval canals the carrier is embedded in a mass of gutta-percha in the coronal two-thirds. A large-diameter H-file is used to eliminate the gutta-percha around the carrier. Once the carrier has been freed, the H-file is rotated into it so the carrier can be pulled and elevated intact. The same technique can be used with rotary nickel-titanium instruments. Large-diameter tapered instruments are used to remove the gutta-percha from alongside the carrier. As the instruments progress apically, the canal walls narrow and the carrier is generally rolled around the rotary instrument and extracted coronally.

In round narrow canals where there is little gutta-percha between the carrier and the canal walls, failure results from inadequate preparation. Solvents are of no use. The technique for removal of the carrier remains the same as for large canal but a smaller-diameter instrument must be used so that it can be inserted between the canal walls and the carrier.

In cases where the carrier cannot be elevated despite being loose, techniques used to remove silver points can be employed; the coronal tip of the carrier is then gently grasped and pulled.

Negotiating the untreated part of the canal

If the initial root filling was short of the apex, after the obturation material is removed there are two possible scenarios: *(1)* the apical portion of the canal can be negotiated and a small-diameter file (08/100 or 10/100) can be introduced relatively easily; and *(2)* there is a blockage at the level where the existing root filling ends, with calcification of the apical portion of the canal, and further preparation of the canal is not possible at this stage.

Negotiating the untreated part of the canal depends on the coronal access preparation, how much obturation material has been successfully removed, the size of the ledge, and the extent of the calcification. The access preparation should provide straight-line access to the apical third, enabling the operator to maintain good control of the instruments while attempting to negotiate the apical portion of the canal.

It should always be assumed that a ledge might be present at the level where the existing root filling ends, and *large-diameter files should never be forced further down the canal* to avoid the risk of transporting the canal and creating a perforation.

Rotary nickel-titanium instruments must not be used to negotiate blocked canals; these instruments cut on the outer part of the curve and may worsen the existing ledge. To bypass the ledge and negotiate the untreated portion of the canal, the coronal portion of the canal must first be enlarged and cleaned; a fine hand file (10/100, 08/100, or 06/100) with a precurved tip is then used with a chelating agent and sodium hypochlorite (Machtou, 1993). In such cases, 18mm or 21mm C+ files (Dentsply-Maillefer) can prove very useful. These files, available in four sizes (06, 08, 10, and 15), are less flexible than traditional files of the same dimension. They are therefore less susceptible to deformation during attempts to negotiate the canal.

Ledges are often created by instruments that work on the outer part of the curve; therefore, the precurved tip of the instrument needs to be directed toward the inner part of the curve, keeping in mind that buccal and lingual curvatures will not be visible radiographically.

Mandibular molar canals

Mesial canals

These canals have a primary distal curvature visible on radiographs (Fig 3-21a) and a secondary curvature not visible radiographically: lingual for the buccal canal, and buccal for the lingual canal (Fig 3-21b). After clearing the obturation material to the level of the ledge (Fig 3-21c), a precurved 08 or 10 C+ file with plenty of chelating agent is introduced into the canal. The file should be oriented distally and lingually for a buccal canal and distally and buccally for a lingual canal (Fig 3-21d).

Once the canal is found, the file must not be withdrawn lest the pathway be lost. This can be one of the most frustrating mistakes made during endodontic retreatment. The file should be advanced several millimeters apically by rotating the instrument in a quarter-turn clockwise/counterclockwise motion (Fig 3-21e). Once the file is past the blockage, it is worked in and out with small, gentle movements; progressively larger movements will eventually free the file.

The next step is to smooth out the walls of the canal and eliminate any ledges created by the blockage. A series of precurved stainless steel hand files of increasing diameter (15, 20, 25, etc) is used to remove dentin shoulders and create a smooth preparation (Fig 3-21f). These files are used with a gentle in-and-out motion. The canal needs regular irrigation and, between successive files, it should be instrumented with a size 10 file to ensure the canal remains patent.

Another technique for elimination of ledges involves the use of the ProTaper Finishing File 1 (F1), which has a tip size of 0.20 mm and a taper of 7% over the first few millimeters of the instrument. A useful feature of this instrument is the large apical taper, which allows dentin ledges to be rapidly eliminated. This instrument must not be used until a stainless steel hand file of diameter 15 or larger has been worked down the canal to create a glide path. For the F1 to enter the apical portion of the canal, it must be precurved until the point of permanent deformation so the tip can enter the already enlarged canal. To achieve this, the instrument is grasped at its tip and curved 180 degrees (the tip needs to practically touch the shaft of the instrument). When released, the instrument will retain a certain amount of deformation that allows it to re-enter the canal. The same effect can be achieved with the Endo-Bender pliers (SybronEndo), which have one flat jaw and one rounded conic jaw that allow the file to be curved to varying degrees depending on where it is positioned in the pliers. However they are bent, the instruments must be initially curved with an exaggerated deformation so that the final curvature is great enough to allow the instrument to enter the canal. Once the ProTaper F1 has advanced beyond the blockage, it is rotated clockwise and counterclockwise, moving progressively further down the canal while removing the obstruction (Fig 3-21g). Small-diameter hand files are used to ensure patency of the canal, and a working-length radiograph can be taken (Fig 3-21h). The canal is then prepared and cleaned.

Distal canal

Although often wide in the coronal region, the distal canal narrows apically and may present with a marked distal curvature that was not prepared during the initial endodontic treatment. After the coronal portion of the obturation material has been removed (Fig 3-21i), a precurved C + file (diameter 08 or 10) should be inserted into the canal with the tip oriented toward the distal aspect so the apical part of the canal can be negotiated. The working length is determined and the apical portion of the canal is prepared manually with a precurved stainless steel hand file to size 15 (Fig 3-21j). Hand nickel-titanium instruments can be used to prepare and clean sharp apical curvatures (Figs 3-21k to 3-21m).

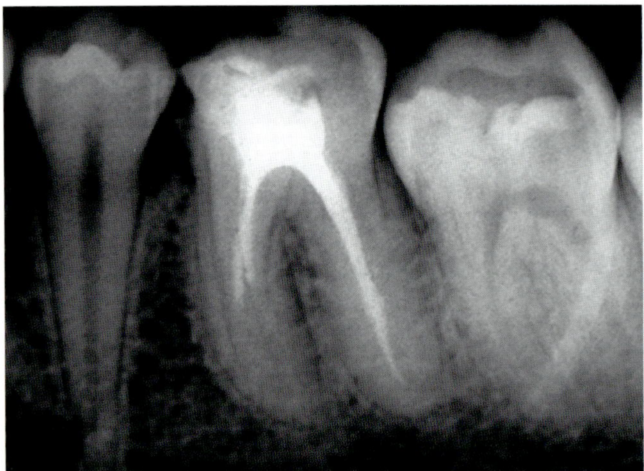

3-21a Preoperative radiograph of a mandibular molar with inadequate endodontic treatment.

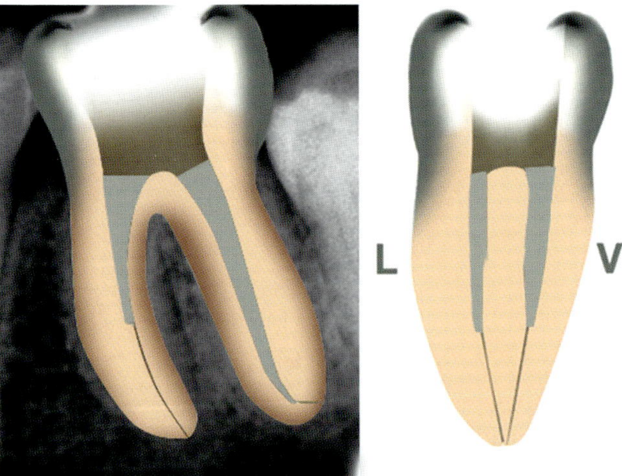

3-21b Diagram highlighting the distal curvature of the mesial root on a radiograph (*left*); the buccal curvature of the lingual canal and the lingual curvature of the buccal canal are apparent in profile, but these are not visible radiographically. Blockages tend to occur at the level of the buccal and lingual curvature.

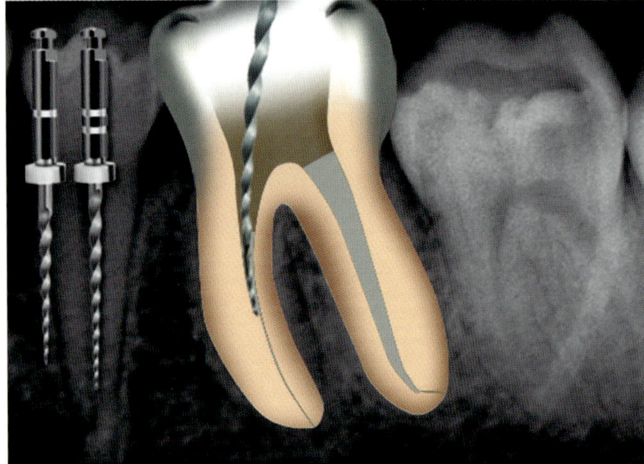

3-21c Obturation material is removed down to the level of the obstruction. A stainless steel file (diameter 10 or 15) is inserted into the canal and a radiograph is taken to check that the obturation material has been successfully removed and to allow the level of the blockage to be assessed.

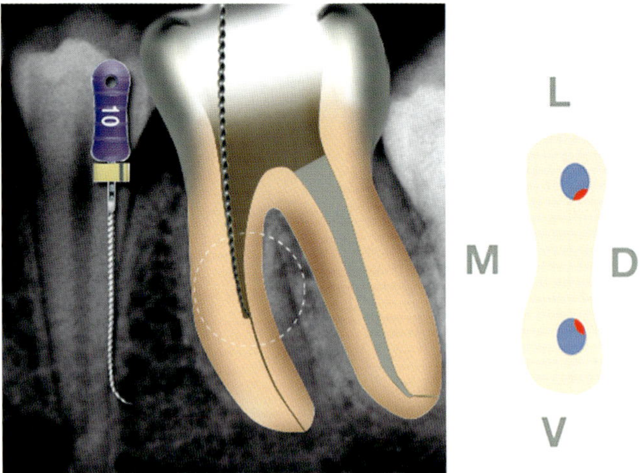

3-21d A precurved stainless steel C+ hand file is inserted into the buccal canal with its tip directed distally and lingually, and into the lingual canal with its tip directed distally and buccally. The diagram depicts a section through the mesial root and shows the blockages (*blue*) and the canals (*red*). The operator must direct the instrument tips toward these red areas when trying to negotiate past the obstructions.

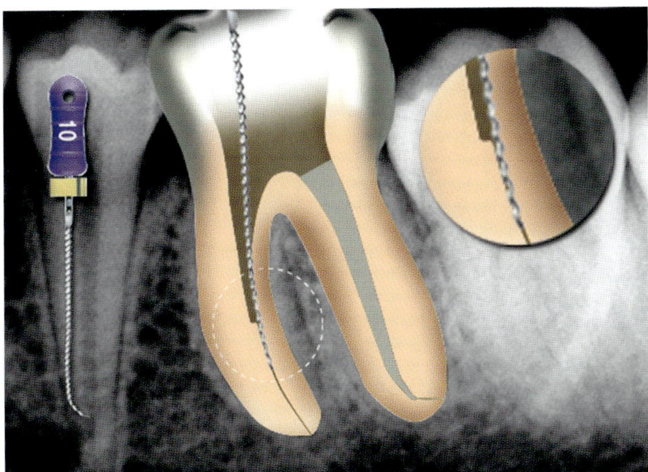

3-21e Once the canal has been located, the file is advanced as far as possible with clockwise and counterclockwise rotational movements, and then a slow in-and-out motion is used.

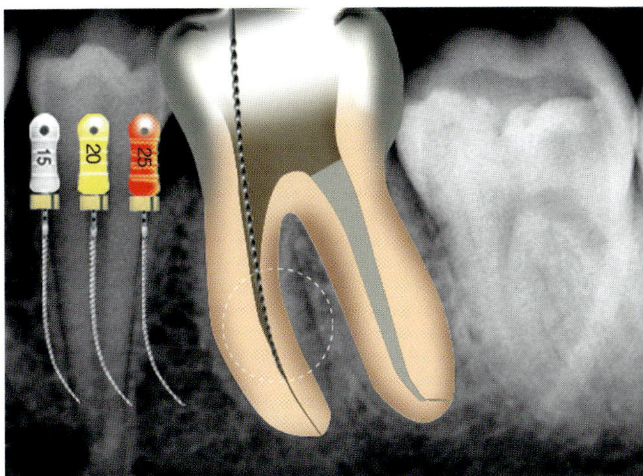

3-21f A series of precurved files of increasing diameter is used to eliminate the shoulder and smooth the canal wall.

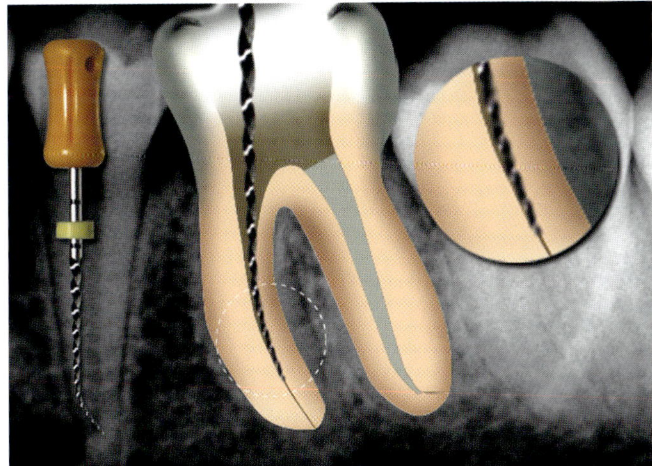

3-21g The canal walls can also be smoothed with a precurved ProTaper F1 hand file used with gentle pulling and rotational movements.

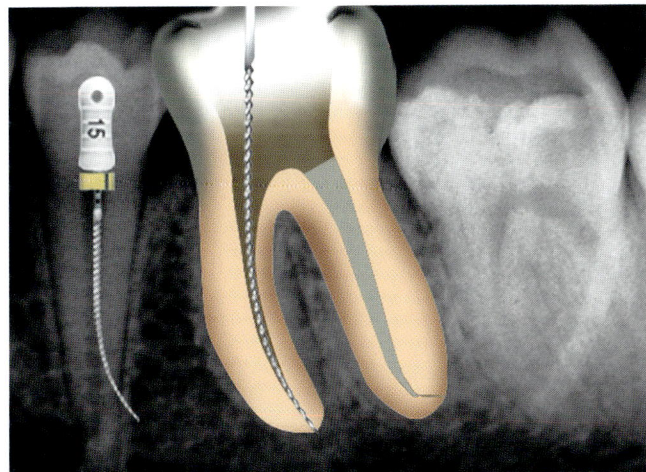

3-21h Patency is achieved and the working length is determined. The apical portion of the canal is then prepared and cleaned.

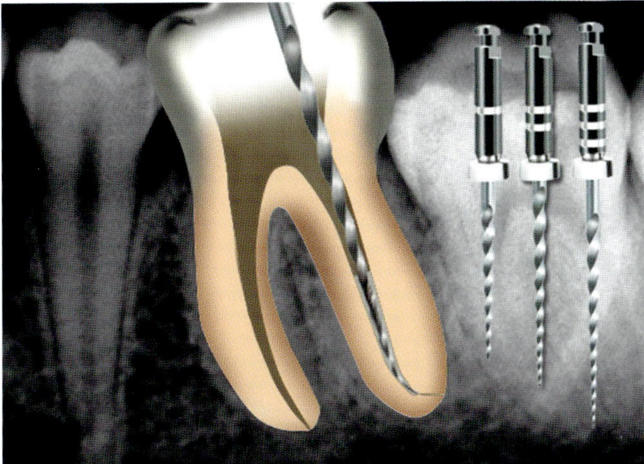

3-21i Removal of obturation material from the distal canal is stopped when an obstruction is encountered.

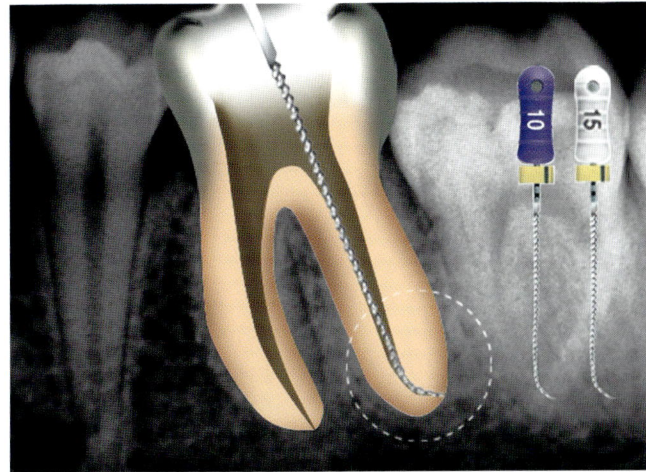

3-21j The tip of a precurved stainless steel C+ hand file is directed distally to attempt to locate the canal. Patency is achieved and working length determined.

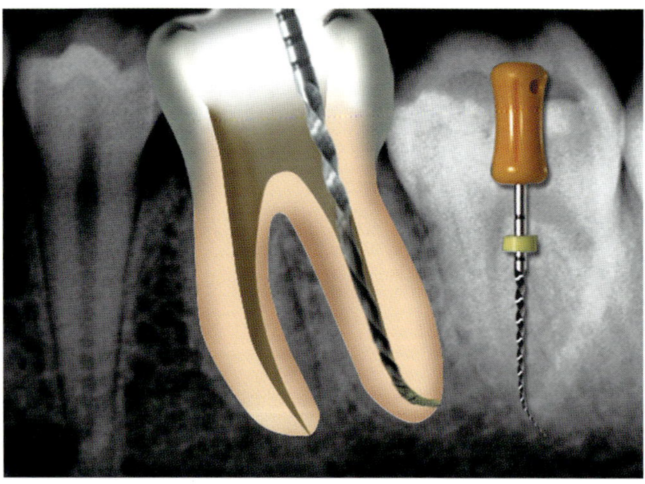

3-21k The apical curvature is prepared with manual ProTaper files.

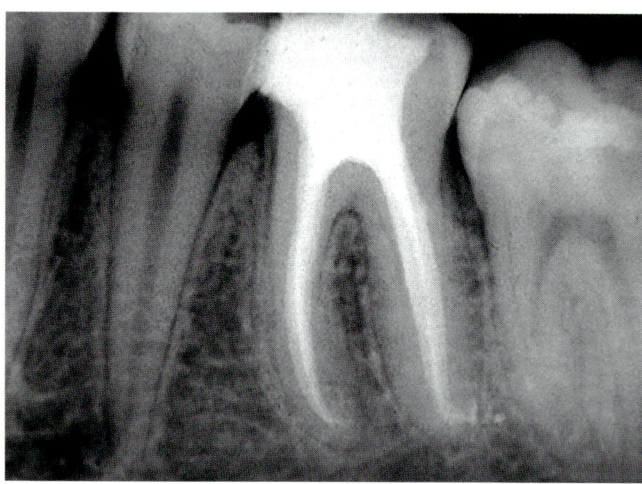

3-21l Postoperative radiograph.

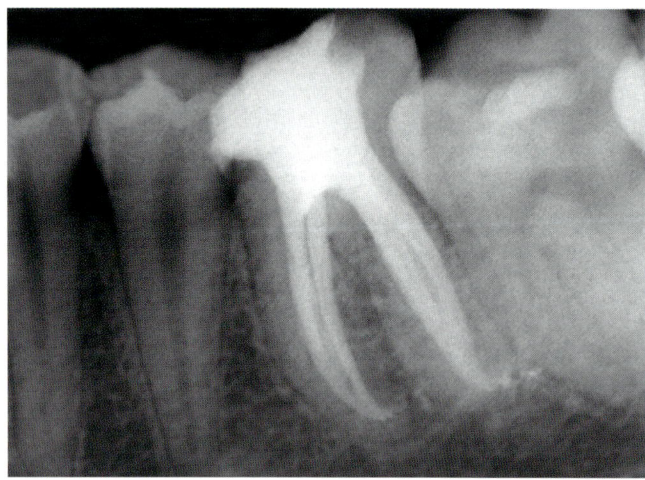

3-21m Postoperative radiograph viewed from another angle.

Palatal canal of maxillary molars

The apical portions of these canals often demonstrate a buccal curvature that is not visible on radiographs. A fine precurved hand file must be oriented buccally to attempt negotiation of the canal.

Once the ledge has been bypassed, it is necessary to evaluate each situation on a case-by-case basis and decide whether or not to remove the obstruction entirely. This depends on the position of the ledge, the size of the obstruction, and the amount of dentin that will need to be removed to clear the obstruction entirely. A significant ledge requiring a large amount of dentin removal may present a considerable risk of weakening the tooth or creating a perforation. In such cases it may be best not to attempt to clear the blockage entirely. Obturating the tooth can therefore prove difficult, since the gutta-percha points may bend when they are introduced into the canal. By marking the coronal aspect of the gutta-percha point, the operator can monitor the point as it enters the canal. The gutta-percha point can be precurved before it is introduced into the canal to facilitate its placement.

Cleaning the canal after removal of obturation material

After the working length has been determined and the canal prepared, any residual obturation material should be removed. Solvent is placed into the canal and agitated with a paper point; this not only cleans the canal walls but also dissolves any sealer that may remain (eg, in isthmuses) after instrumentation. At this stage, if the paper point comes out stained by debris, the canal is not clean. Copious irrigation with sodium hypochlorite disinfects the canal and removes all traces of solvent from the root canal system.

Cases in which a canal cannot be negotiated

In cases where, despite all efforts, the apical portion of the canal cannot be negotiated, only the accessible part of the canal can be prepared, cleaned, and obturated. The tooth must be monitored radiographically at regular intervals. If there was no lesion preoperatively and aseptic techniques were employed, the probability of a lesion appearing is extremely low, despite the apical portion of the canal remaining untreated. In these cases the reported success rate is high (Friedman, 1998 and 2002). Even if a lesion is present preoperatively, healing is still seen in 60% of cases (Akerblöm, 1984) (Figs 3-22a to 3-22c).

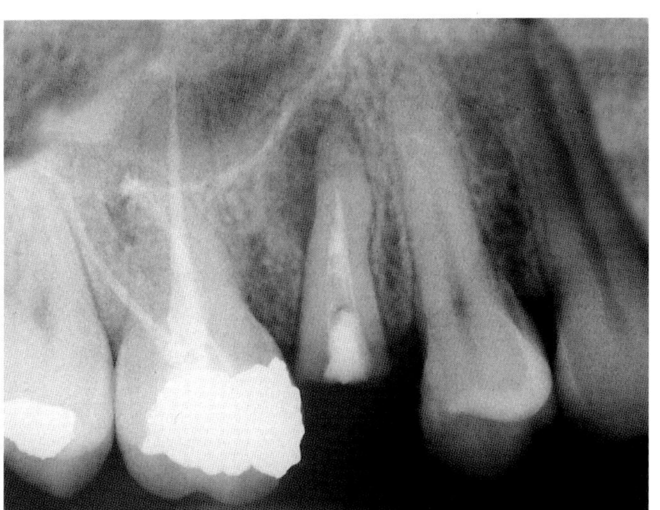

3-22a Preoperative radiograph of a maxillary premolar with a lateral and periapical lesion.

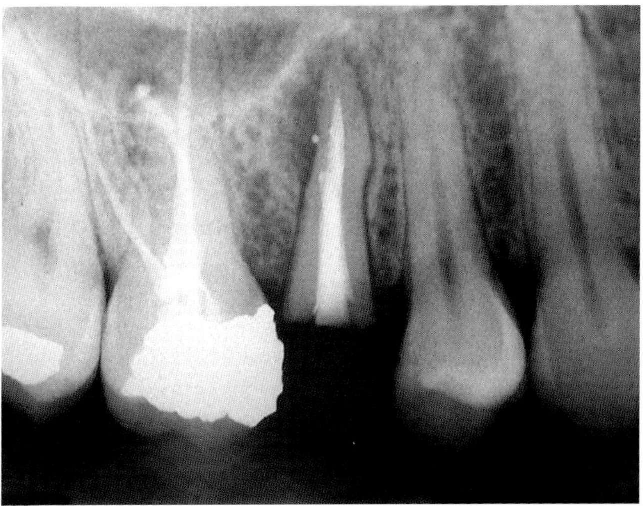

3-22b Immediate postoperative radiograph. Despite all efforts, the apical portion of the canal could not be negotiated. Note the obturation of the lateral canal.

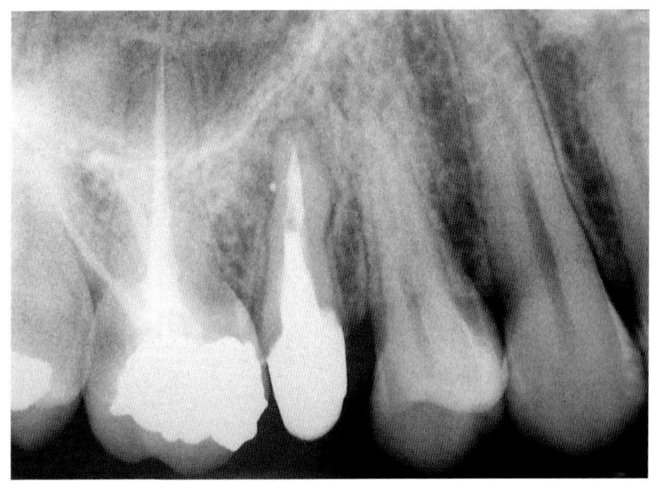

3-22c Radiograph taken 6 months postoperatively showing healing.

In effect, removal of a leaking coronal restoration and a failing root filling under copious irrigation cleanses the root canal system and sufficiently reduces the bacterial load so healing can take place.

Thus, endodontic retreatment should not be considered a failure simply because the apical portion of the canal was left untreated. Postoperative monitoring is essential. Adjunctive treatment should not be offered unless the lesion increases in size, does not disappear, or becomes symptomatic (Figs 3-23a to 3-23e).

A definitive coronal restoration must be placed immediately. Delaying the placement of a coronal restoration compromises the healing process because of the risk of bacterial penetration and reinfection. A provisional post-retained crown does not provide a good seal; however, a post and core or a bonded core in conjunction with a provisional crown is acceptable and recommended.

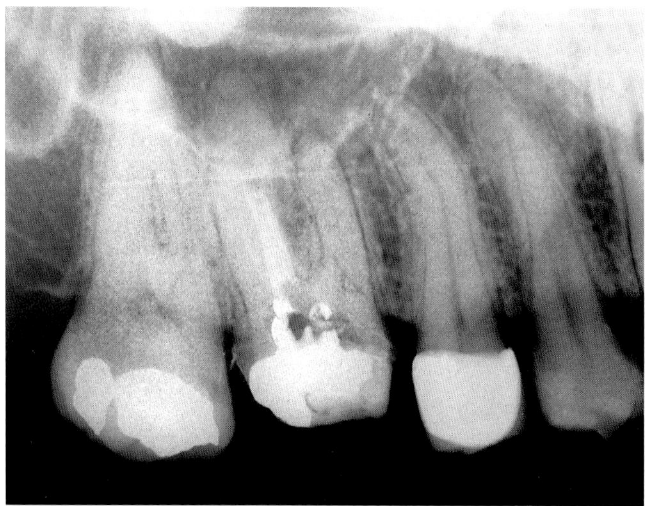

3-23a Preoperative radiograph of a maxillary molar in need of endodontic retreatment. There is a periapical lesion associated with the mesiobuccal root.

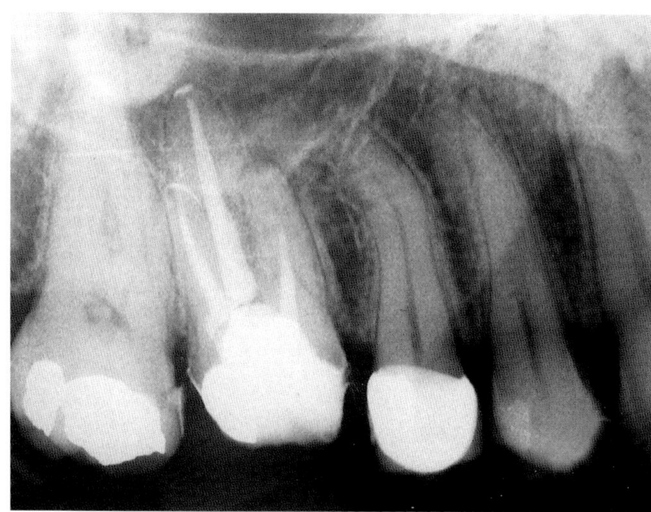

3-23b Postoperative radiograph showing incomplete obturation of the mesial root because the apical portion of the canal could not be negotiated.

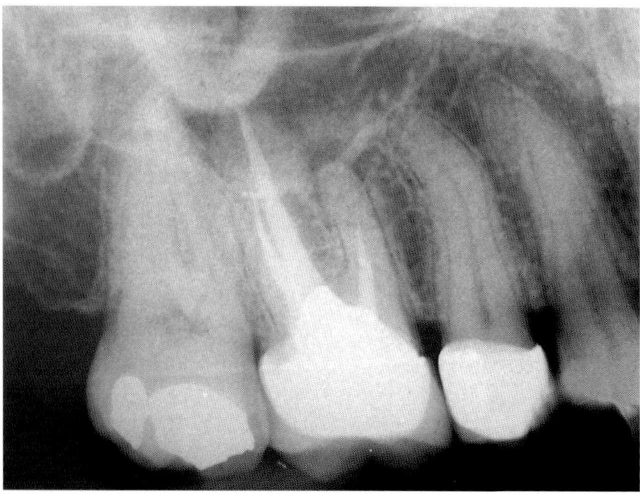

3-23c Radiograph taken 6 months postoperatively demonstrating the persistent lesion associated with the mesial root.

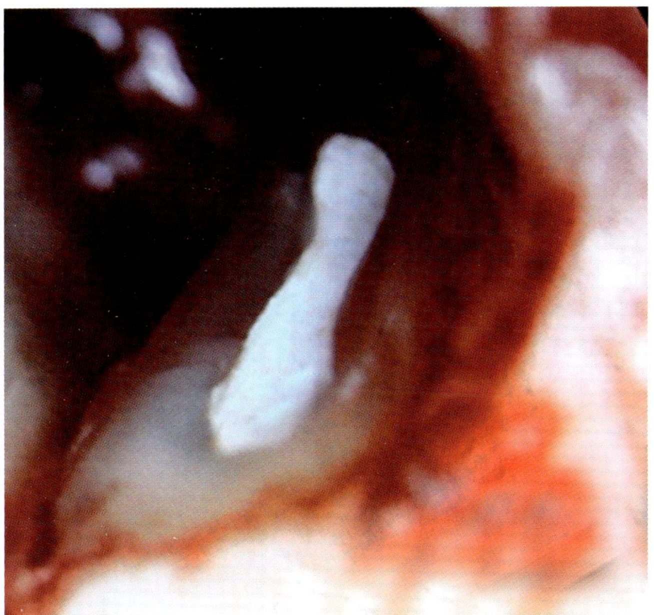

3-23d Clinical photograph of the retrograde obturation of the mesial root. Note the oval shape of the cavity; this enabled the clinician to prepare and obturate the two canals in this root and the isthmus which connects them.

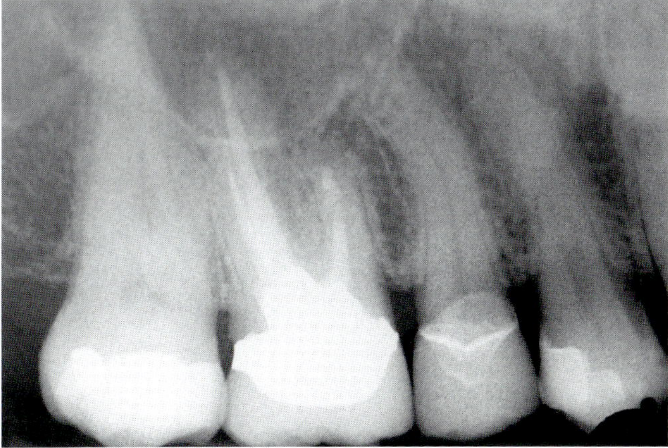

3-23e Radiograph taken 7 years postoperatively.

If the problem was clearly endodontic in origin and the retreatment has been conducted properly, there is no justification for not placing a definitive restoration. If the conventional retreatment should fail, a surgical approach will be necessary and the coronal restoration will be left untouched.

Management of Fractured Instruments

Fractured instruments are a problem commonly encountered in endodontic treatment and can occur with any instrument, including barbed broaches, stainless steel hand files, rotary nickel-titanium instruments, Lentulo spiral fillers, and thermomechanical compaction devices, among others. Advances in technology (eg, ultrasonics, IRS) and the introduction of the operating microscope in particular now make it possible to remove instrument fragments that would in the past have been impossible to retrieve. Nevertheless, despite these developments, it is still not possible to remove all fractured instruments. The clinician should attempt to retrieve the fragment using the techniques and equipment available, but determined efforts to do so may result in a weakened root or a perforation.

Factors influencing the removal of fractured instruments

A variety of factors affect the prognosis for the retrieval of a fractured instrument; these must be taken into consideration so the chance of success and the limitations of treatment can be evaluated. If a proper assessment is performed and the right equipment is available (most importantly an operating microscope), the chance of retrieving the fractured instrument nears 87% (Suter et al, 2005).

Canal anatomy
The possibility of accessing and then bypassing a fractured instrument depends on the shape of the canal, its diameter, the presence of any curvatures or concavities, and the thickness of the dentin.

Location of the fragment
The chance of retrieving a fractured instrument is higher if it lies in the coronal part of the tooth and in a straight portion of the canal. An instrument lodged around a curve can be retrieved if it is possible to bypass or if at least one-third of the instrument is accessible. If a fractured instrument lies apical to a curvature, the only possibility is to try to bypass it; the chance of successful retrieval is very low.

Type of instrument
The level of difficulty of the procedure will depend partly on the instrument that fractured. In general, a stainless steel hand file is easier to retrieve than a rotary nickel-titanium instrument, which may have threaded into the canal walls.

Cause of fracture
This may be difficult to ascertain initially but may help the operator decide on the best approach.

More than with the other aspects of retreatment, the probability of retrieving a fractured instrument is linked to clinician skill and available equipment. Some techniques for removal of fractured instruments can be performed without any specialized equipment (eg, negotiating past the fragment); other removal techniques (eg, ultrasonic vibration) risk further complications such as perforations and therefore necessitate the use of an operating microscope.

Techniques for the removal of fractured instruments

The length of time needed to remove a fractured instrument is highly variable and depends on the type of instrument, the size of the fragment, and whether the instrument has threaded into the dentin. Careful analysis of conventional and angled radiographs will allow the following to be determined:

- Canal in which the fragment is located
- Size of the fragment
- Nature of the instrument (eg, hand file or rotary instrument)
- Position of the fragment within the canal
- Root anatomy (length, curvature, thickness of dentinal wall)
- Defects in the initial access preparation

Retrieval of a fractured instrument should never be attempted with rotary nickel-titanium instruments, which may themselves fracture and complicate the problem.

First step
The first step, irrespective of what type of instrument has fractured, is to modify the access cavity to create straight-line access to the fragment. This stage is fundamental: it prevents instruments from binding in the coronal portion and allows good instrument control to be maintained. It also ensures direct vision of the fractured instrument unless the fragment is situated beyond a curvature. This step is completed with manual nickel-titanium instruments and/or Gates Glidden burs (Figs 3-24a and 3-24b).

Second step
The goal of the second step is to pass a stainless steel hand file laterally alongside the fragment; a small-diameter (08 or 10), precurved hand file should be used with copious amounts of chelating agent. If the canal is oval in section, it is relatively easy to move the file later-

ally past the fragment. However, if the canal is round in section and the instrument blocks the entire lumen, this can be difficult to achieve. In canals that are oval in their coronal two-thirds (eg, premolars), fractured instruments tend to lodge in the center of the canal, and the clinician must attempt to introduce the file along one side of the fragment.

If it is possible to pass a file the length of the fragment, hand files of increasing diameter are used with copious irrigation to widen the opening (Fig 3-24c). One of these instruments is then held in place with gentle pressure, and ultrasonic vibration is applied to it in an attempt to elevate out the instrument fragment by vibration (Fig 3-24d). The same result can be achieved with an ultrasonic file of diameter 15/100 (Satelec or EMS) which can be introduced into the canal alongside the fragment and vibrated gently under copious irrigation.

Before using the ultrasonic instruments in multi-rooted teeth, it is advisable to place cotton pledgets in the other canal orifices to ensure that if the fractured instrument is retrieved it is prevented from dropping into another canal (Fig 3-24e).

In the majority of cases, fractured instruments can be retrieved by this technique. Endodontic treatment can then be completed as normal (Figs 3-24f to 3-24h). In cases where a file has been negotiated past the fractured instrument but the fragment still cannot be retrieved after ultrasonic vibration is used, the canal is prepared and obturated. Thus the fractured instrument becomes embedded in a mass of gutta-percha during the obturation and rarely poses further problems.

Third step

If the fractured instrument cannot be bypassed, the next step involves freeing the coronal 2 to 3 mm of the fragment by using ultrasonic instruments to create a gutter in the surrounding dentin. An attempt is then made to remove the fragment by applying ultrasonic vibration.

If ultrasonic vibration is not effective, specialized instruments designed for instrument removal must be used to grip the fragment. *These steps are difficult and must be performed with caution. Use of an operating microscope is essential to ensure good vision, and the tip of the ultrasonic instrument must be visible as it is introduced into the canal to avoid further complications such as perforations.*

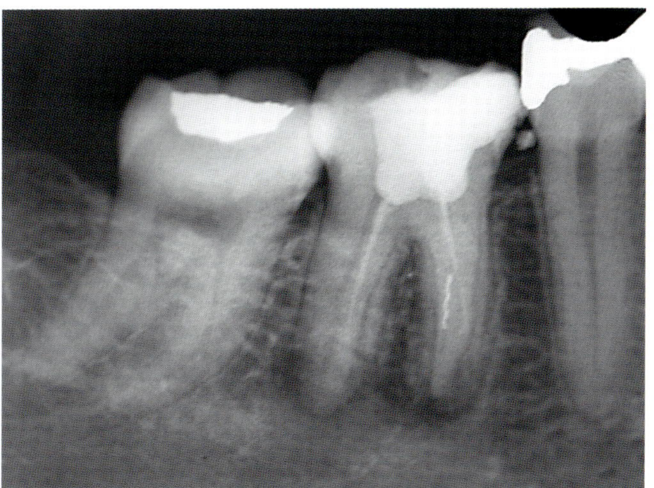

3-24a Preoperative radiograph of a mandibular molar with a fractured Lentulo spiral filler in the mesial canal and periapical lesions associated with both mesial and distal roots.

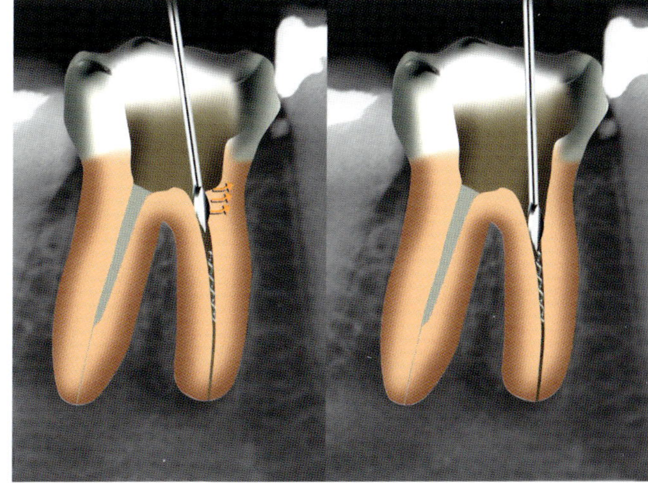

3-24b The first step involves modifying the access cavity to ensure straight-line access.

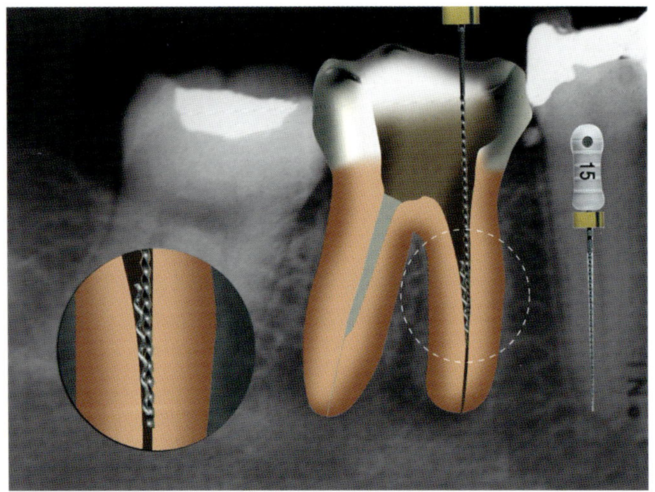

3-24c An attempt is made to negotiate past the fractured instrument with precurved hand files (diameter of 08 or 10). If this succeeds, the pathway is then widened with larger files.

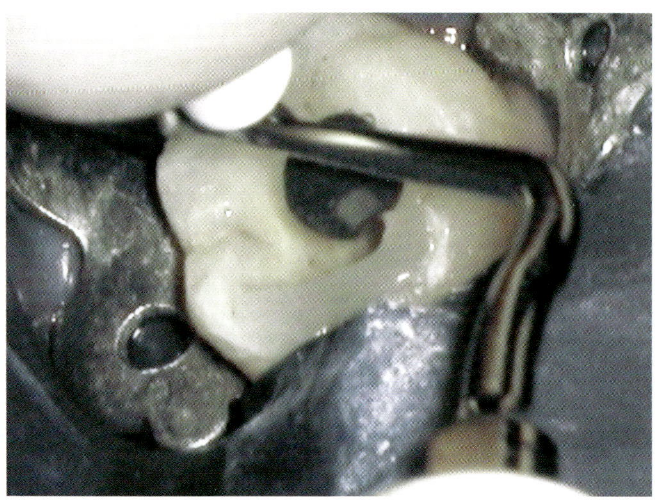

3-24d A hand file is held in place and ultrasonic vibration is applied. An ultrasonic file could also be used along the length of the fractured instrument.

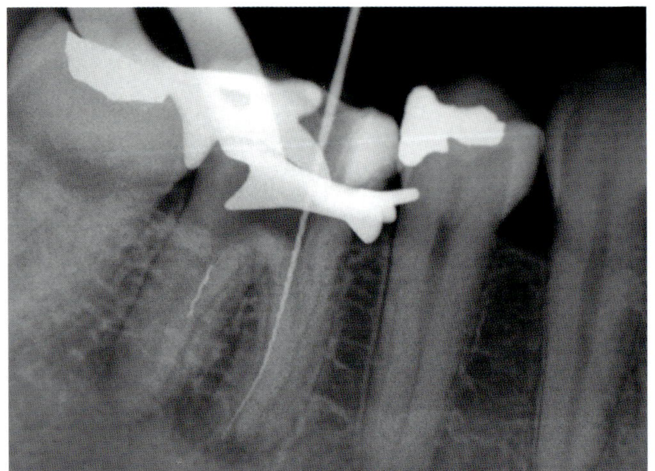

3-24e During this maneuver the other canal orifices must be protected by cotton pledgets to prevent the retrieved fragment falling into another canal, as happened in this case.

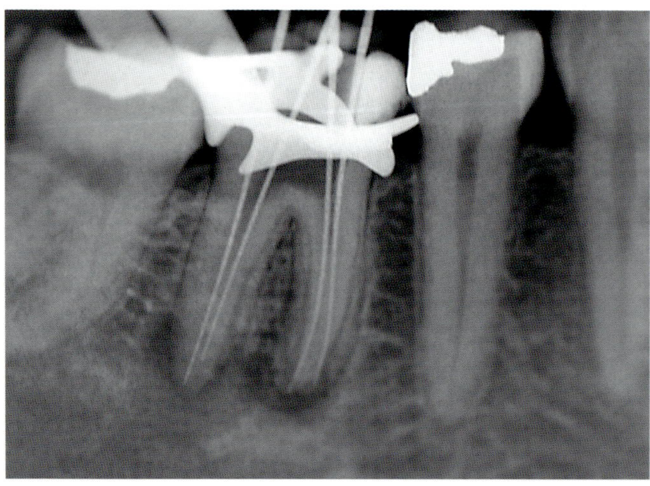

3-24f Once the fractured instrument has been retrieved, the working length can be determined and the canals are then prepared.

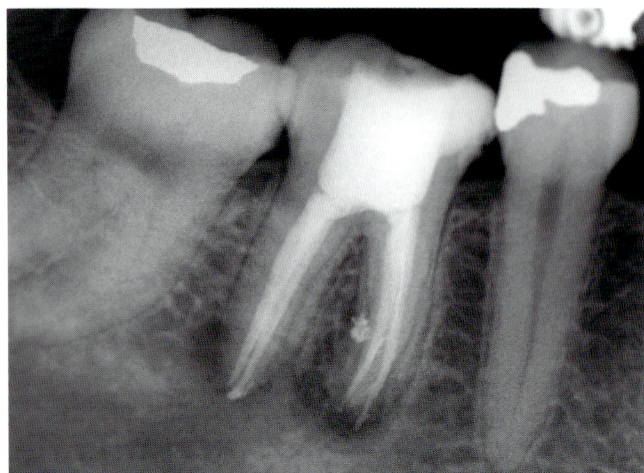

3-24g Immediate postoperative radiograph.

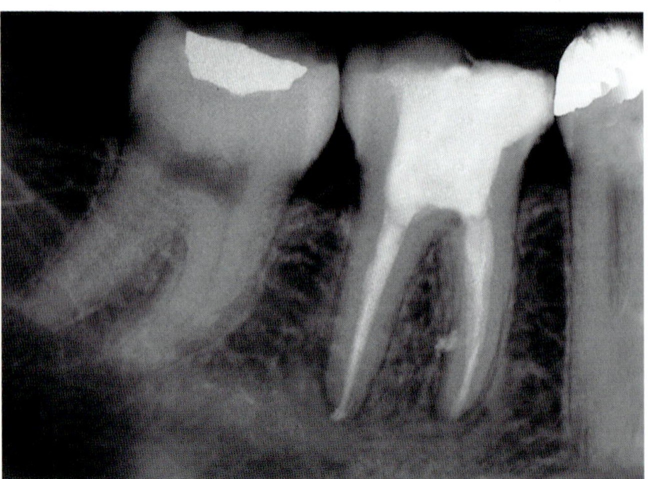

3-24h Healing 6 months postoperatively.

The canal is first enlarged coronally with Gates Glidden drills 2, 3, and 4 (Figs 3-25a and 3-25b) until the tip of the drill can penetrate the canal enough to contact the fractured instrument. A second Gates Glidden drill, which has been modified to remove the cutting tip, is used at low speed to create a ledge or shelf at the level of the fractured instrument (Fig 3-25c). Once access has been achieved and the fragment is visible (Fig 3-25d), titanium ProUltra Endo tips (Dentsply) or ET20 and ET25 (Satelec) are used to create a gutter around the fragment (Fig 3-25e). Aggressive cutting tips are not advised other than in the coronal portion of a wide root because they may remove excessive dentin and risk destroying the coronal part of the instrument fragment, thus compromising access to the remaining apical part. Once a gutter has been created in the dentin, the ultrasonic tip is vibrated (while in contact with the fragment) and rotated in a counterclockwise direction (Fig 3-25e). In certain cases the vibrations are enough to free the fractured instrument. The ultrasonic tip also can be gently wedged between the fractured instrument and the canal wall, which sometimes causes the fragment to suddenly free itself. Once the canal is opened endodontic treatment can be continued (Figs 3-25f and 3-25g).

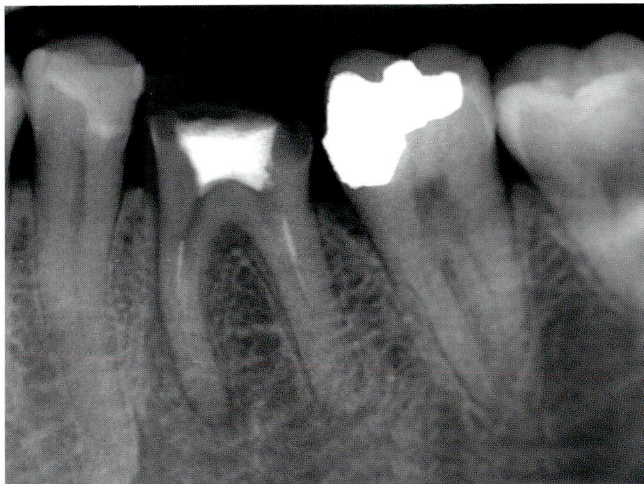

3-25a Preoperative radiograph of a mandibular molar with a fractured instrument in the mesial root.

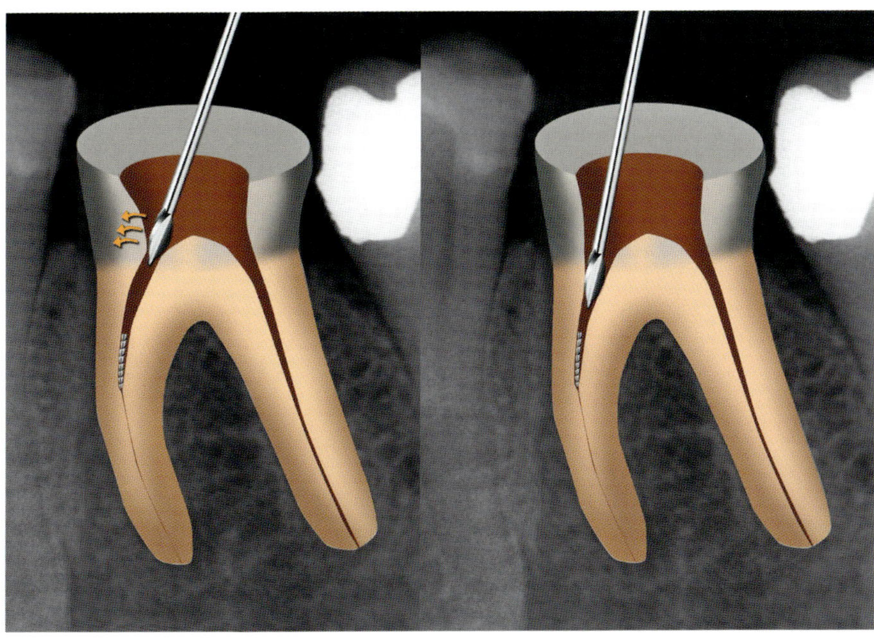

3-25b The coronal access cavity is enlarged to improve visibility and ensure straight-line access to the fragment.

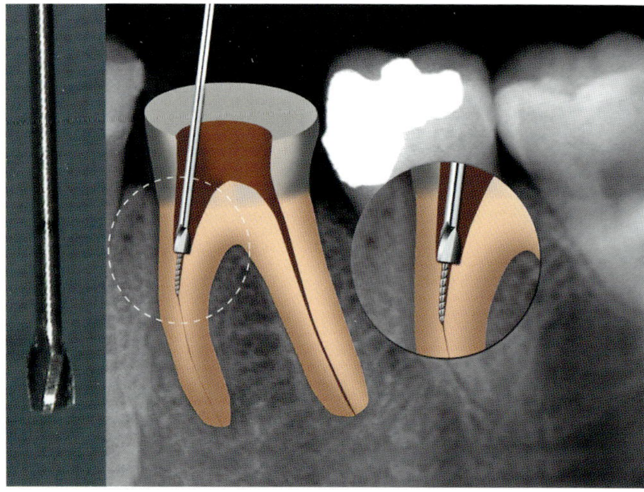

3-25c A Gates Glidden drill whose cutting tip has been removed is used at low speed to create a ledge at the level of the fractured instrument.

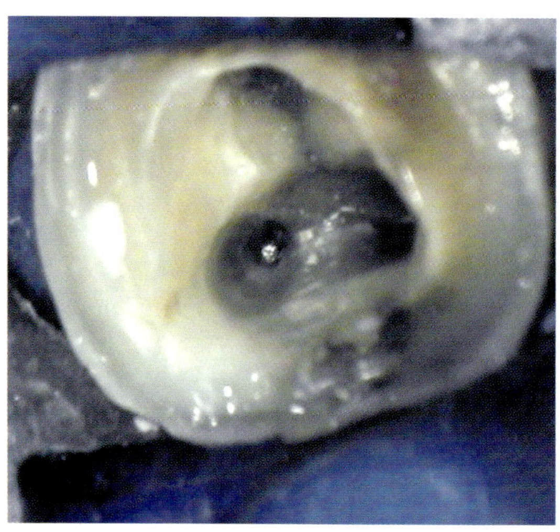

3-25d Before using the ultrasonic instruments, direct access to the fragment must be achieved.

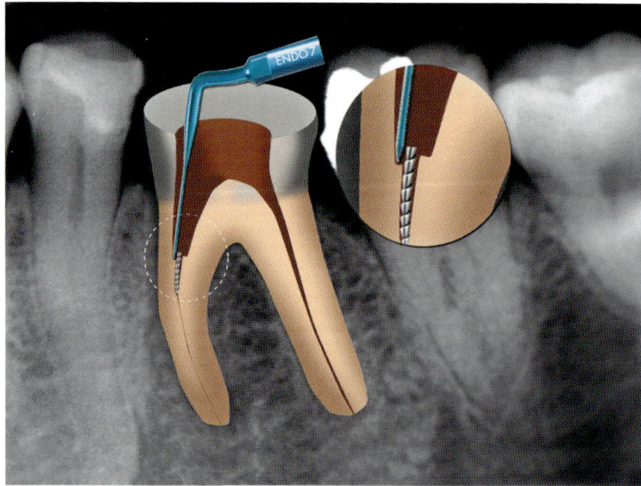

3-25e Ultrasonic tips (ET20 or ProUltra 6, 7, or 8) are then used to create a gutter around the fragment and free the coronal aspect of it.

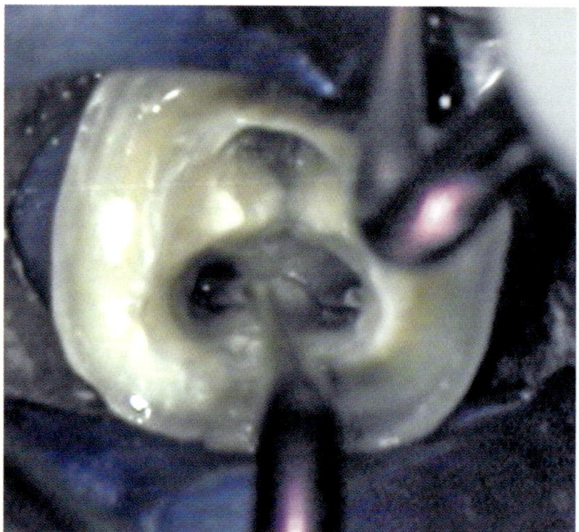

3-25f This procedure must not be performed other than under direct vision, or a perforation may occur. The ultrasonic vibrations are sometimes sufficient to expel the fragment from the canal.

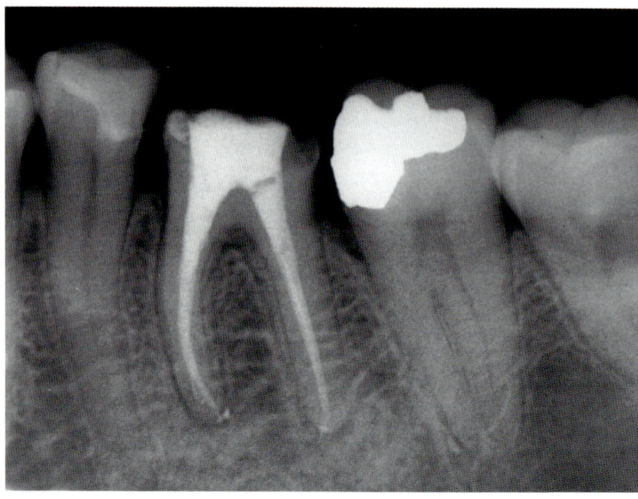

3-25g Postoperative radiograph.

The ultrasonic instruments must be used without water irrigation so that visual control can be maintained throughout the step. Water spray can be used to remove any debris that is generated, but its use is not advised while the instrument is active because the operator loses sight of the working tip. In some cases, although the tip of the fragment may be successfully freed, the ultrasonic vibration does not dislodge the fractured instrument. The final possibility for retrieving the fragment consists of using a dedicated instrument removal and retreatment system.

Using the instrument removal system

Most of these retreatment systems consist of a hollow tube that is placed over the coronal tip of the fractured instrument. Once the fragment has been grasped the whole assembly is twisted and the fragment is unscrewed and removed from the canal.

- The "homemade" system uses a hypodermic needle (21 or 25 gauge) with the bevel removed; it may need to be shortened. The needle is placed in the canal over the fractured instrument so that the coronal aspect of the fragment sits within the lumen of the needle. An H-file of appropriate length and diameter is introduced from the other end of the needle and then rotated and twisted until it locks into the fractured instrument. The fractured instrument can then be lifted out of the canal.
- A variation of this technique involves placing a chemically cured composite (eg, Core Paste XP, Den-Mat) down the needle or using the composite with the Cancelier system (series of hollow tubes of varying diameters). The needle or tube is left in place for 5 minutes and not moved. Once the composite has set, the whole ensemble is twisted and unscrewed to remove the fragment. Some authors have recommended the use of cyanoacrylate adhesive in place of the composite, but this method is less reliable and more difficult to control.
- The Masserann kit (Micro-Mega) is an instrument removal device that works on a concept similar to the needle technique. This system consists of a hollow extractor tube, a wedge, and a series of trephines that allow a gutter to be created around the fractured instrument. The hollow extractor tube is placed into the root canal to cover the exposed coronal tip of the fragment. The wedge is screwed into the tube, trapping the fractured instrument against the wall of the tube and allowing its removal. A large amount of tooth tissue is destroyed when the Masserann extractor is used; it should therefore not be used unless the fractured instrument is situated in a wide root and is located coronally. *For the fractured instrument to be retrieved, the diameter of the tube must be greater than that of the fragment. If the diameter of the tube matches that of the fractured instrument, the inserted wedge will act to push the fragment further into the canal rather than to engage and secure it.* Thus it is strongly advised that the Masserann extractor not be used in narrow, oval canals unless the tip of the fractured instrument extends up into the access cavity.
- The Dentsply's IRS (Fig 3-26) is similar to the Masserann extractor but has certain advantages. Like the Masserann device, the IRS consists of two hollow tubes into which wedges can be inserted, but the IRS tubes have thinner walls and smaller diameters than the Masserann tubes (1 mm for the black microtube and 0.8 mm for the red microtube). This allows them to be advanced further down the root canal and causes less destruction of tooth tissue. The distal end of each tube has a bevelled edge to help it slide over the edge of the fractured instrument, guiding the fragment into the lumen of the tube. This is particularly important in cases of canal curvature where the fragment tends to be wedged against the outer wall of the curve. The tube is also designed with a cut-out window in the distal end, which allows the tip of the fractured instrument to be displaced out through the window when the wedge is inserted and tightened against the fragment.

Before the IRS can be used, the coronal access must be improved (Figs 3-27a to 3-27c), and a trench should be created around the fragment with the ultrasonic tips so that at least 3 mm of the fractured instrument is exposed. The exposed fragment is then vibrated with ultrasonic instruments (Fig 3-27d). An appropriately sized tube is selected and gently introduced into the canal to prevent any damage; it should slide passively into the canal and fit over the fractured instrument. The fine, narrow walls that allow the tube to penetrate further into the root canal may otherwise fracture. In curved canals, the long part of the bevelled edge of the tube should be oriented against the outer wall of the curve. The wedge is inserted into the tube and twisted in a counterclockwise direction, thus engaging and securing the fragment by wedging it within the lumen of the tube. The tube-and-wedge assembly is then removed from the canal (Fig 3-27e), allowing root canal treatment to be continued (Fig 3-27f).

This system is difficult to use when retrieving fractured instruments; it is better suited to the removal of Lentulo spiral fillers or silver points.

Fractured Lentulo spiral fillers

As with silver points, it is imperative that the operator resist the temptation to pull on the visible portion of a Lentulo spiral filler. Tugging on the fragment without any preliminary

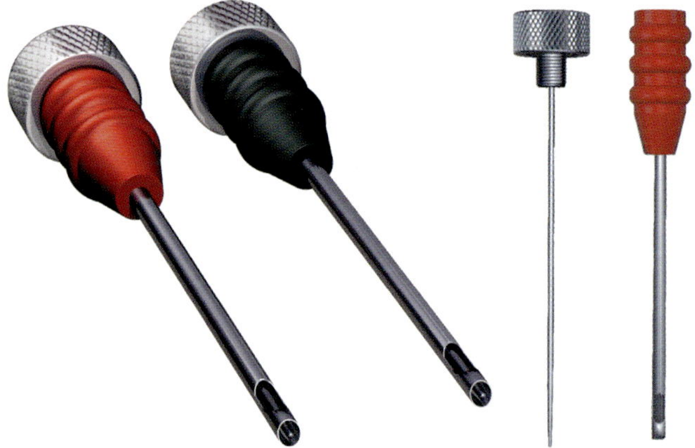

3-26 The IRS is designed to remove fractured instruments. Like the Masserann system, it employs a hollow tube and a wedge to insert into the tube; however, the IRS tubes are narrower and finer than those in the Masserann kit.

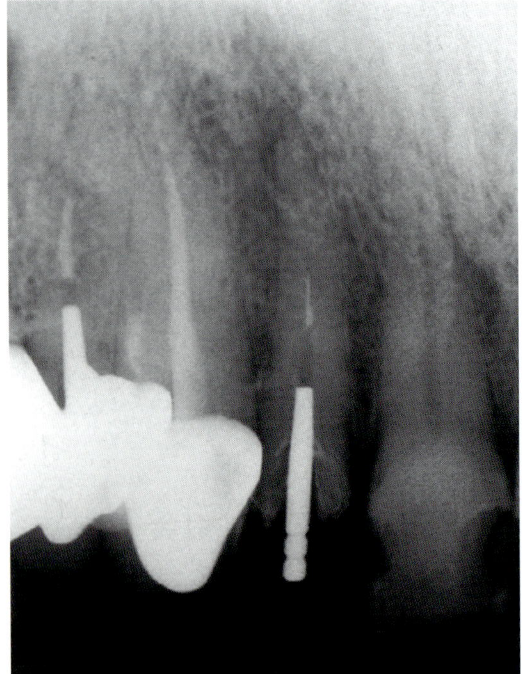

3-27a Preoperative radiograph of a maxillary lateral incisor with two fractured instruments (a barbed broach and a nickel-titanium instrument).

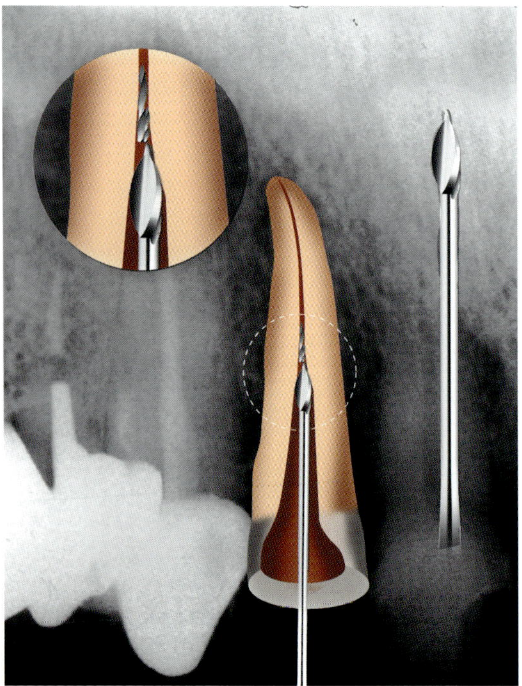

3-27b A Gates Glidden drill is used to widen the canal for instrumentation.

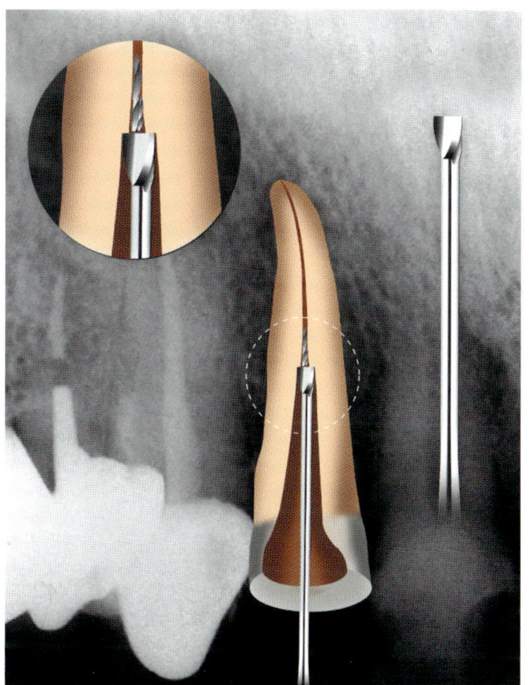

3-27c A modified (shortened) Gates Glidden drill is used to establish a ledge around the fragment.

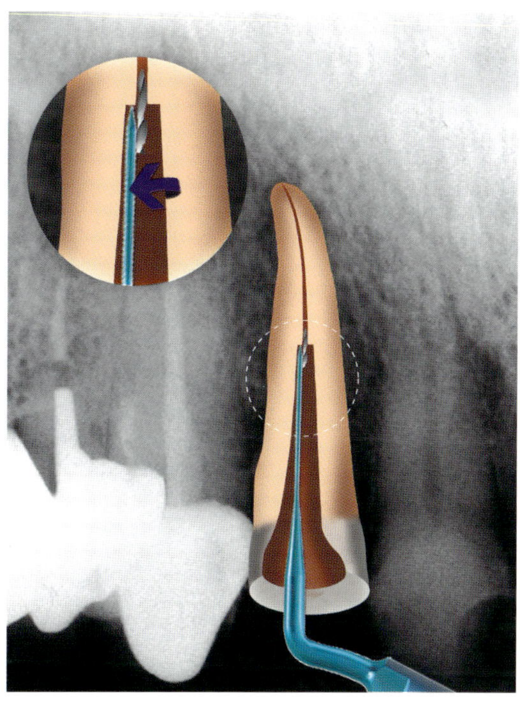

3-27d Ultrasonic tips are used to create a gutter and free the coronal 3 mm of the fragment so it can be vibrated. In this case, vibration alone was sufficient to remove the fractured nickel-titanium instrument.

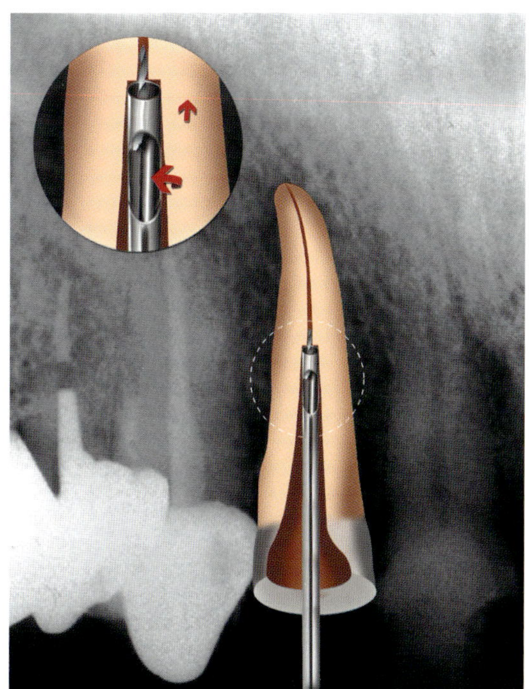

3-27e An IRS tube is selected and inserted passively into the canal until it covers the exposed coronal tip of the fractured instrument. The wedge is inserted and twisted counterclockwise; the entire assembly can then be removed from the canal.

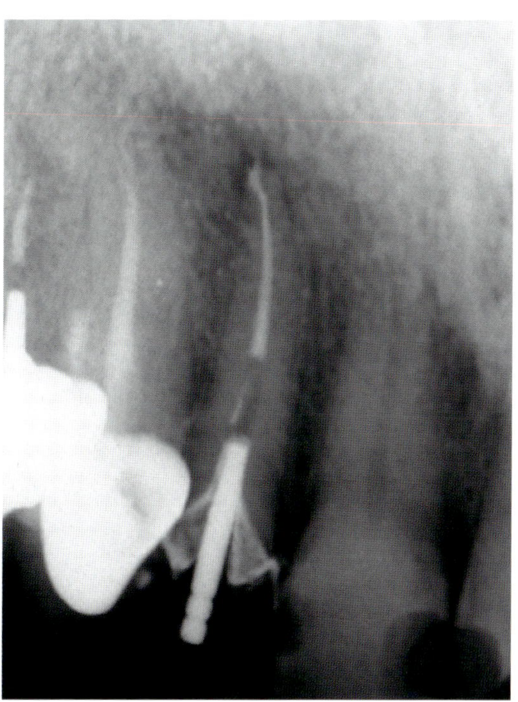

3-27f Immediate postoperative radiograph.

preparation risks fracturing the instrument further. Even if the coronal aspect of the fractured instrument appears to be free, the fragment may be trapped apically. Moreover, as Lentulo spiral fillers are used in the obturation stage of endodontic treatment, the fractured instrument is likely to be well coated in sealer.

Once the access cavity has been modified as necessary, an H-file of appropriate diameter is used along with a solvent to eliminate as much sealer as possible from within the canal and from the threads of the spiral filler. An H-file of diameter 25, 30, or larger (if possible) is inserted between the fractured instrument and the canal walls or passed between the threads of the spiral filler to engage the fragment and attempt to remove it (Figs 3-28a and 3-28b). After the sealer is cleared and as many threads of the spiral filler as possible have been freed, either a Masserann extractor (if the fragment is situated coronally) or an IRS can be used to grasp the fractured instrument and remove it with a clockwise rotational movement. Unlike other instruments, which are removed with a counterclockwise "unscrewing" motion, Lentulo spiral fillers are removed with a "screwing" motion (Figs 3-28c and 3-28d).

Thermocompaction devices

- If a length of only a few millimeters has fractured off the instrument tip, possibly from excessive pressure or cyclic fatigue, the fragment is likely to be embedded in the gutta-percha and will be easy to remove once the gutta-percha is removed.
- If the device broke because it was rotated in the wrong direction, a large portion of the instrument may have threaded itself into the canal walls and/or penetrated the periapical region. In such cases it is difficult if not impossible to retrieve the fractured instrument. The coronal aspect of the fragment must be freed and then vibrated for a considerable period of time with the ultrasonic instruments. The Masserann kit can then be used with a clockwise rotational movement, similar to the technique used for Lentulo spiral fillers. This is one of the few indications for using the Masserann kit rather than the IRS device, as the IRS is too fragile to withstand the forces needed to retrieve a thermocompaction device.

Summary

The likelihood of successfully retrieving a fractured instrument should be evaluated on a case-by-case basis. The clinician's own skill must be considered in addition to the value and function of the tooth, the amount of dentin remaining, the location of the fragment, and the nature of the fractured instrument. None of the techniques for removing fractured instruments guarantee successful retrieval, and several different methods may need to be attempted in an effort to remove the fragment.

If a fractured instrument that cannot be bypassed or removed blocks a canal, the apical part of the canal must be left untreated (Figs 3-29a and 3-29b). The coronal aspect is prepared and straight-line access is created; after copious irrigation, the canal is dried and obturated (Fig 3-29c). A coronal restoration is placed to ensure the root canal system is well sealed, and the tooth is monitored (Fig 3-29d). If strict aseptic techniques have been employed and an aseptic working environment was maintained, the results are likely to be favorable (Fig 3-29e).

Endodontic treatment is not an end in itself. In some cases the decision should be made not to retreat, especially if previous attempts have been unsuccessful. Retreatment procedures risk weakening the tooth significantly and endangering its long-term survival.

A recent study (Spili et al, 2005) compared the success rates of 158 endodontically treated roots, some containing fractured nickel-titanium or stainless steel instruments and some with no fractured instruments; the overall success rate 1 year (or more) postoperatively was 93.7%.

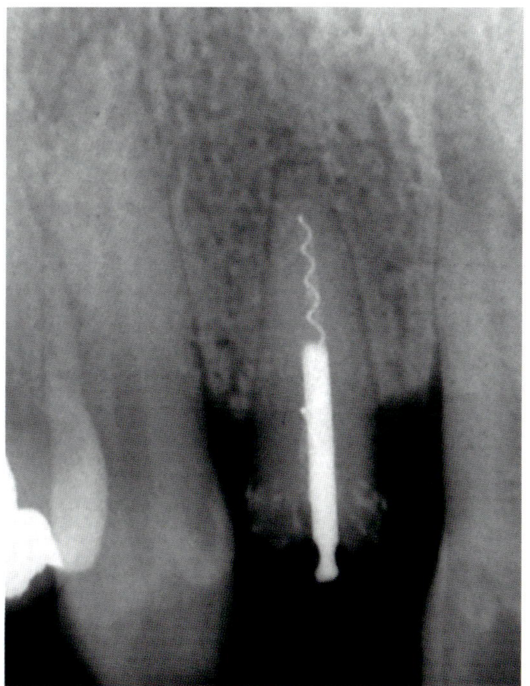

3-28a Preoperative radiograph of a fractured Lentulo spiral filler in a lateral incisor. Even if the coronal aspect of the spiral filler is visible, it is imperative to resist the temptation to grasp it and pull.

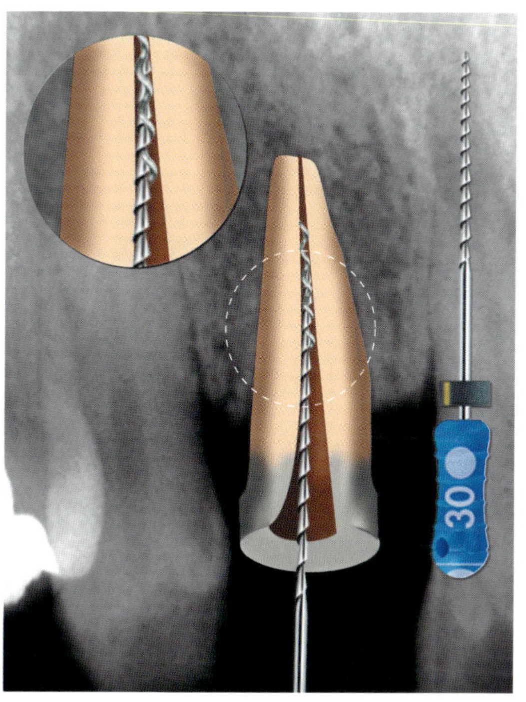

3-28b An H-file is used with a solvent to clean the canal and disengage the threads of the spiral filler.

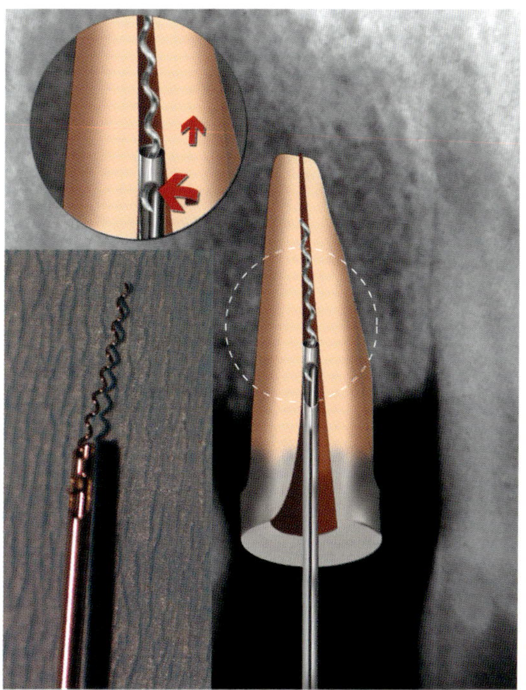

3-28c A tube from the IRS is placed passively into the canal so the spiral filler sits within the lumen of the tube. The wedge is then inserted and screwed into place with a counterclockwise rotation. The whole assembly is subsequently removed with a clockwise rotation.

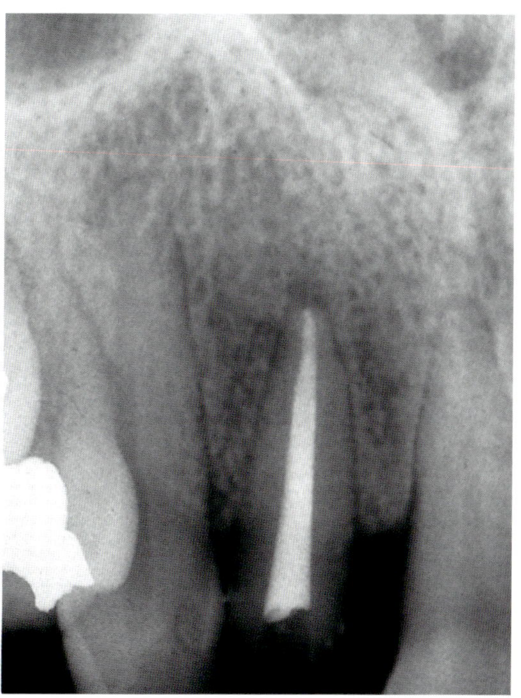

3-28d Postoperative radiograph.

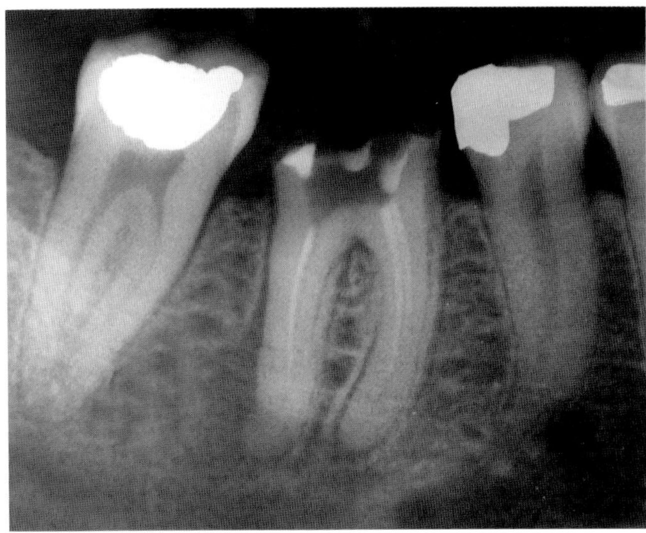

3-29a Preoperative radiograph of a mandibular molar with periapical lesions associated with both roots.

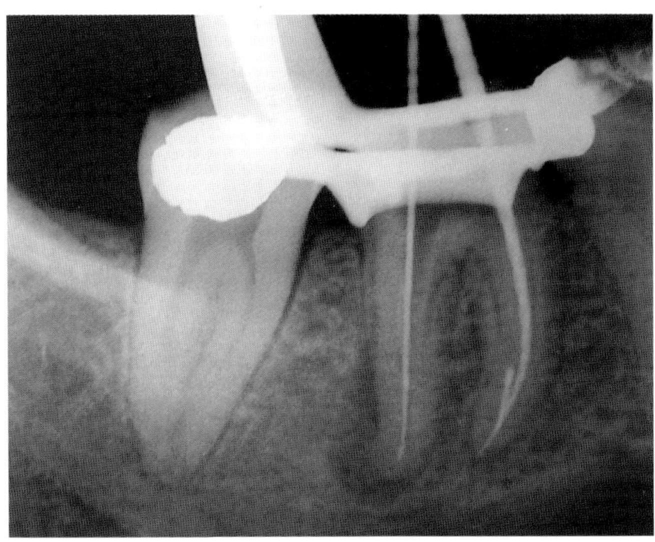

3-29b Radiograph taken during treatment shows a fractured instrument in the apical region of one of the mesial canals.

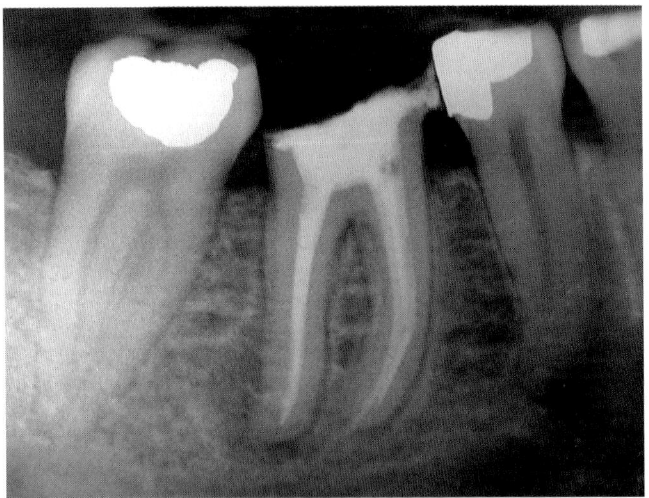

3-29c An attempt to bypass the instrument was unsuccessful, so the coronal part of the canal has been prepared, cleaned, and obturated.

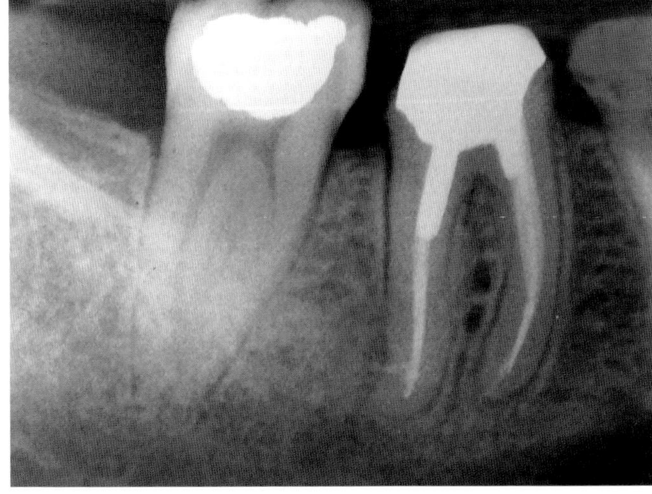

3-29d Radiograph taken 6 months postoperatively demonstrates healing. Note the post and core that has been placed during this monitoring period.

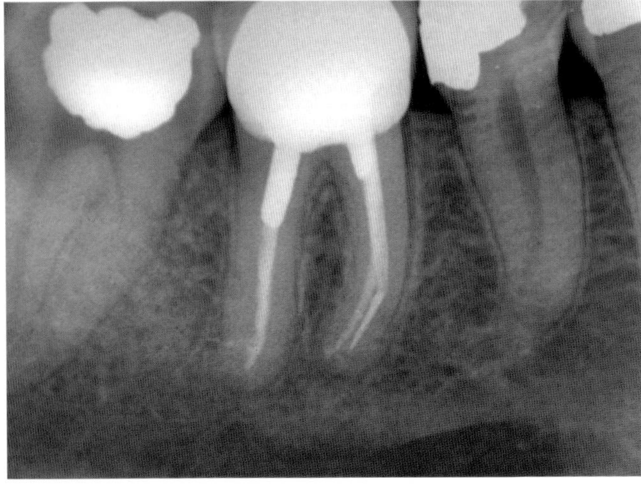

3-29e Radiograph taken 3 years postoperatively.

In the absence of preoperative periapical lesions, the success rate for teeth containing fractured instruments was 98.4% compared to 96.8% for teeth without any fractured instruments; this difference was not statistically significant. In the presence of preoperative periapical lesions, the success rate for teeth containing fractured instruments was 86.7% compared to 92.9% for teeth without any fractured instruments; this difference was again not statistically significant. Therefore, the presence of a fractured instrument does not affect the success rate for treatment on a tooth without a preoperative lesion. The success rate declines only slightly for treatment on a tooth with a preoperative lesion, *as long as strict asepsis has been maintained before (sterilizing instruments), during (use of rubber dam, copious irrigation), and after (restoration and coronal seal) endodontic treatment*. Nevertheless, in cases where radiographic or clinical signs appear or persist, the clinician must consider a surgical approach.

Unlike conventional endodontic treatment, for which there is an established protocol to follow, retreatment cases have no set treatment protocol because of the huge variation from case to case. The most rational approach to retreatment is to adopt basic guidelines that are always followed. The clinician should be familiar with various methods of retreatment, so if one technique should prove unsuccessful, alternative techniques can be employed. Each case must be judged independently of others. The different treatment options discussed in this chapter are summarized in Figs 3-30a to 3-30e. Even when the retreated canal cannot be negotiated to its full length, if general guidelines are followed, the retreatment procedure will improve the prognosis of the tooth by reducing the bacterial load in the root canal system.
It is the responsibility of all clinicians to acknowledge their individual limitations according to abilities, experience, and the equipment available. The aim of retreatment is to provide a service to the patient by improving the existing situation.

3-30a Algorithm for retreatment involving nonsoluble materials (ie, silver points or hard paste).

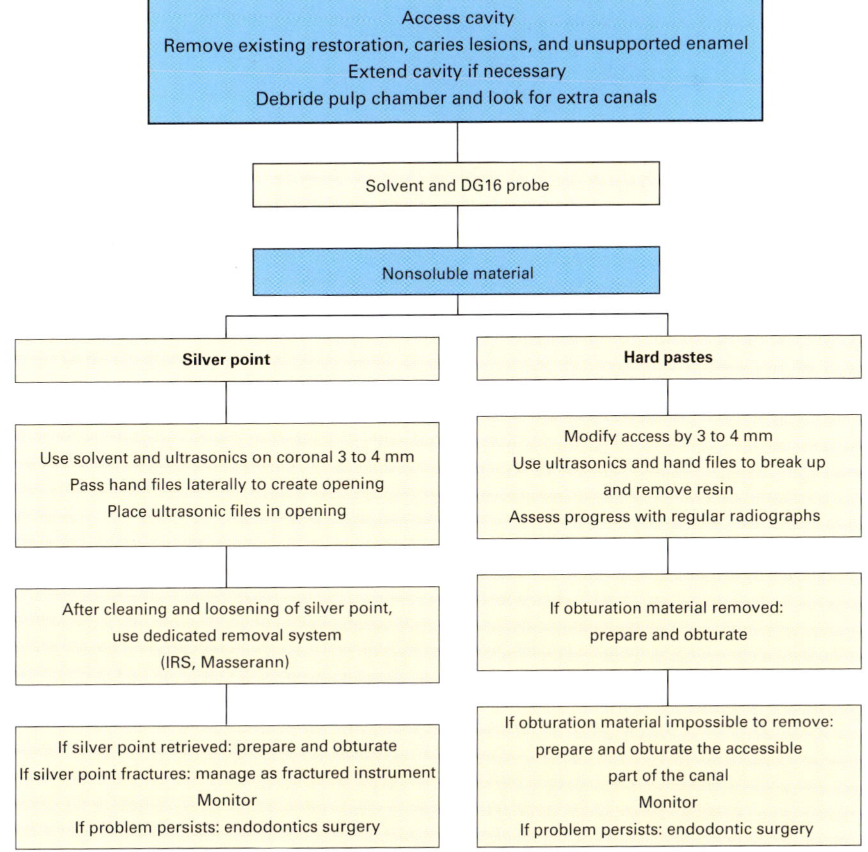

3-30b Algorithm for retreatment involving soft paste, gutta-percha, or Thermafilo.

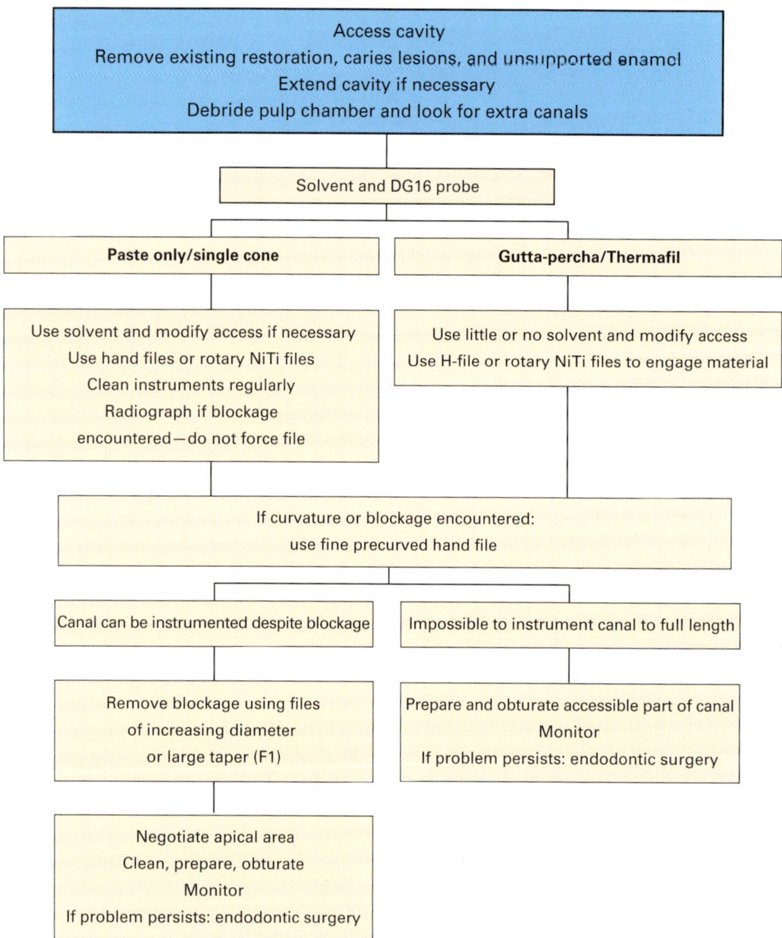

3-30 c Algorithm for retreatment involving a fractured instrument that *can* be bypassed laterally.

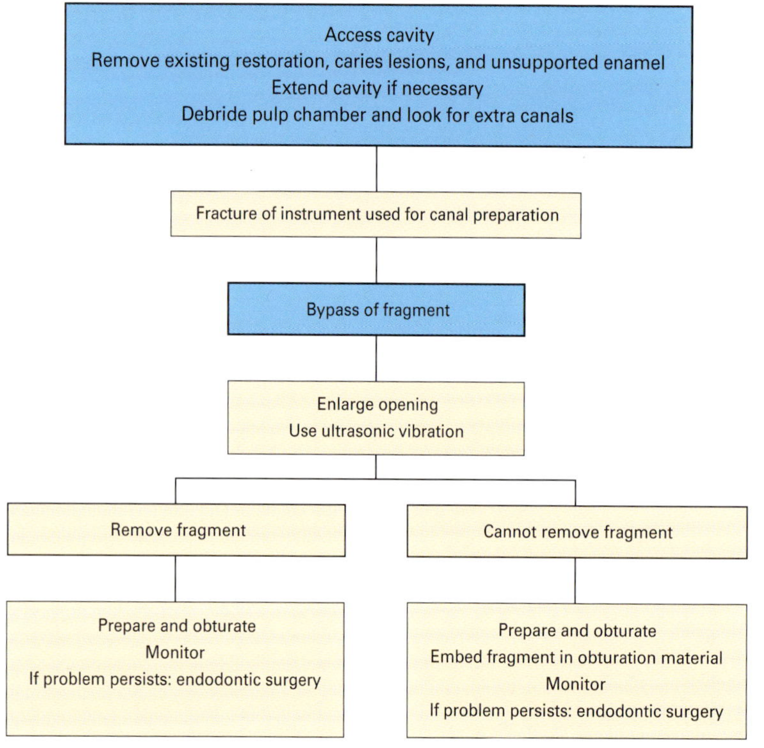

3-30d Algorithm for retreatment involving a fractured instrument that *cannot* be bypassed laterally.

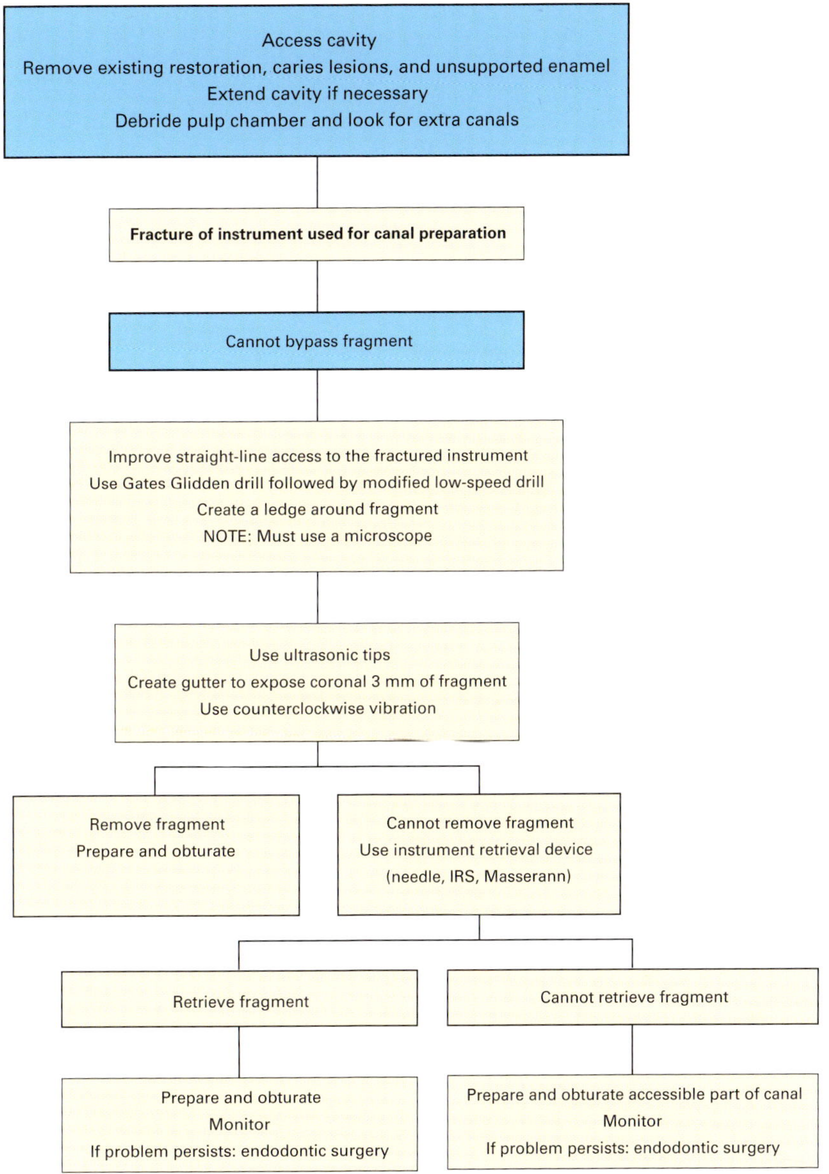

3-30e Algorithm for retreatment involving a fractured Lentulo spiral filler.

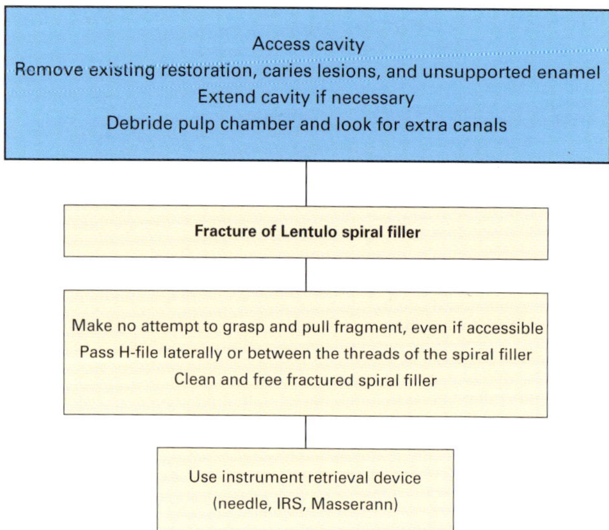

Management of Perforations

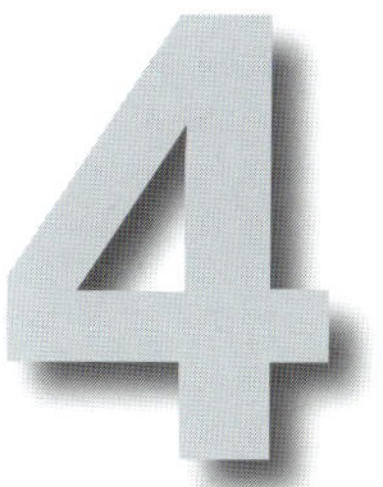

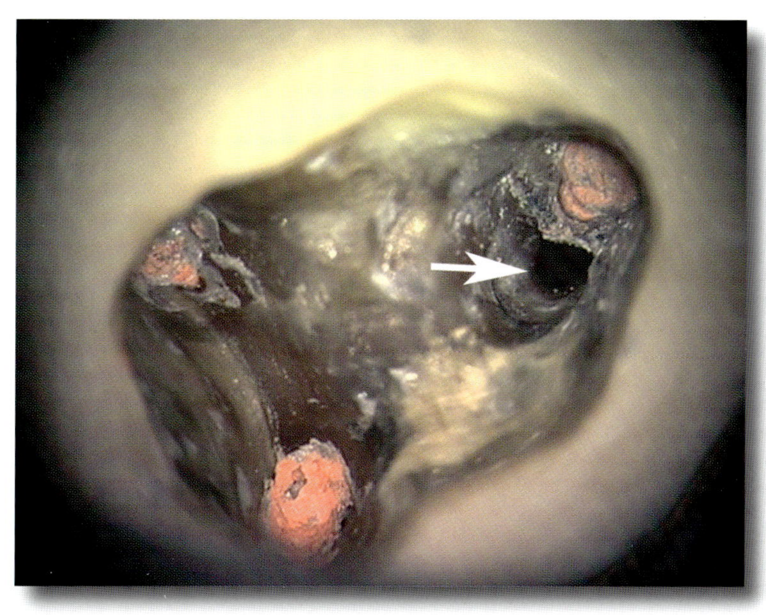

A perforation in endodontics is defined by the American Association of Endodontics as "a mechanical or pathologic communication between the root canal and the external tooth surface." The resulting communication causes inflammation and loss of the adjacent tissues. Resorption of the surrounding tissues is induced by bacteria, which is also the case with periapical lesions.

Perforations originate from one of two etiologies: *(1)* pathologic, following internal/external resorption or dental caries, or *(2)* iatrogenic, caused by clinician error during endodontic treatment. Only iatrogenic perforations are considered in this chapter.

Iatrogenic perforations occur in first-time endodontic treatment from poor angulation during access cavity preparation or from the clinician searching for canals. More frequently, they occur in endodontic retreatment while modifying the access cavity, debriding the pulp chamber, searching for canals, using rigid instruments in an uncontrolled manner to remove obturation material from the canal without checking the angulation of the instruments, or attempting to force an instrument further to overcome a blockage. In each of these cases, the perforations result from cutting instruments (drills or ultrasonics) used blindly or from excessive pressure exerted on inflexible files that are incorrectly angled in the canal.

There is no universal protocol for the treatment of perforations. Different materials can be employed and different approaches can be adopted: surgical, nonsurgical, or a combination of both. A thorough clinical and radiographic assessment should be performed before choosing the most appropriate technique for a particular case.

Factors Influencing Prognosis and Type of Treatment

Treatment of perforations and the subsequent prognosis of the affected teeth depend on many factors (Fuss and Trope, 1996).

Age of lesion and degree of bacterial contamination

These two factors are unquestionably the most important in terms of the prognosis. Healing is far less likely around a long-standing, contaminated perforation with associated bone resorption than around an uncontaminated perforation that is obturated immediately. Regardless of the cause of the perforation, it must be isolated and obturated as quickly as possible to avoid any bacterial contamination.

Site of perforation

The level and the site of the perforation affect the chance of bacterial contamination and the accessibility of the perforation for treatment.

Likelihood of bacterial contamination

The prognosis for perforations situated between the base of the gingival sulcus and the bony crest is generally poor. The larger and more coronal the perforation is (ie, perforations caused by poor bur angulation during access cavity preparation), the higher the chance of contamination and resultant attachment loss.

For this reason the periodontal state of the tooth, which is evaluated by probing and periodontal indices (eg, bleeding, plaque index), plays an important role in determining the prognosis of a perforation repair. A communication between the perforation and the base of a periodontal pocket compromises the chance of success. The prognosis is far worse if the lesion has been present for some time (Fig 4-1).

Access for treatment

The more coronal a perforation, the more visible and the more accessible it is; the more apical the perforation, the more limited the access.

Size and shape of perforation

A large oval perforation (eg, one created on the mesial surfaces of single-rooted teeth when a bur is angled incorrectly during access cavity preparation) is more difficult to obturate and seal than a round perforation (eg, one created in the pulp chamber floor of a molar) (Fig 4-2a and 4-2b).

Presence or absence of cortical bone

A perforation resulting in complete destruction of the bony cortex (eg, a buccal perforation on a maxillary anterior tooth where the bony cortex is very thin, almost non-existent) creates direct contact between the perforation and the overlying gingiva. This should not be treated in the same way as a perforation that is within bone, even if some bone resorption has occurred.

Choice of material for perforation repair

The choice of material depends on the clinical situation. The main aim is to provide a long-lasting repair that creates a good seal using a biocompatible material.

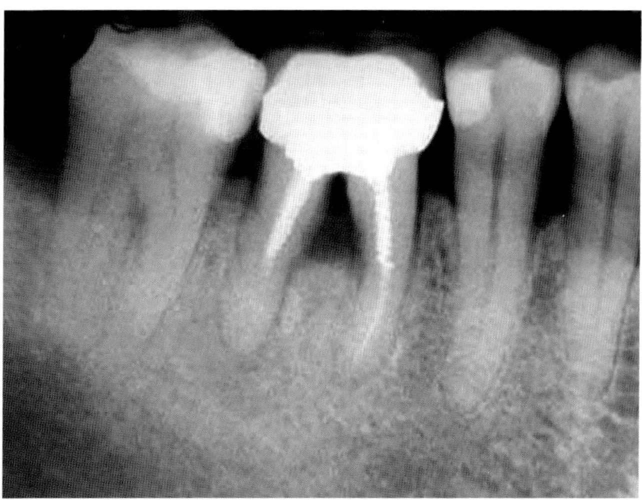

4-1 A large perforation through the pulp chamber floor has resulted in significant bony resorption in the furcation area. In this case the only sensible treatment is extraction.

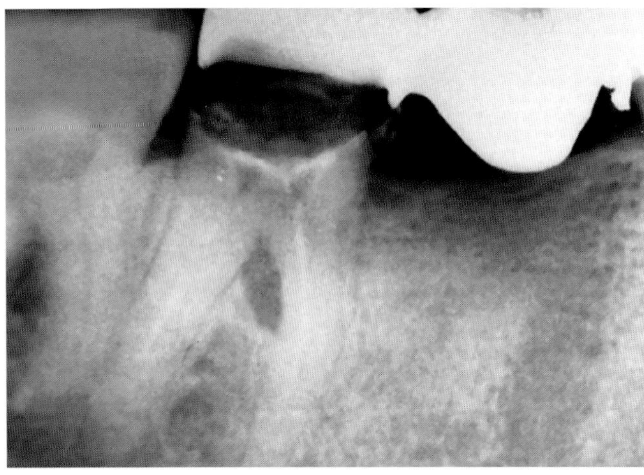

4-2a Perforation through the pulp chamber floor of a mandibular molar. Despite the presence of a lesion, periodontal probing confirmed there was no communication between the base of the gingival sulcus and the furcation. This type of lesion has a favorable prognosis.

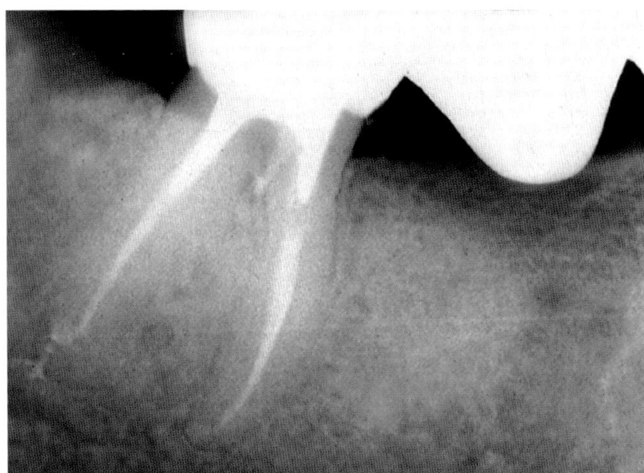

4-2b Radiograph taken 5 years postoperatively demonstrates healing of the furcation after retreatment and perforation repair with ProRoot MTA.

Materials Used for Perforation Repair

A variety of different materials can be used to repair perforations; the choice depends on the site of the perforation and the type of treatment to be performed. For surgical treatment of a buccal perforation at the level of the bony crest, where hemostasis can readily be achieved, use of an adhesive material such as glass ionomer may be indicated. However if the perforation occurs in the pulp chamber floor, mineral trioxide aggregate (ProRoot MTA, Dentsply) is more appropriate. A small root perforation situated in the apical third of a canal can be dealt with as a lateral or accessory canal. After being cleaned it is obturated with gutta-percha exactly as if it were another canal.

In some situations a surgical approach is required, and the perforation should be obturated with a nonadhesive material (adhesive materials are affected by moisture contamination). In these cases, Intermediate Restorative Material (IRM, Dentsply) or SuperEBA (Harry J. Bosworth) may prove more suitable than ProRoot MTA, which requires a deeper cavity for retention.

The material that is currently favored for the treatment of perforations, especially those in the pulp chamber floor, and for the treatment of teeth with open apices is mineral trioxide aggregate (ProRoot MTA). This material, which is entirely mineral in composition, is a form of Portland cement. It has been shown to be very biocompatible and to form a good seal, though its mechanism of action remains unclear. The powder is dispensed in sealed sachets of 1 g and is available in grey or white; the latter allows for a more esthetic result when performing pulp capping or pulpotomies in anterior teeth. Although the manufacturers advise discarding any unused powder once a sachet has been opened, it can be stored in a clean container (eg, an empty film canister) and sealed to prevent moisture contamination. When mixed with water, this powder produces a colloidal gel that will take approximately 4 hours to set completely. This setting time affects the way in which it is used. During placement and while it is not fully set, the MTA can be easily washed out of the cavity. Thus, any procedures for which irrigation is necessary should be completed before the MTA is placed. After the MTA has been placed, it is sometimes advisable to cover it with a moist cotton pledget (squeezed to remove excess water) to hydrate the material as necessary to achieve a full set. In most cases, the moisture provided by the adjacent tissues is sufficient. Enough powder is mixed with water to obtain a relatively thick paste with a consistency similar to that of a temporary cement.

If the mix is too thin or the material is covered with a wet rather than a moist cotton pledget, the setting reaction is compromised.
The ProRoot MTA has an alkaline pH (approximately 13), and its setting reaction is compromised by the presence of pus. Copious irrigation with sodium hypochlorite and a temporary calcium hydroxide dressing in the defect should resolve the inflammation and allow the pH to return to normal.

The usual working time of the material is approximately 5 minutes, but it can be increased by covering the mix with damp gauze.
Studies have been published that clearly demonstrate the superior biocompatibility and sealing ability of ProRoot MTA compared with other conventional materials used for the treatment of lateral perforations and perforations of the pulp chamber floor (Lee et al, 1993; Nakata et al, 1998). The periodontal tissues that contact the ProRoot MTA regenerate with the formation of a cementum-like tissue or an epithelial attachment with direct contact (Pitt Ford et al, 1995; Torabinejad et al, 1997; Holland et al, 2001). One of the advantages of this material lies in its hydrophilic nature; this property allows the material to produce a good seal even in a cavity contaminated by blood or moisture (Torabinejad et al, 1994). MTA is currently considered the material of choice for the treatment of perforations, provided the indication for its use has been correctly identified.

Perforations in the Coronal Third

Perforations in the coronal third are generally easier to access, but the prognosis can prove less favorable than in more apical perforations. This discrepancy is linked to two factors: *(1)* size and shape of the defect and *(2)* location of the defect.
These perforations are generally large and are created when rotary instruments (burs, Gates Glidden drills) are used for access cavity preparation. Furthermore, since the perforation is created laterally, the instrument will not have been angled perpendicular to the root surface. The resultant perforation tends to be oval in shape, and placement of obturation material in a defect like this is difficult to control.
If the perforation is suprabony, there may be a communication between the perforation and the base of the gingival sulcus or a periodontal pocket. A multidisciplinary approach, including orthodontic traction and/or periodontal surgery, may be necessary.

The clinician should routinely check for a communication with the sulcus by probing the affected area before any decision about retreatment is made.

Anterior teeth

Perforations in maxillary incisors and canines tend to occur on the buccal aspect when an instrument has been angled poorly during access cavity preparation or post-hole preparation. A defect may be suprabony, infrabony, or lie partially above the bony crest and partially in communication with the sulcus. Treatment is different in each case, so periodontal probing is essential to determine the nature of the perforation.

Suprabony perforation

In the instance of suprabony perforation, repair of the defect is integrated into the coronal restoration, with prior crown lengthening if necessary.

Infrabony perforation

The buccal cortex of bone must be assessed. This is done by insertion of a long, blunt instrument (eg, an amalgam plugger) into the perforation while the clinician places a finger over the buccal aspect of the tooth in the cervical region. If the instrument is palpated beneath the gingiva, bony destruction has occurred. The extent of the bony destruction determines the type of treatment chosen and the obturation material used.

- If there is no communication with the gingival sulcus and the buccal bone has not been destroyed (Fig 4-3a), it is necessary to adopt a coronal approach and obturate the perforation with ProRoot MTA. The canal is first identified, prepared, and cleaned (Fig 4-3b). Perforations generally occur on the buccal aspect, so the clinician should look for the canal palatally. The perforation is cleaned with a small excavator and ultrasonic instruments, then isolated with a cotton pledget. After drying the canal, a prefitted gutta-percha point covered in sealer is placed into the canal and sectioned just beneath the level of the perforation (Fig 4-3c). This is then condensed to ensure the obturation of the apical part of the canal (Fig 4-3d).

  The cotton pledget is removed and the perforation is obturated. ProRoot MTA is mixed with enough water to obtain a paste with a consistency similar to that of Cavit (3M ESPE). The material is loaded into the MTA Gun (Dentsply), a device similar to an amalgam carrier with a range of small-diameter straight and curved tips (Fig 4-3e). The ProRoot MTA is dispensed into the perforation and delicately condensed, bringing the material into contact with the adjacent periodontal tissues; this stage can be done using either a plugger or the butt end of a paper point (Fig 4-3f). *The aim is not to obtain a perfect seal by condensing the material as if it were gutta-percha but simply to bring it into contact with the tissues.* This maneuver is repeated with one or two further additions of MTA to complete the obturation, which can be checked radiographically (Fig 4-3g). The tooth can then be restored during subsequent appointments (Fig 4-3h).

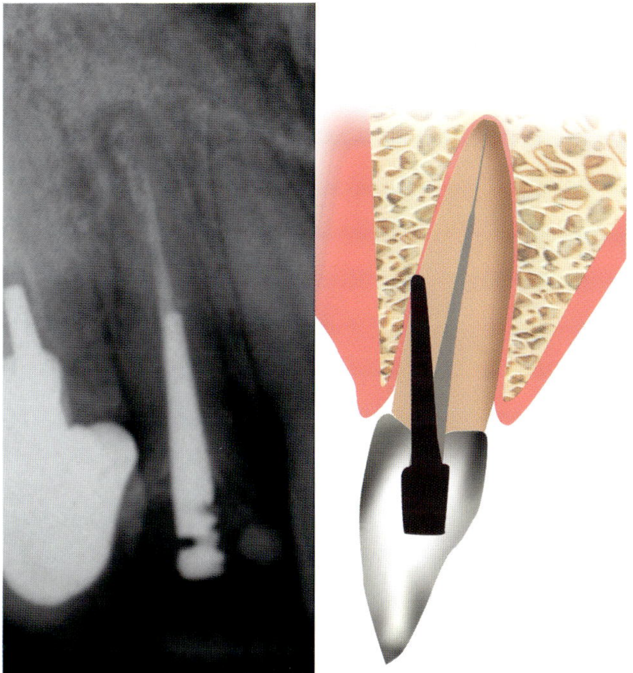

4-3a Preoperative radiograph and diagram demonstrating a maxillary lateral incisor with a buccal perforation created during post-hole preparation. Conventional right-angled radiographs of buccal perforations can be misleading and may not reveal the defect.

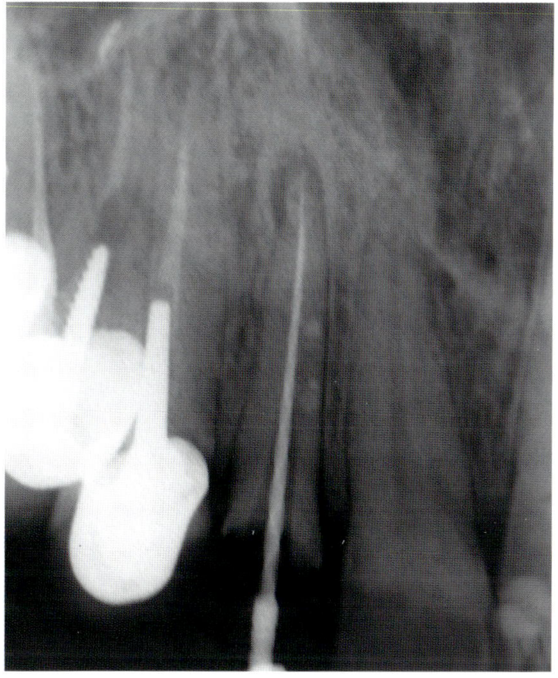

4-3b The canal is located and existing obturation material is removed. The canal is then prepared and cleaned. Rubber dam has been secured with Wedjets (Coltène/Whaledent) placed beneath thc contact points of the adjacent teeth; resin is used to bond the dam to the tooth undergoing treatment.

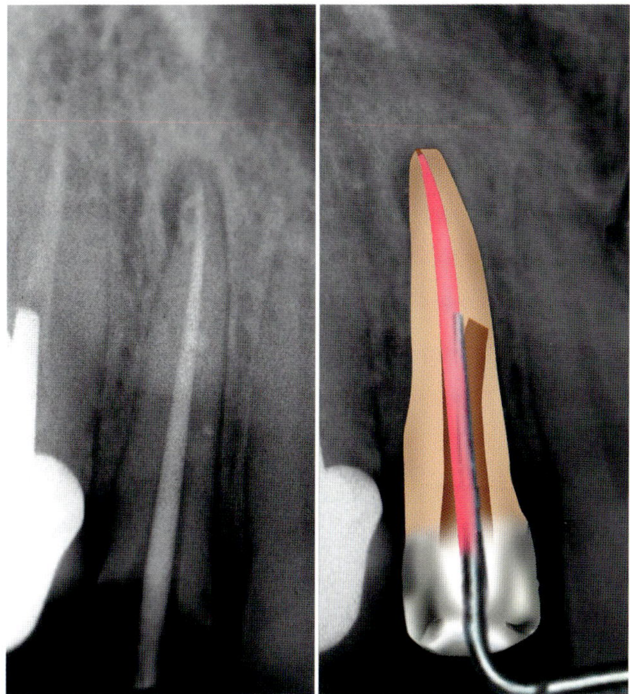

4-3c A gutta-percha point is prepared and a radiograph (*left*) is taken to check that it reaches to the full length of the canal. Once the canal has been dried, the gutta-percha point is covered in sealer and inserted into the canal. It is sectioned just below the level of the perforation using a heated instrument such as a Buchanan System B Plugger (SybronEndo).

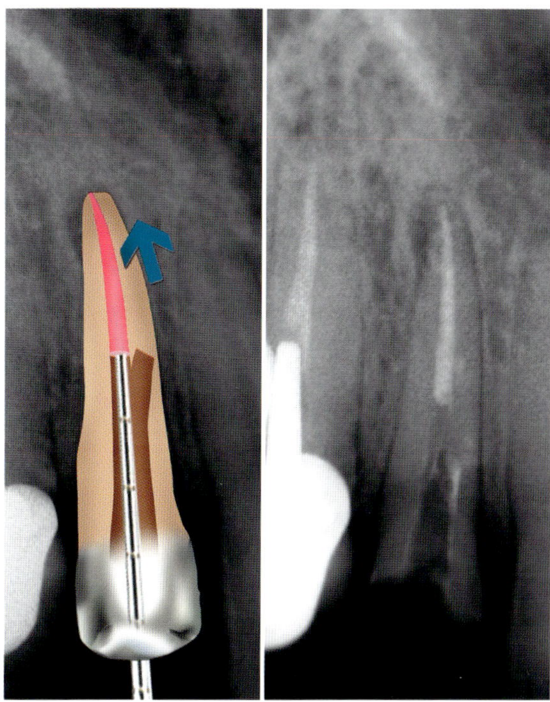

4-3d The gutta-percha point is then condensed with a heated instrument to ensure that the apical portion of the canal is well sealed.

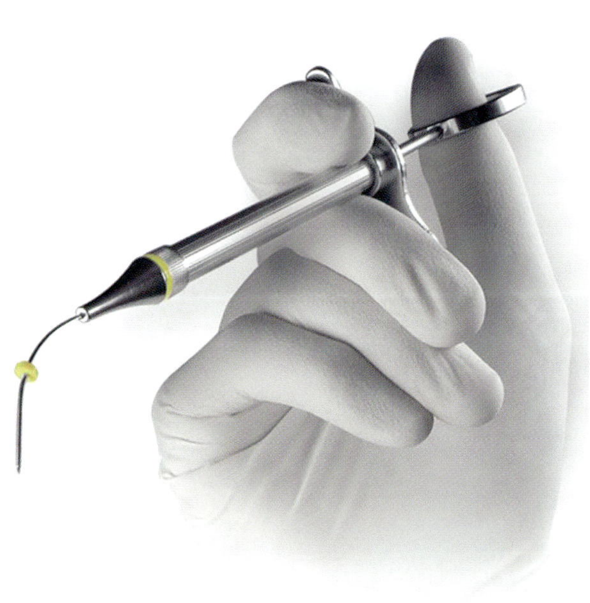

4-3e ProRoot MTA is loaded into the MTA Gun.

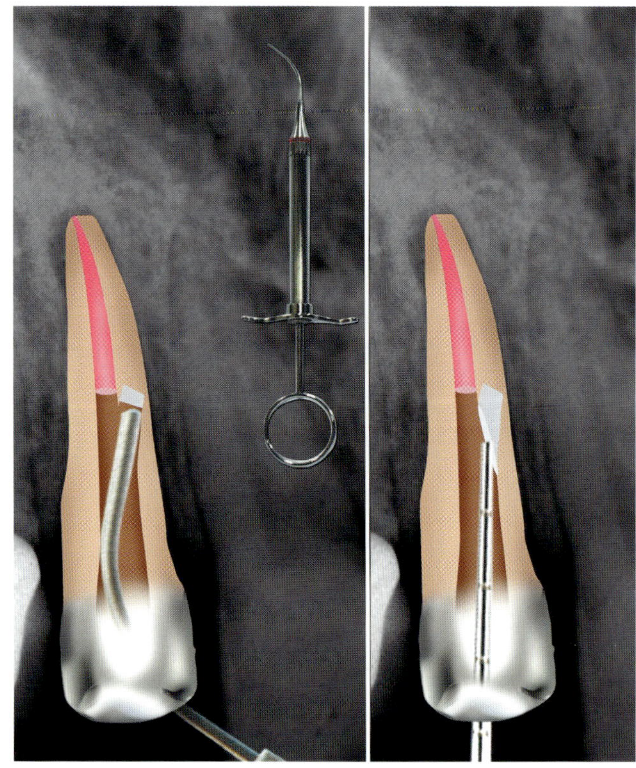

4-3f ProRoot MTA is dispensed into the perforation (*left*) and then delicately brought into contact with the tissues with the aid of a plugger. This maneuver is repeated until the obturation is complete and the perforation defect is sealed.

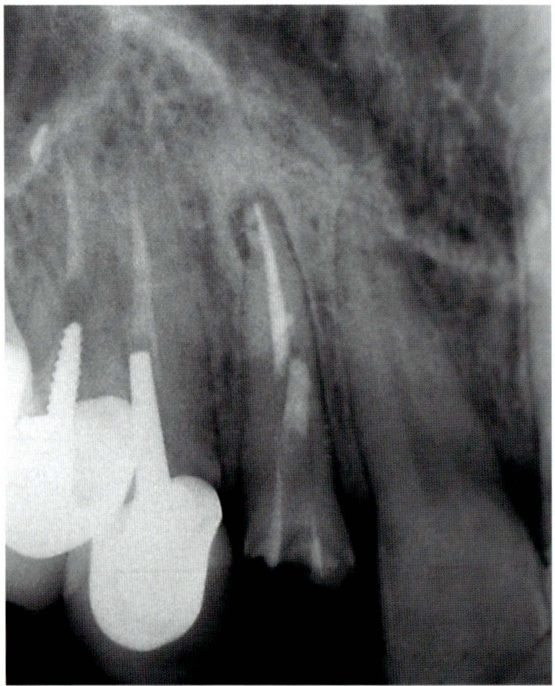

4-3g A radiograph is taken to check the placement of the material.

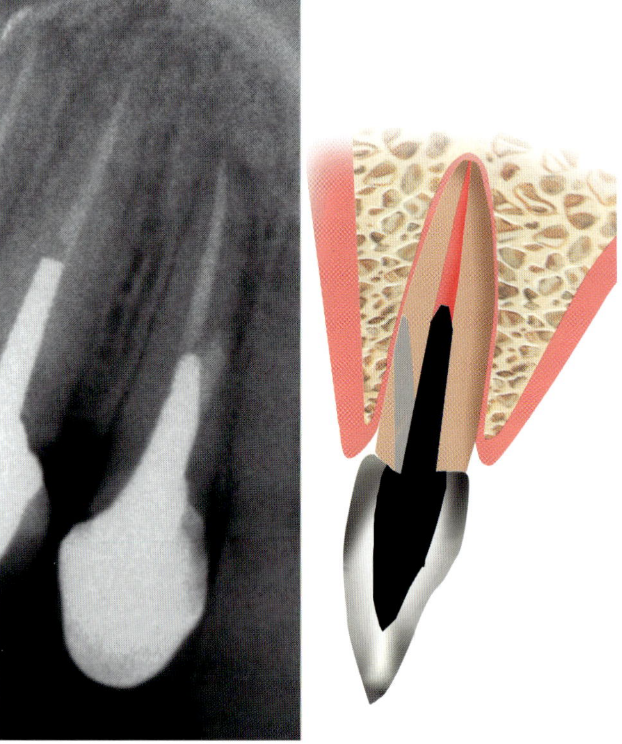

4-3h Radiograph taken 1 year postoperatively. Clinical examination reveals that the tooth is functional and periodontally sound.

- In cases where the perforation is in communication with the sulcus or lies partly above and partly below the bony crest, obturation from the coronal aspect is difficult (Fig 4-4a). Depending on the length of the root, the mesiodistal dimensions of the affected tooth, and the anticipated esthetic result, rapid orthodontic traction may be indicated to position the perforation above the bony crest. Alternatively, a surgical approach may be adopted, in which the perforation is exposed with a full-thickness flap and bone is removed to allow good access to the perforation. Once good hemostasis has been achieved (Fig 4-4b), the perforation is sealed with an adhesive material (Figs 4-4c and 4-4d) to provide an immediate seal. Regular clinical and radiographic monitoring is essential (Figs 4-4e and 4-4f).

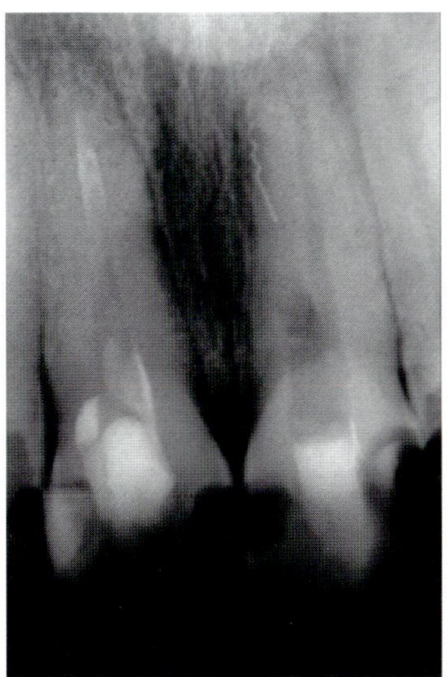

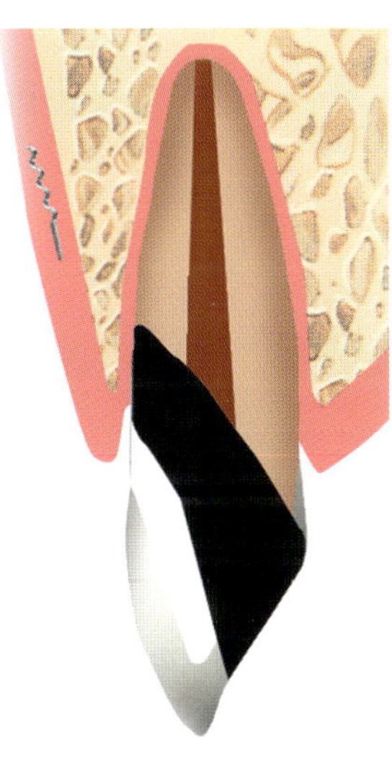

4-4a Preoperative radiograph and diagram demonstrating a central incisor with a buccal perforation and fractured Lentulo spiral filler. Clinical examination revealed destruction of the buccal cortex and a perforation lying partly above and partly below the bony crest, communicating with the sulcus.

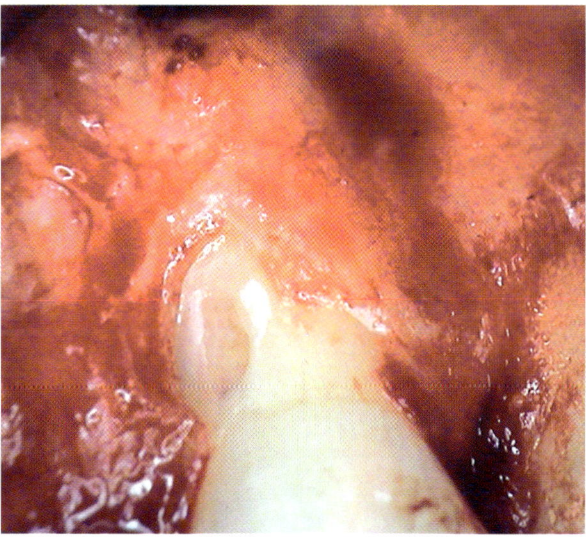

4-4b View of the perforation once granulation tissue has been curetted away, bone removed, and hemostasis achieved.

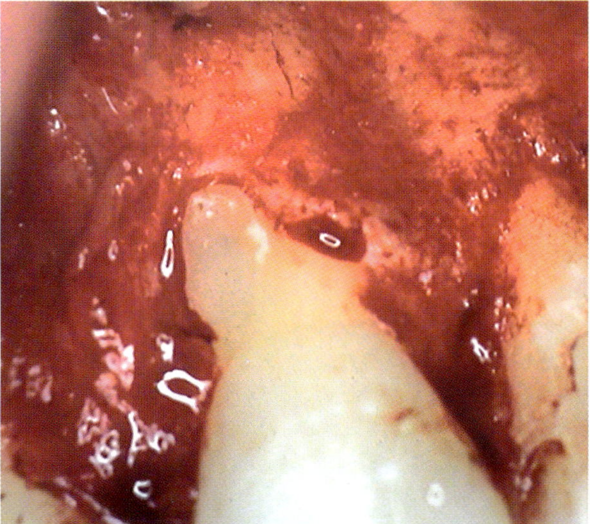

4-4c View of the perforation after obturation with an adhesive material (Dyract, Dentsply). The material was polished after placement.

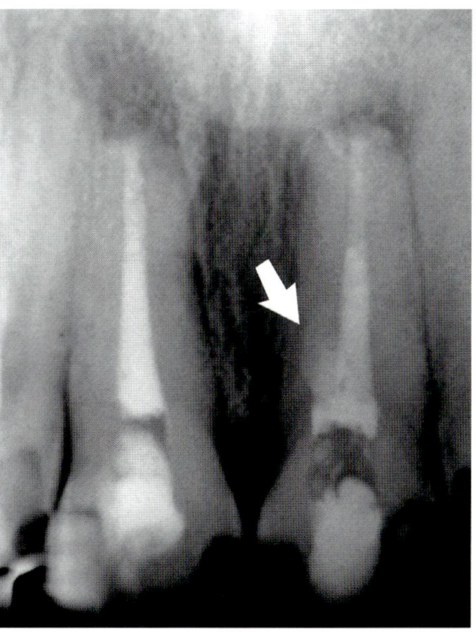

4-4d Immediate postoperative radiograph. The repaired perforation is visible *(arrow)*.

4-4e and 4-4f Clinical photograph and radiograph taken 8 years postoperatively. The right central incisor, extracted 4 years previously because of trauma, has been replaced with a fixed partial denture.

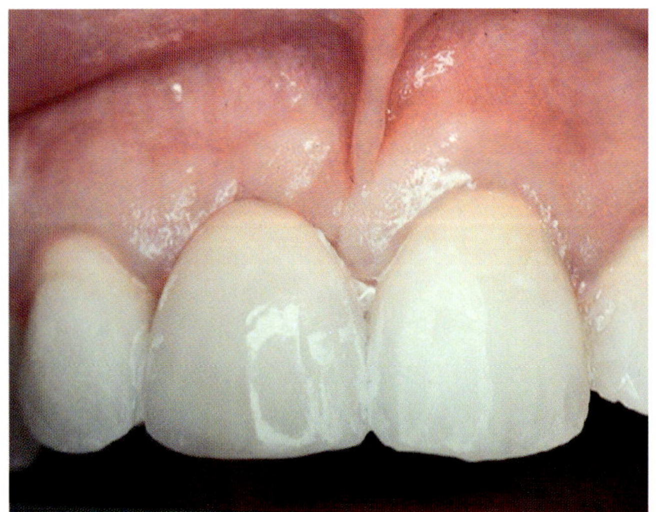

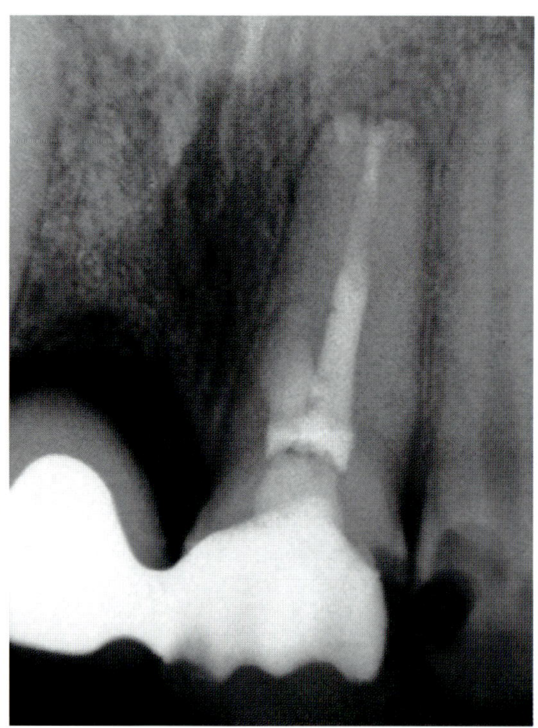

In the absence of a bony cortex and where a direct communication exists with the buccal aspect, use of ProRoot MTA is not recommended because it may crumble and wash away before it is fully set.

Posterior teeth

In posterior teeth, perforations in the coronal third are dealt with in the same way as they are in anterior teeth. Access is more difficult, and surgical or orthodontic treatment is complicated by the risk of furcation involvement.

After the perforation is identified on a preoperative radiograph (Fig 4-5a), it is cleaned and irrigated (Fig 4-5b). ProRoot MTA is dispensed into the perforation a little at a time from the MTA Gun; with the help of a plugger or the butt end of a paper point, the MTA is delicately brought into contact with the adjacent tissues (Figs 4-5c and 4-5d). A moist cotton pledget, squeezed to remove excess water, is placed over the material, and a temporary filling is placed in the tooth. It is advisable to prepare and obturate the canals before repairing the perforation defect. In this way, the perforation is disinfected by the hypochlorite bathing the access cavity during canal preparation. Obturating the canals before repairing the defect also prevents any ProRoot MTA from falling into the canals during the perforation repair. Nevertheless, in certain cases in which it is impossible to dry the root canal system adequately, the canals cannot be obturated first. The entrances to the prepared canals must be protected with cotton pledgets during the placement of the ProRoot MTA. The canals are then obturated at a later visit (Fig 4-5e). A coronal restoration should be placed as soon as possible after completion of the endodontic treatment. Regular clinical and radiographic examination is necessary to monitor the tooth (Fig 4-5f).

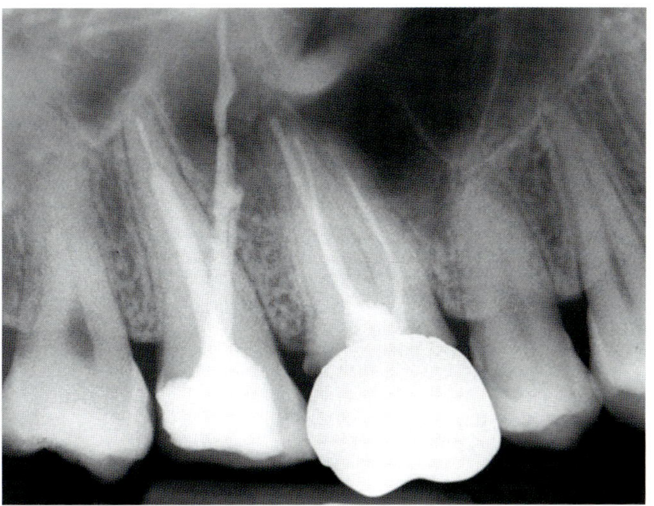

4-5a Preoperative radiograph of a maxillary molar with a buccal perforation through which a large amount of obturation material has been extruded.

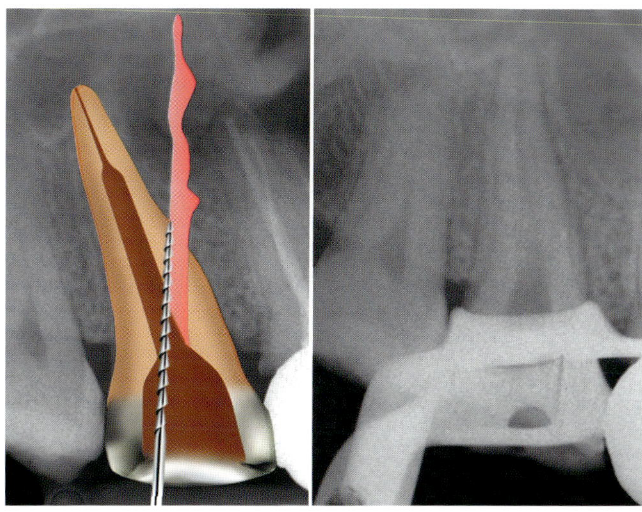

4-5b A large-diameter H-file was used to remove the extruded gutta-percha. The palatal canal was also cleared of obturation material.

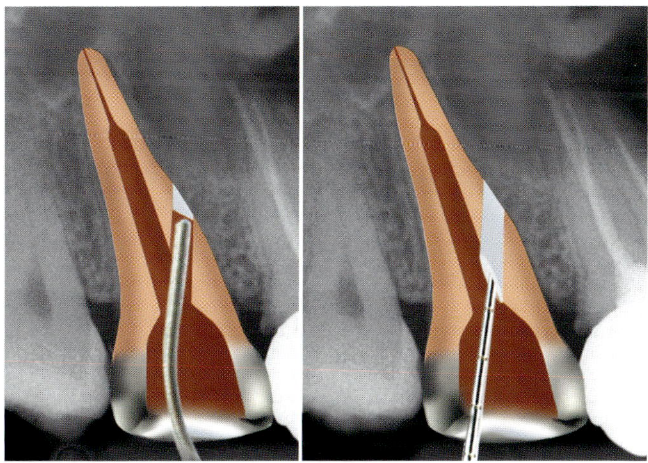

4-5c The ProRoot MTA is loaded into the MTA Gun, dispensed into the perforation (*left*), and placed in contact with the adjacent tissues. In this case, the perforation was repaired before the canals were obturated because of difficulties with moisture control.

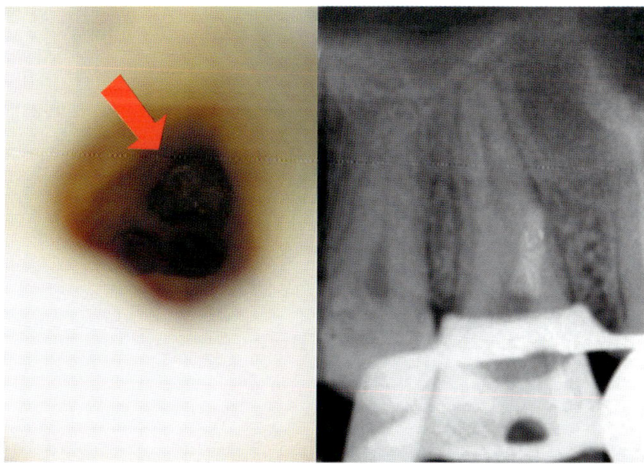

4-5d The perforation repair is verified radiographically. In this case, the perforation was created buccal to the two buccal canals *(red arrow)*.

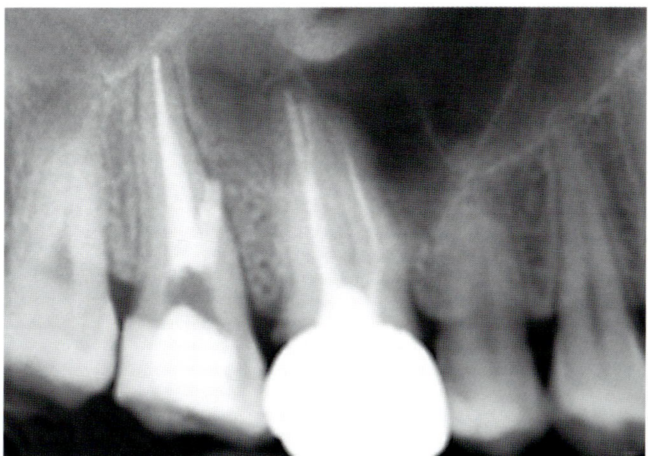

4-5e Postoperative radiograph after obturation of the canals (completed at a subsequent visit).

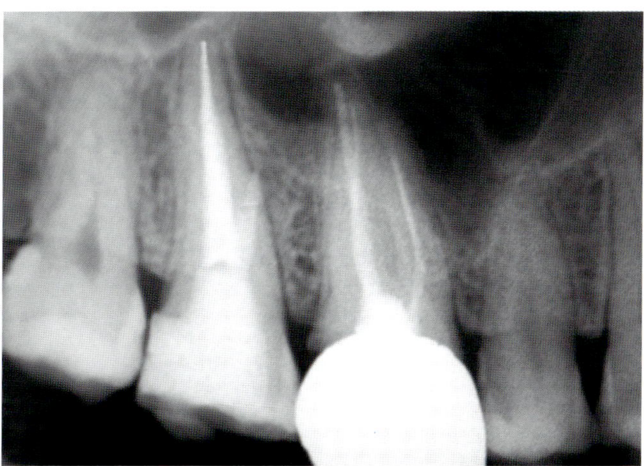

4-5f Radiograph taken 3 years postoperatively.

Furcation or Strip Perforations

Lateral perforations in the furcation region occur after over–instrumentation of the inner furcal wall of the canals. Known as *strip perforations*, these can occur in any root. Mesial roots of molars are most frequently affected (Fig 4-6) because of their specific anatomy, which includes a concavity that is not evident radiographically and canals that are off-center in relation to the furcation. Uniform removal of dentin during canal preparation may lead to perforations in the interradicular walls.

Strip perforations are difficult to treat because the edges of the defect are irregular. These perforations tend to be relatively large with thin, jagged edges resembling a tear or a rip in the canal wall. If the defect is not repaired, the resulting interradicular bone loss will inevitably lead to eventual loss of the tooth.

A strip perforation can often go unnoticed during canal preparation. It may become evident only after the canal is dried, when a drop of blood may be seen on a paper point after contact with the perforation site. Treatment should be attempted as follows: hemostasis is obtained and the canal is obturated by placing a gutta-percha point into the apical portion of the canal, sectioning it just below the level of the perforation and then condensing it. In this way, the apical part of the canal is obturated with gutta-percha up to the level of the perforation. The rest of the canal is obturated with ProRoot MTA.

In other cases, the inner furcal wall of the canal, weakened during the preparation stage, can give way under the pressure of obturation; sealer and dentin debris pass through the perforation and enter the furcation region. Often, only when the postoperative radiograph is taken does it become apparent that a strip perforation has occurred and the root canal system is not adequately sealed. Some authors recommend immediate surgical intervention to seal the defect, thus avoiding periodontal inflammation and resultant bone loss. Surgical treatment has a better prognosis if completed while the tooth is periodontally sound. After a coronal restoration has been placed, a full-thickness flap is raised. Preserving a cervical band of bone, interradicular bone is removed to allow the area to be accessed and cleaned. Dentin chips and sealer are curetted away, and the gutta-percha is burnished against the wall of the root canal.

Treatment results from strip perforations remain unpredictable, and there are few guidelines available. Treatment options include repairing the defect and restoring the tooth, sectioning the affected root, or extracting the tooth and placing an implant. These should be discussed with the patient, and the advantages and disadvantages of each must be clearly explained.

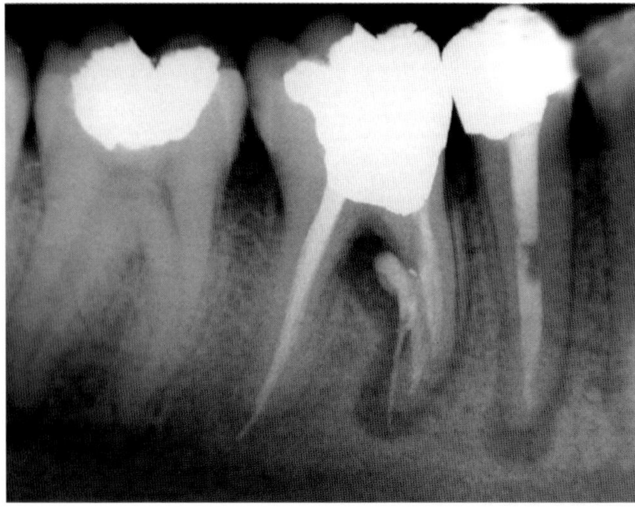

4-6 Strip perforation in the furcation region of a mandibular molar.

Perforations of the Pulp Chamber Floor

Unlike lateral perforations, which tend to be oval in shape, perforations of the pulp chamber floor are generally round and therefore easier to obturate. The prognosis is nevertheless dependent on the proximity of the sulcus and the presence of a communication between the perforation and the oral cavity.

As with all perforations the main goal is to prevent bacterial contamination. Thus, if a perforation is created during access cavity preparation, repair should be made at the same visit and not delayed until a subsequent appointment. In the case of a pre-existing perforation, the goal of obtaining a good seal remains the same, but the procedure may vary depending on the clinical scenario (Fig 4-7a). After rubber dam has been placed and the access cavity modified, the stages outlined below should be followed (Box 4-1).

Box 4-1 Stages of treatment for repairing the pulp chamber floor

1. The canals are located and the perforation identified.
2. The canals are prepared under copious irrigation with sodium hypochlorite and then obturated (Fig 4-7b); a cotton pledget is used to protect the perforation and prevent sealer being extruded through the defect.
3. The perforation is obturated with ProRoot MTA. The material is loaded into the MTA Gun, dispensed into the perforation (Fig 4-7c), and then carefully packed into the defect using an amalgam plugger or the butt end of a paper point (Fig 4-7d). The plugger selected for use must be of approximately the same diameter as the perforation to enable the operator to pack the MTA properly against the tissues. If the plugger is too small, there is a risk of forcing the material into the furcation region. Because of the excellent biocompatibility of MTA, extrusion of the material will not compromise healing, but the excess material serves no purpose and therefore should be avoided as much as possible.
4. Once the perforation has been obturated, a moist cotton pledget is placed over the site of repair, and the canal is covered with a temporary dressing (Fig 4-7e).
5. Between appointments, the ProRoot MTA has time to reach a full set, but a coronal restoration must be placed as soon as possible to ensure a good seal. Regular clinical and radiographic monitoring is necessary (Fig 4-7f).

In some situations the perforation must be repaired before the canals are obturated. If the canals are not ready for obturation at the end of the appointment (eg, existing root canal filling remaining, tooth symptomatic, moisture control difficult), the perforation repair should nevertheless be completed rather than being delayed until the next visit; this allows the material to reach a full set between appointments. In these cases it is prudent to protect the entrances to the canals before placing the MTA. Once set, ProRoot MTA is very difficult to remove.

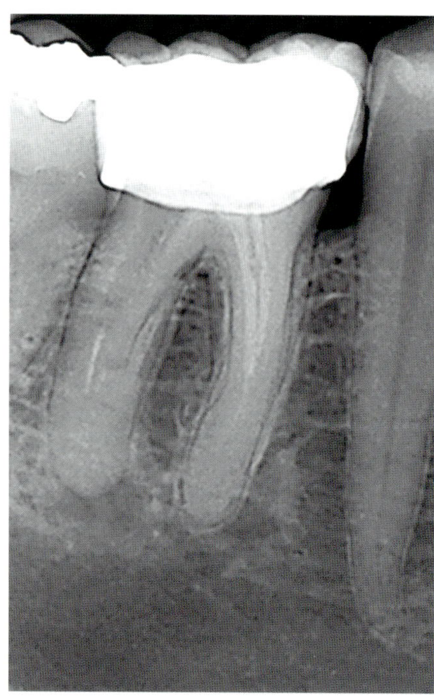

4-7a Preoperative radiograph of a mandibular molar with a perforation of the pulp chamber floor, which is not evident radiographically. Periodontal probing revealed a normal sulcus depth.

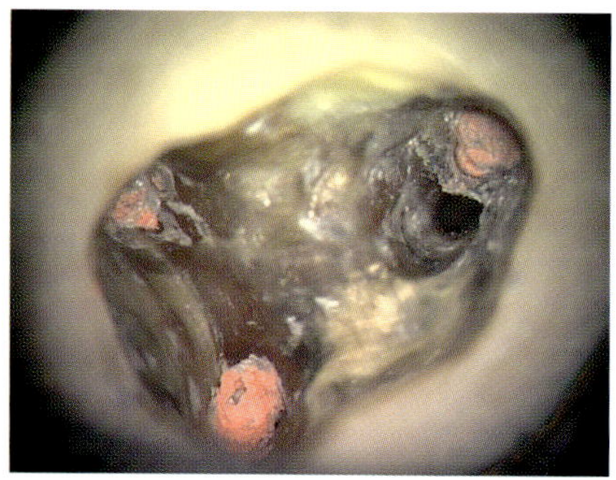

4-7b Clinical photograph of the perforation close to the entrance of the distal canal. The canals have been cleaned and obturated.

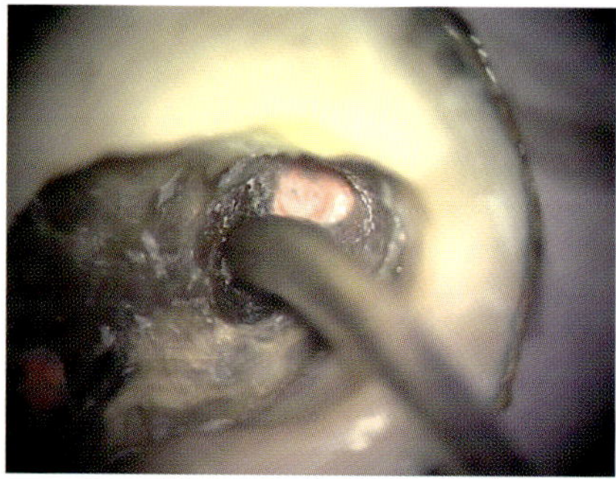

4-7c ProRoot MTA is dispensed into the perforation with the help of the MTA Gun and then delicately packed into the defect.

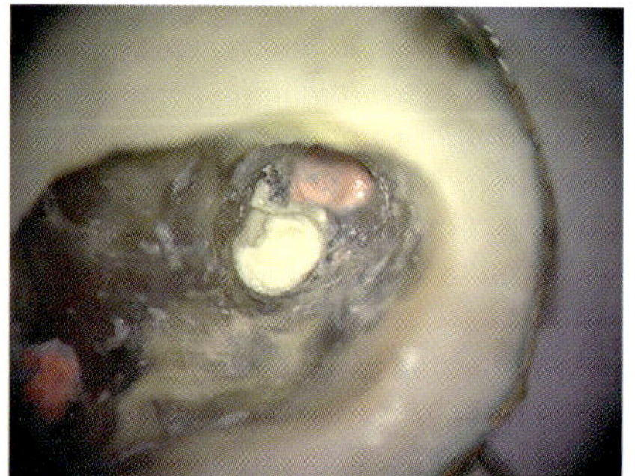

4-7d Clinical photograph of the perforation after obturation.

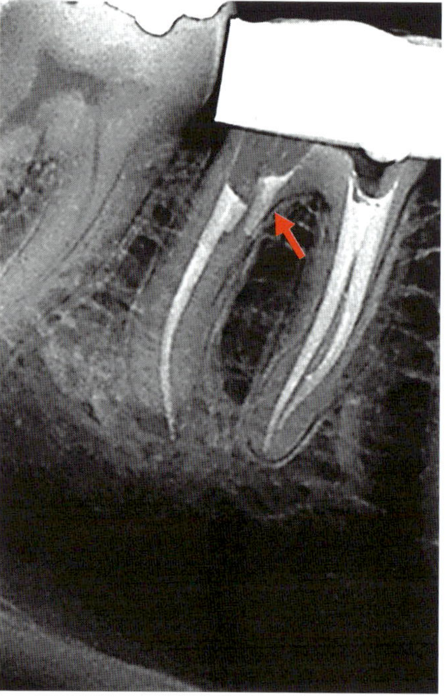

4-7e Postoperative radiograph demonstrating the perforation repair (*arrow*) and the obturated canals.

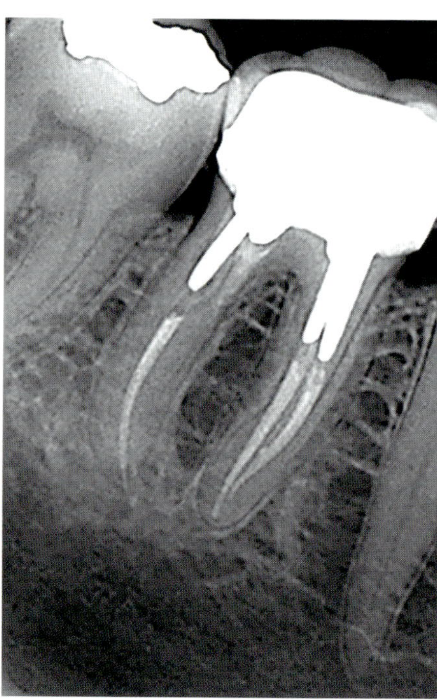

4-7f Radiograph taken 2 years postoperatively.

Perforations of the Middle and Apical Thirds of the Canal

Perforations in the middle third of the canal tend to occur on the buccal or lateral aspect of the root during inappropriate post-hole preparation, as the clinician searches for canals or, more commonly, when an instrument is forced apically in an attempt to negotiate a blocked or calcified canal. The choice of treatment depends on the size and site of the perforation, the presence of a post, and the nature and quality of the coronal restoration.

When attempting retreatment via a coronal approach, two problems are likely: difficulty in (1) identifying the site of perforation and (2) locating the "true" canal. Identifying the site of the perforation can be difficult because it may be located on any of the tooth's surfaces. A radiograph provides only limited information, and an additional angled view can be helpful. The "true" canal is elusive because the perforation is often accompanied by a blockage in the true, anatomic canal. As a result, instruments tend to enter the perforation site ("false" canal) rather than the unprepared or previously obturated true canal.

The technical difficulty in treating perforations in the middle and apical thirds via a coronal approach stems from poor visibility and the fact that the true and false canals will follow a common path for several millimeters and then bifurcate in a region where access and vision are severely limited. Furthermore, if the perforation was created during an attempt to negotiate a blocked or calcified canal, finding the path of the original canal can prove to be very difficult or even impossible.

However, when a perforation results from overpreparation of a canal, during post-hole preparation for example, finding the path of the true canal is relatively easy because the canal will have already been enlarged during initial preparation. If coronal access is feasible, the access cavity is modified and the coronal part of the canal enlarged so the true canal can be located. The treatment that follows depends on the diameter of the canal and the size of the perforation.

Small perforations

A small-diameter perforation can be treated in two ways:

1. *As an additional canal.* The working length of the perforation is determined, and the false canal is prepared, cleaned, and filled exactly as if it were an ordinary canal.
2. *As a lateral canal or an apical delta.* In this case, once the true canal is located (Figs 4-8a and 4-8b), it is prepared and cleaned (Fig 4-8c). The perforation is filled as if it was a lateral canal, and when gutta-percha is condensed into the main canal, sealer is forced along the path of the lateral canal or perforation defect (Figs 4-8d and 4-8e). This procedure is much more difficult if the perforation is located apically (Fig 4-9a). In the case of a curved canal, finding the true canal can prove particularly difficult if not impossible.

After the existing root canal filling has been removed from the coronal part of the canal, the perforation is cleared of any obturation material. A precurved small-diameter stainless steel hand file is used to search for and locate the apical path of the true canal (Fig 4-9b). Once found and negotiated, the canal is prepared to its full length and copiously irrigated. All the instruments used in this sequence should be precurved so that they can be placed directly into the canal without risk of entering the false canal and widening the perforation. The gutta-percha point must also be precurved to allow its fitting in the canal. The gutta-percha point is covered with sealer and inserted into the canal; if there is any doubt about its position, a radiograph can be taken to check that the gutta-percha point is in the correct position. It is then compacted using vertical compaction. Hydraulic pressure is sufficient to allow obturation of the perforation (Fig 4-9c). Postoperative follow-up allows the tooth to be assessed and monitored (Fig 4-9d).

In cases where the true canal cannot be negotiated despite several attempts, the perforation is measured and then prepared and filled like a normal canal. Surgical intervention with retrograde filling may be indicated if clinical or radiographic signs develop and further retreatment becomes necessary.

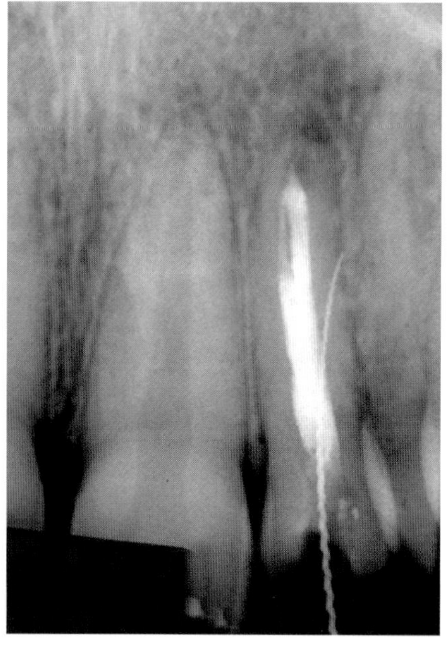

4-8a Radiograph (provided by the referring practitioner) demonstrating a small-diameter file in a buccal perforation that had been accidentally created during efforts to remove the existing obturation material.

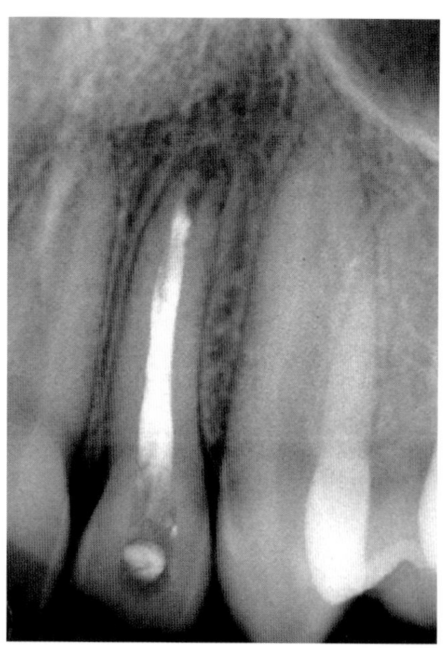

4-8b Preoperative radiograph.

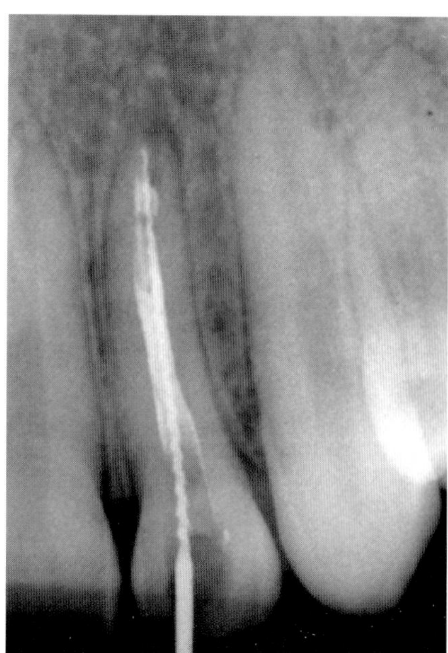

4-8c Radiograph demonstrating the path of the canal that was found. Rubber dam is held in place with Wedjets.

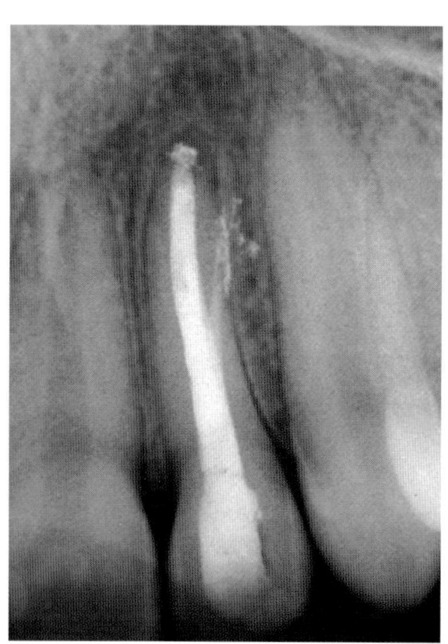

4-8d Radiograph of the obturated canal and the obturated perforation. In this case the perforation was treated like a lateral canal. Only the main canal was prepared, under copious irrigation, and obturated with gutta-percha.

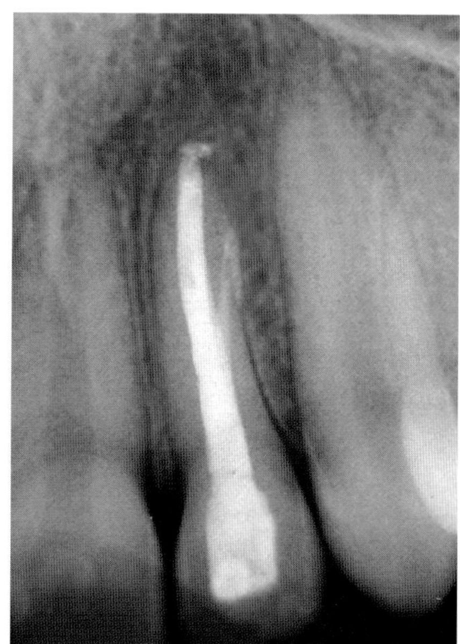

4-8e Radiograph taken 5 years postoperatively.

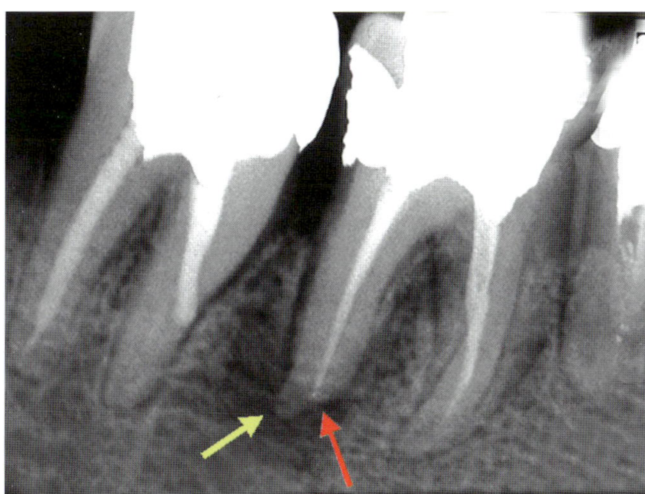

4-9a Preoperative radiograph demonstrating an apical perforation *(red arrow)* probably created as a result of a large-diameter stainless steel hand file being used with excessive pressure. The true apical opening of this mandibular molar in fact lies distal to the perforation *(yellow arrow)*.

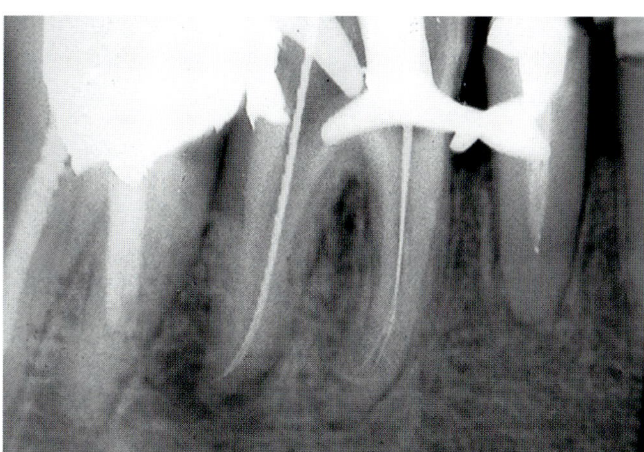

4-9b After the existing root canal filling has been removed, precurved small-diameter hand files are used to find the true pathway.

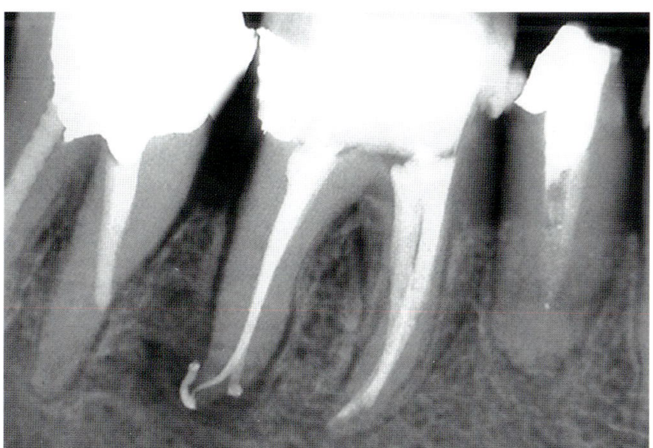

4-9c A series of precurved instruments is used to prepare the apical part of the canal, and the canal is then obturated with gutta-percha using warm vertical condensation. The perforation is obturated by hydraulic pressure in the same way that an apical delta would be.

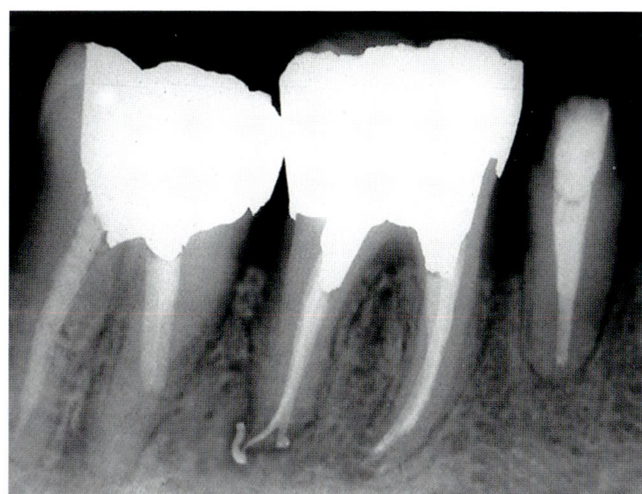

4-9d Radiograph taken 3 years postoperatively.

Large perforations

Larger perforations should be obturated with ProRoot MTA. These bigger defects are often caused by excessive post-hole preparation (Fig 4-10a). Before treatment starts, periodontal probing must be performed to check that there is no communication between the perforation, the lesion, and the base of the gingival sulcus. The post is removed as described in chapter 2.

Box 4-2	Clinical protocol for obturating perforations

1. The portion of the canal coronal to the perforation is cleaned and disinfected.
2. A fine, precurved hand file is used to find the path of the apical part of the canal. The canal is prepared and disinfected in the conventional manner (Fig 4-10b).
3. A gutta-percha point is adjusted to the working length, and the apical part is covered with sealer before being inserted into the canal. The gutta-percha point is sectioned just below the level of the perforation (Fig 4-10c) and then condensed (Fig 4-10d).
4. The perforation is obturated with ProRoot MTA. This is dispensed from the MTA Gun (Fig 4-10e) and then carefully packed into the defect with a plugger or the butt end of a paper point (Fig 4-10f).
5. A moist cotton pledget is placed in the access cavity and covered with a temporary dressing.
6. A definitive coronal restoration must be placed as soon as possible. Regular clinical and radiographic follow-up allows healing to be assessed and will help determine if further adjunctive treatment is needed (Fig 4-10g).

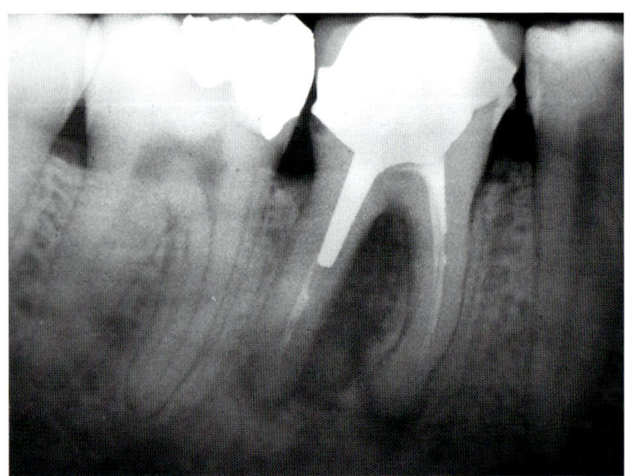

4-10a Preoperative radiograph demonstrating a furcation defect that corresponds to a perforation created during preparation for the post in the distal canal. Clinical examination revealed the integrity of the epithelial attachment and confirmed the absence of a communication between the oral cavity and the lesion. A coronal approach was decided.

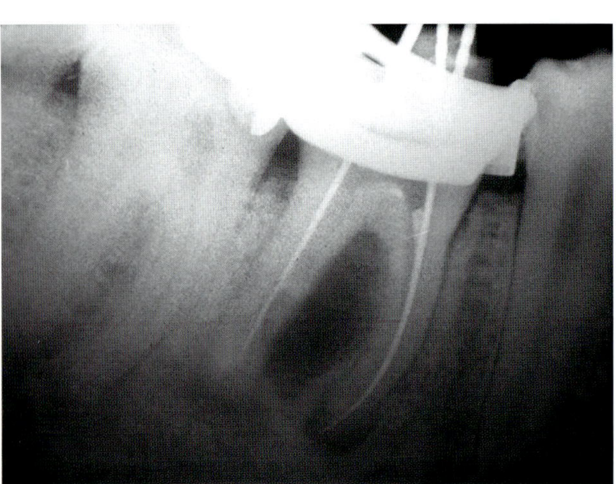

4-10b After removing the post, the canals are located, existing obturation material is removed, and canal preparation is completed under copious irrigation.

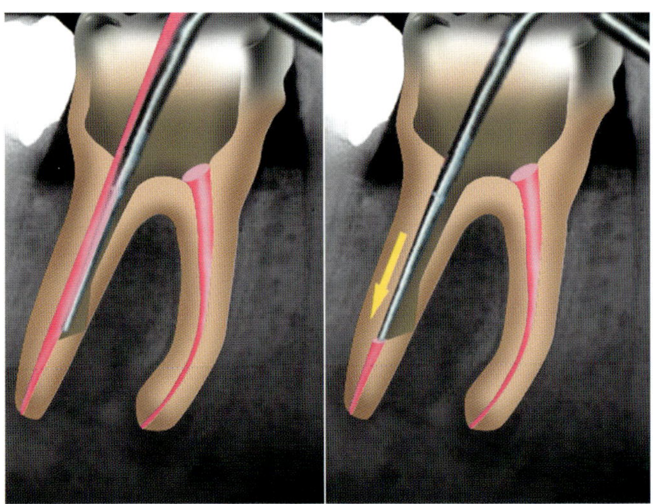

4-10c The canal is dried and a prepared gutta-percha point with sealer on the apical aspect is inserted into the canal. It is then sectioned just below the level of the perforation *(left)* and condensed apically.

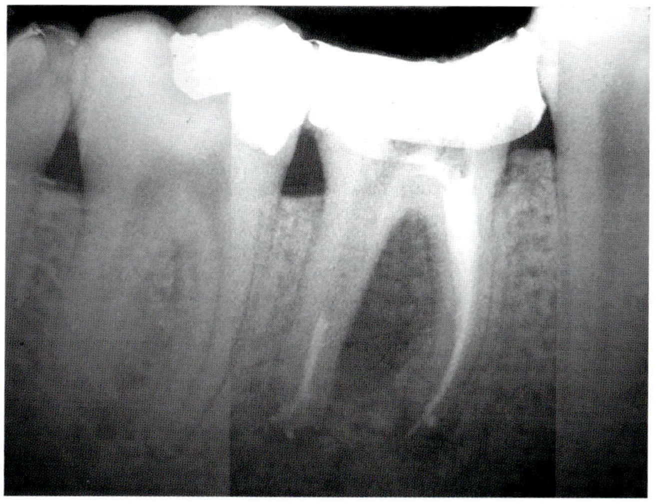

4-10d Radiograph to assess the apical obturation of the distal canal.

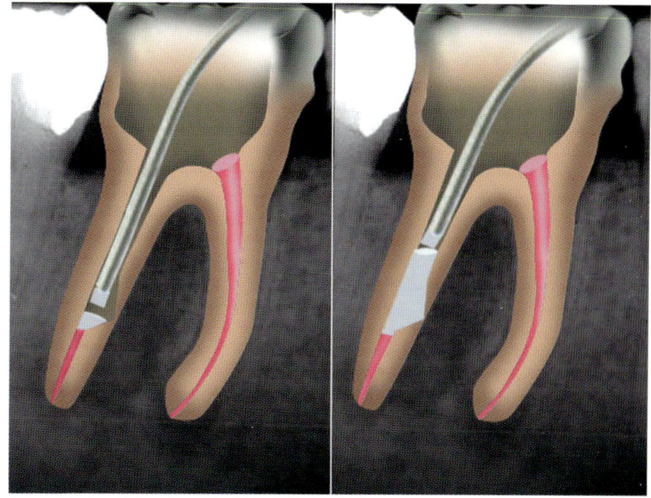

4-10e ProRoot MTA is placed into the perforation with the MTA Gun.

4-10f Additional ProRoot MTA is placed into the canal and gently packed into the defect using a plugger or the butt end of a paper point. A radiograph allows the obturation to be assessed.

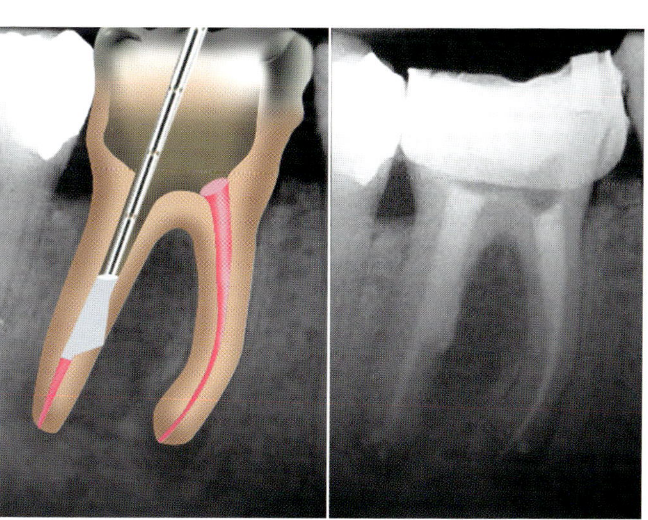

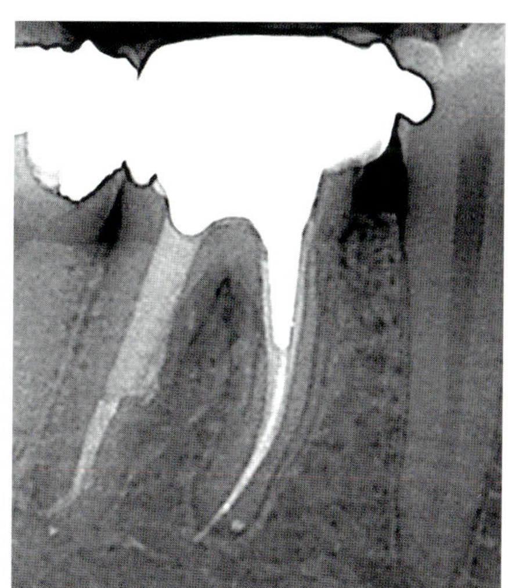

4-10g Radiograph taken 2 years postoperatively.

In cases where post removal looks difficult and there is a high risk of fracturing the root by attempting to dislodge the post, a surgical approach may be indicated for first-line treatment (Fig 4-11a). A full-thickness flap is raised to provide access to the lesion. Granulation tissue is removed by curettage. The defect is prepared with surgical ultrasonic tips and then obturated. If the root filling in the apical part of the canal is inadequate, this can be dealt with at the same time by resecting the root end and placing a retrograde filling. The bony cavity is cleaned and debrided and the flap sutured in place. Postoperative radiographs allow healing to be monitored (Figs 4-11b and 4-11c).

Such clinical situations can be difficult to manage, especially if the post extends to the level of the perforation. In these cases it is difficult, if not impossible, to create a cavity deep enough and retentive enough to ensure a good seal. This must be taken into consideration when treatment options are being discussed.

Iatrogenic perforations occurring during endodontic treatment are particularly displeasing for the clinician and can have significant implications for the patient. Fear of creating a per-

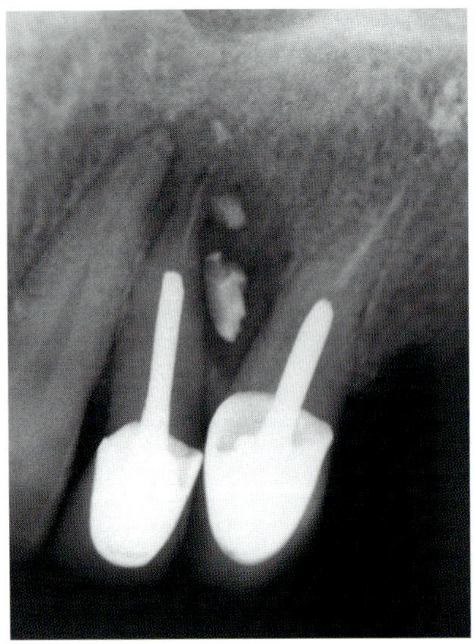

4-11a Preoperative radiograph of a lateral incisor with a distal perforation at the base of the post. In this case, it was decided that, given the size of the post and the amount of remaining root structure, the treatment would be performed from a surgical approach.

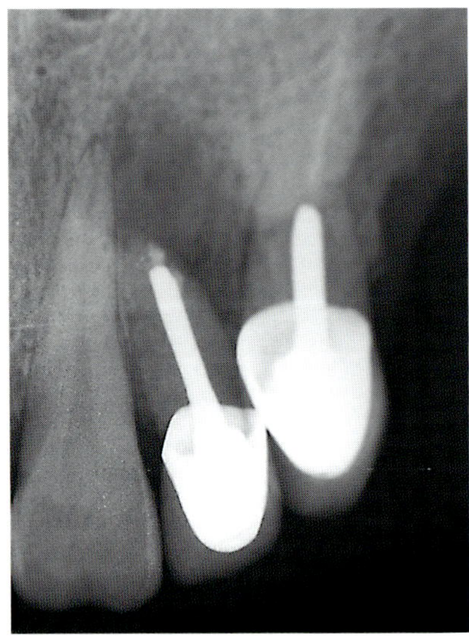

4-11b Immediate postoperative radiograph showing the perforation repair and the retrograde obturation.

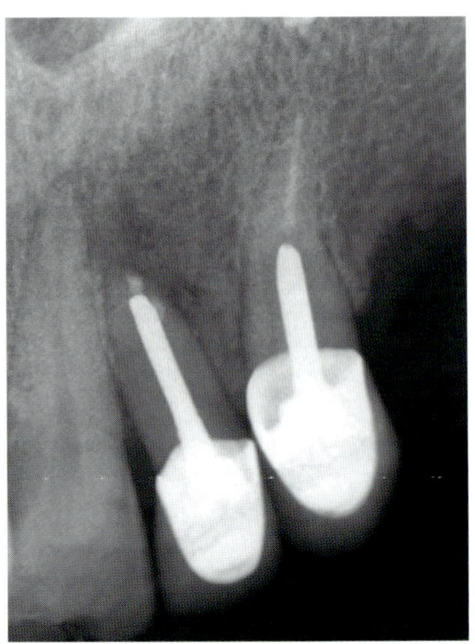

4-11c Radiograph taken 1 year postoperatively.

foration often prevents practitioners from undertaking retreatment when it is indicated. It is imperative that every effort be made to avoid a perforation by following the simple guidelines (Box 4-3) that are often neglected.

Box 4-3	**General guidelines**
Preoperative radiographs allow the clinician to determine the angulation of the tooth for correct positioning of instruments, the shape and contents of the pulp chamber, and the possibility of any blocked canals.	
Additional lighting and magnification vastly improve operating conditions; the operator must maintain direct visual access to cutting instruments in the pulp chamber. Useful aids include loupes or a microscope, long-shank burs so the head of the handpiece does not restrict vision, and ultrasonic instruments dedicated to endodontic retreatment.	
During removal of obturation material, instruments must never be forced apically if resistance is encountered. Radiographs taken during this stage of treatment will allow assessment of the cause of the blockage.	

If a perforation should occur during treatment, the main goal is to prevent bacterial contamination.
With a pre-existing perforation, the extent of damage to the tooth and the periodontal tissues must first be assessed; a treatment plan can be devised after a thorough clinical and radiographic examination. The ultimate aim is to obtain a good seal using whichever techniques and materials are deemed most suitable in that particular case.

Treatment of Teeth with Open Apices

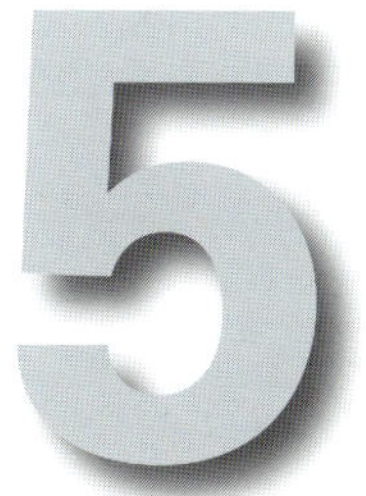

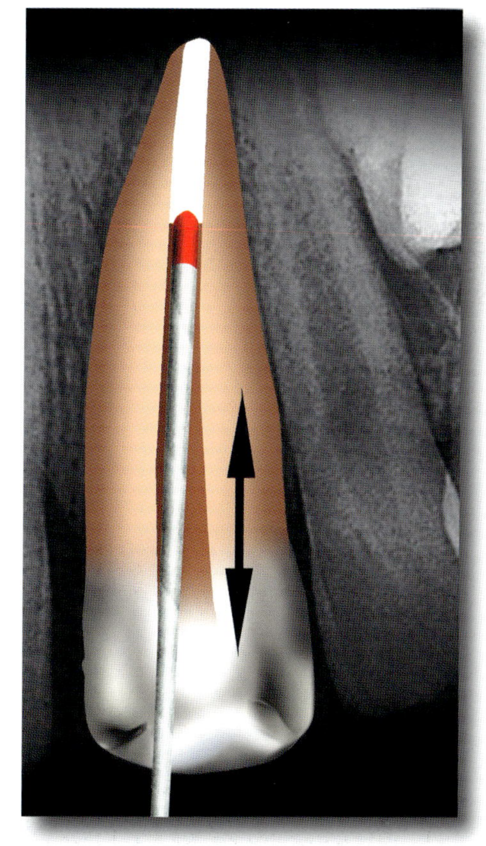

Teeth with open apices are particularly complex to manage. The width of the root canal, the large apical opening, and the thin root canal walls make the preparation, cleaning, and gutta-percha obturation of these teeth more difficult than treatment of a tooth in which root formation is complete.

Immature Teeth

Roots are formed by odontoblasts in a healthy pulp. Dentin is laid down in a coronal-apical direction and in a centripetal manner, thus progressively reducing the size of the canal lumen. If the tooth is subjected to trauma, the neurovascular bundle that is situated apically may be damaged. The result is one of two possible clinical scenarios: *(1)* the foramen is large enough that over a period of several weeks revascularization occurs between the surrounding periapical tissues and the pulp tissue; or *(2)* the vascular supply is lost, the pulpal tissue becomes necrotic, and loss of the dentin-forming cells causes root formation to cease.

After trauma it is often difficult to determine the pulp's status. Application of a thermal stimulus may be felt by the patient, but this is not a guarantee that the pulp will retain long-term vitality. Vitality testing, particularly thermal stimulation, evaluates pulpal response and the integrity of nerve fibers but does not assess the vascularization of the pulp tissue. Immediately after trauma, nerve fibers may persist even though the vascular supply has been interrupted. In the absence of blood flow within the tissues, the fibers will rapidly become hypoxic and disappear. It is only at this stage, sometimes several days after the incident, that the vitality tests will be negative and the diagnosis of necrosis can be made. It is therefore important in the days and weeks after trauma to perform repeat vitality tests and check the reproducibility of results, before making a decision about the tooth's vitality.

Furthermore, following a traumatic episode the nerve fibers in a tooth may be unable to transmit nerve impulses for a short period. This phenomenon is known as *pulpal shock* and does not signal loss of pulp vascularization. This is commonly seen in immature teeth; the neuronal network is incompletely established at this age, and therefore a disordered response to a stimulus may occur that does not indicate true necrosis. *It is therefore crucial that the practitioner does not perform a pulpectomy on the day of the incident purely on the basis that thermal stimulation does not elicit a response.* Emergency treatment should be completed only as necessary; the patient should be evaluated several days later and then again after a period of several weeks to repeat the vitality tests.

Electric pulp tests are the most reliable diagnostic tool. The level at which the stimulus evokes a response can be noted and results compared over a period of time, which gives an idea of the evolution of the pulpal state:

- If the value or reading falls over time, the nerve fibers are becoming more easily stimulated and the prognosis is good.
- Conversely, if the value increases, the nerve fibers are becoming hypoxic and there is a high chance that necrosis will ensue.

Monitoring (short-, medium-, and long-term) is essential in such a situation. A pulpectomy should be considered only in the following situations:

- Significant pain indicating a pulpitis (rare)
- Absence of clinical signs but continued negative thermal tests after a monitoring period of several weeks, and/or increased electric pulp test readings from month to month until there is no response at all
- Discontinuation of root formation (determined radiographically over several months) signaling the loss of dentin-forming cells
- Clinical signs of infection (eg, abscess, fistula).

- Appearance of an apical radiolucency, suggesting a lesion of endodontic origin. This must be approached with caution, however, because the radiographic appearance of normal trabecular bone around the apex of an immature tooth is very similar to the radiographic appearance of a lesion of endodontic origin.

Treatment by Apexogenesis

Apexogenesis is the biologic process responsible for the formation of the root on the apex of the tooth and the completion of the apex's growth. Treatment by apexogenesis refers to a procedure that allows the root tip of an immature tooth to continue forming after trauma; this is done by protecting and conserving the dentin-forming cells by keeping the pulp vital if possible. In cases of pulp exposure through coronal fracture, a superficial partial pulpotomy should be completed as soon as possible; this must be followed up by direct pulp capping to prevent bacterial contamination and necrosis.

A number of materials have been proposed for use in pulp capping. Calcium hydroxide has long been recognized as a suitable material that is capable of stimulating the formation of a dentin bridge to protect the underlying pulp. Currently, ProRoot MTA appears to be the material of choice for direct pulp capping. It stimulates the formation of a hard tissue bridge that, in terms of structure and sealing ability, is superior to those induced by other materials (Aeinehchi et al, 2003).

Despite the development of new materials such as MTA, with its wide range of possible uses, a superficial partial pulpotomy and pulp capping should not be performed on an inflamed pulp (Figs 5-1a to 5-1f). This treatment should therefore not be performed on a carious, symptomatic tooth; Pulp capping should be limited to the treatment of pulpal exposures following trauma with an associated coronal fracture. As soon as the pulp comes into contact with the oral cavity, the superficial pulpal layer is contaminated and inflammatory processes are activated in response. A partial pulpotomy to a depth of 2 mm is sufficient to remove this superficial layer of contaminated pulp tissue. This pulpotomy is performed with a round tungsten carbide bur on a contra-angle handpiece or with ultrasonic surgical instruments combined with water irrigation. The bur selected for use should be slightly larger than the pulp exposure to allow simple removal of the infected pulp tissue; care must be taken not to catch the pulp on the rotating instrument and cause complete pulp extirpation. A large paper point with a butt end dipped in 2.5% sodium hypochlorite is used to apply light pressure to the pulp for 5 minutes to achieve hemostasis. MTA is placed directly over the pulp and gently packed into place using large dry paper points. The coronal restoration must be placed as soon as possible.

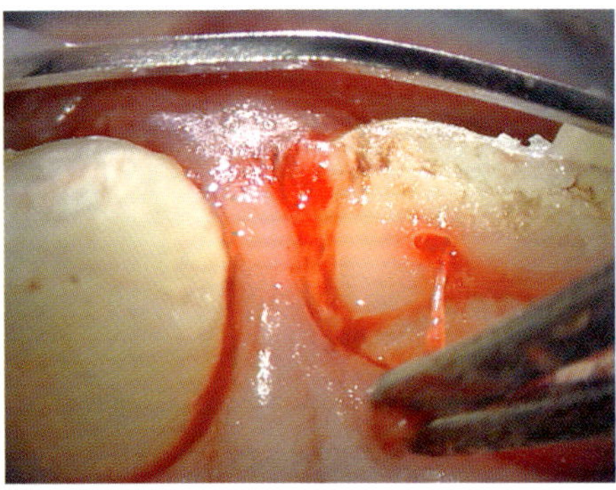

5-1a This 7-year-old child suffered trauma to the right maxillary central incisor (seen in a mirror), resulting in a coronal fracture with pulpal exposure. The concomitant luxation has been reduced and a splint placed. Rubber dam could not be used, so the operating field is kept dry with cheek retractors and aspiration.

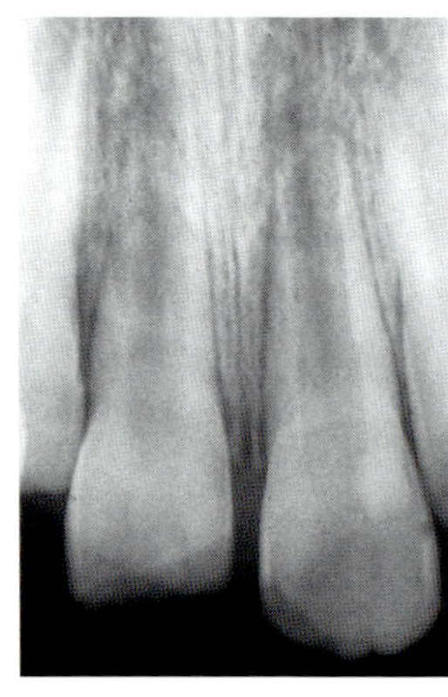

5-1b Radiograph showing that root formation of the maxillary central incisors, particularly that on the right side, is incomplete.

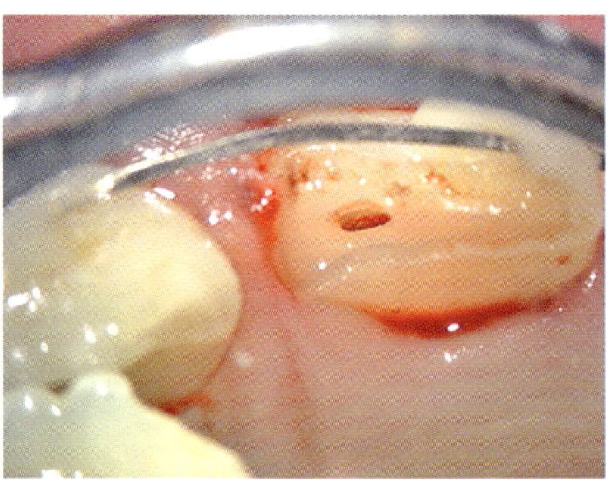

5-1c Partial pulpotomy performed with surgical ultrasonic instruments combined with water irrigation.

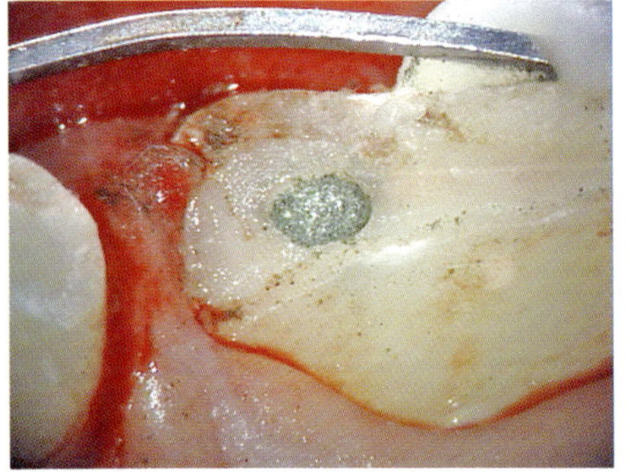

5-1d ProRoot MTA placed directly over the pulp and condensed with a large-diameter paper point. Glass ionomer cement is then used to provide a good coronal seal until a definitive restoration can be placed.

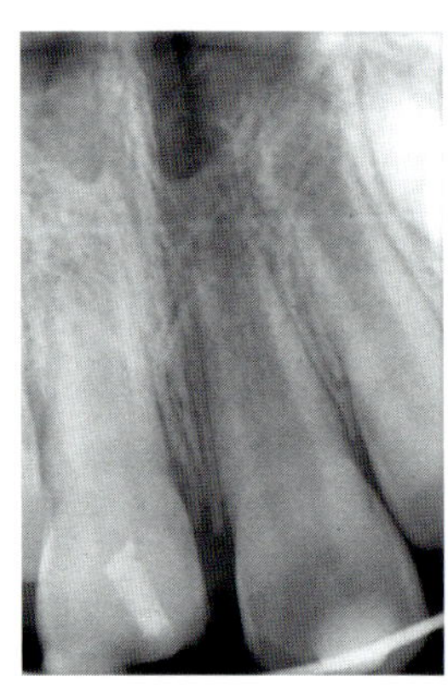

5-1e Postoperative radiograph.

5-1f Radiograph taken 18 months postoperatively shows that root formation continued normally (possibly even slightly quicker than the adjacent nontraumatized in tooth). Prompt treatment and the use of a biocompatible material with good sealing properties allowed the vitality of the tooth to be maintained.

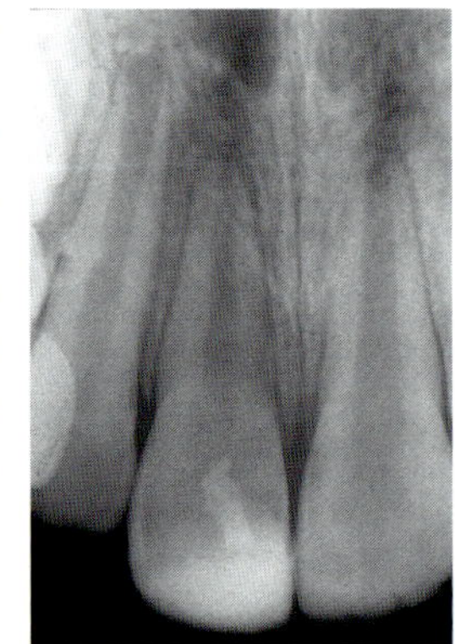

Treatment by Apexification

In cases where the tooth's vascular supply has been interrupted, the pulp becomes necrotic and endodontic treatment is indicated. Endodontic treatment of immature teeth has long been considered a challenge. Differences in morphology cause inherent difficulties: the presence of thin dentinal walls and therefore reduced mechanical resistance of the tooth; the size of the canal lumen and foramen, and the absence of an apical constriction, which makes it difficult to create an apical taper and achieve the desired resistance form to facilitate obturation; and the sometimes divergent nature of the canal walls, depending on the stage at which root formation ceased.

Numerous techniques and materials have been proposed to induce apical closure, a process known as *apexification* (Webber, 1984). These are based on either of the following:

- The use of certain materials, primarily calcium hydroxide, which directly induce apical closure. Once apical closure has been achieved by the formation of a mineralized tissue barrier, the canal can be obturated. These procedures are time consuming and the results unpredictable.
- The placement of an apical plug (eg, collagen, tricalcium phosphate, and more recently ProRoot MTA), which enables the operator to obturate the canal at the same visit and restore the tooth without further delay. Apical closure occurs naturally over time.

The principal factors for successful apexification include

- Thorough debridement and disinfection of the root canal system.
- Good obturation of the root canal system and a good apical seal.
- The position of the root apex. Apexification is impossible if the apex of the tooth is not situated within the bony cortex. In such cases a surgical approach is necessary to resect the root end so a good seal can be created; the formation of a healthy periodontal membrane indicates healing.

Apexification with calcium hydroxide

This technique is the most commonly described in the literature. A temporary calcium hydroxide dressing is placed in the root canal and then changed at regular intervals until a hard tissue barrier has formed. Once this canal closure occurs, the canal is obturated conventionally with gutta-percha.

Rubber dam is fitted and the canal is disinfected. The canal must be instrumented to remove the superficial infected layer of dentin and predentin; large-diameter H-files are used on each of the canal walls. The working length is determined radiographically. Copious irrigation with 2.5% sodium hypochlorite is essential to ensure that the canal is properly disinfected; this must be done with care to avoid forcing sodium hypochlorite through the apex. The canal is dried with large paper points and dressed temporarily with a calcium hydroxide–based medicament.

Pure calcium hydroxide

Pure calcium hydroxide is produced by mixing the powder with sterile water; the mixture is then wrapped in gauze to remove excess water. The material has a paste-like consistency and can be placed into the canal using an amalgam carrier. It is then condensed with a large paper point or a plugger that has been dipped in the calcium hydroxide powder. Further paste is added until the canal is filled with calcium hydroxide to the cementoenamel junction.

Commercial preparations of calcium hydroxide

Many laboratories now produce calcium hydroxide–based root canal medicaments (eg, Pulpdent paste, Pulpdent; Calasept, Nordiska Dental; Hypocal, Ellinan; Calxyl, OCO-Präparate). Generally dispensed in a syringe, the material is deposited directly into the canal and then gently condensed with the butt end of paper points. The consistency and ease of use of the material makes the overall manipulation of the material far easier. Nevertheless, the concentration of calcium hydroxide varies between manufacturers, depending on the amount of additives such as methyl cellulose. This must be taken into consideration when choosing a product. The action of these products relies on the material having direct contact with the tissues. It is therefore important to establish, by whatever means possible, that the calcium hydroxide is in contact with the apical tissues but is not being forced through the apical foramen. The alkaline pH of the substance could be harmful to the surrounding tissues if large amounts are extruded through the apex. The access cavity is then obturated. The coronal seal is an important factor in determining the success of treatment; if it is inadequate, bacterial contamination will follow and the calcium hydroxide dressing will dissolve, inevitably leading to failure. Because the next stage of treatment will not be performed for several weeks, a simple temporary dressing is not sufficient. It is preferable to use composite or a glass-ionomer cement. Because calcium hydroxide has a radiographic appearance similar to that of dentin, a radiograph taken midtreatment allows verification that the canal has been well obturated with calcium hydroxide (Figs 5-2a and 5-2b).

Follow-up

The length of time necessary to achieve apical barrier formation depends on the stage of development of the tooth, the divergence of the radicular walls, and the presence of any apical pathology.

Regular follow-up of the patient is important and allows the clinician to monitor the coronal seal of the provisional restoration. Radiographs permit assessment of the apical barrier formation; if the calcium hydroxide appears to be dissolving, which will be radiographically evident, it will need to be replaced.

Replacing the temporary calcium hydroxide dressing

The calcium hydroxide is replaced every 3 months until an apical barrier forms. At each appointment rubber dam must be placed and the coronal restoration removed. The canal is carefully rinsed and cleaned to remove all of the existing dressing; an ultrasonic endodontic file can be used but must be kept clear of the canal walls.

With a small-diameter file adjusted to the estimated working length, the formation of an apical barrier is carefully assessed. If apical closure has occurred and is evident radiographically, replacement of the calcium hydroxide is not necessary and the canal can now be obturated. If this is not the case, the dressing is replaced and the access cavity sealed. Histologically the hard tissue barrier appears to be made up of osteoid-like and cementoid-like tissue. It does not provide a complete seal, and a degree of permeability remains. It is therefore imperative to complete the treatment by obturating the canal with gutta-percha (Fig 5-3).

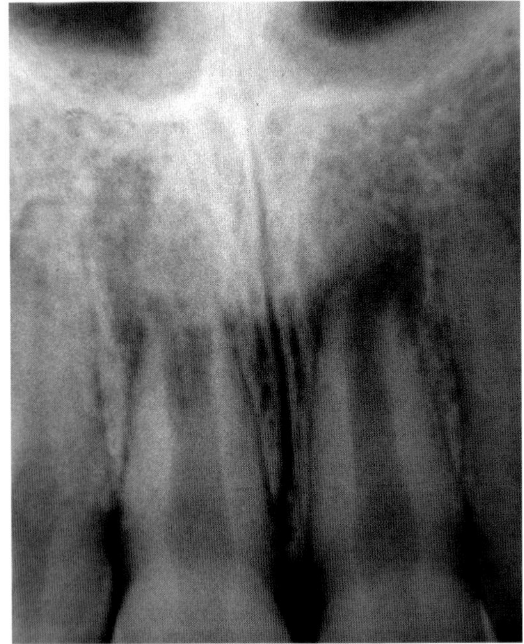

5-2a Preoperative radiograph.

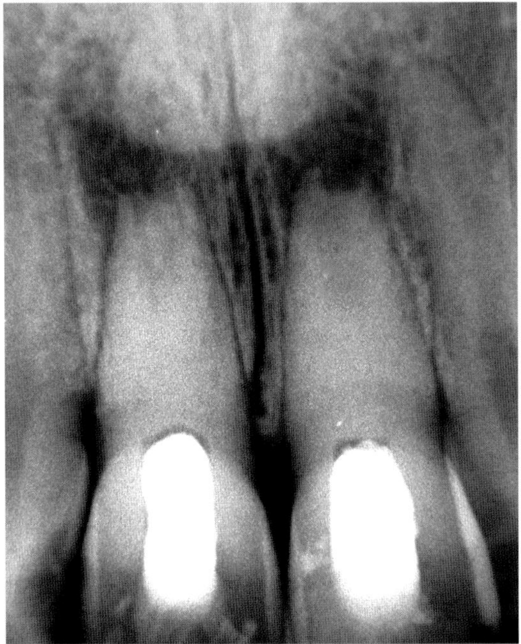

5-2b Calcium hydroxide has a similar radiographic appearance to dentin, so once the canal is filled it is no longer visible radiographically.

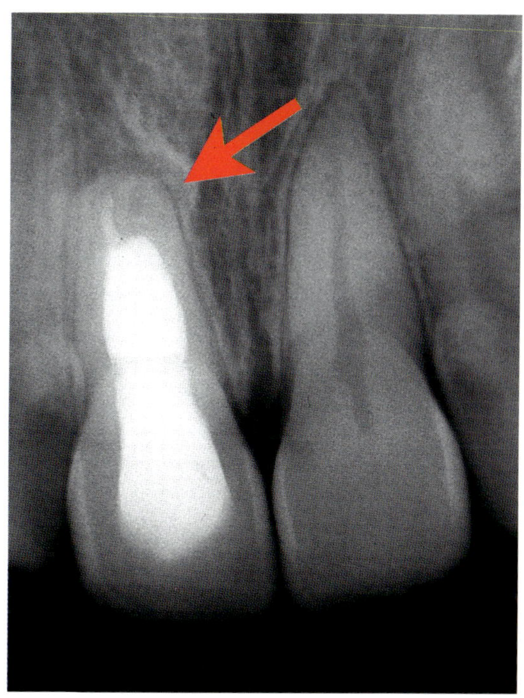

5-3 Regular replacement of the calcium hydroxide dressing in the root canal of this maxillary incisor has allowed the formation of an apical barrier approximately 3 mm thick (*red arrow*). The remainder of the canal was then obturated with gutta-percha.

If any clinical signs develop between appointments, the dressing is removed, the canal is disinfected, and the dressing is replaced. If orthodontic treatment is underway, the calcium hydroxide treatment must be continued to avoid the risk of root resorption, and definitive obturation cannot be considered until the orthodontic retention phase.

Difficulties associated with this technique

Placing regular calcium hydroxide dressings to induce a hard tissue barrier is a well-recognized form of treatment and has been used for more than 30 years. Despite the reliability of this form of treatment, the technique has some drawbacks:

- The calcium hydroxide changes must be done over several months, if not years. The cooperation of the patient is therefore a key factor in the success of the treatment.
- Until the apical barrier appears, definitive obturation cannot be completed, and the canal therefore remains empty and very fragile for the duration of the treatment. Moreover, in the absence of a definitive coronal restoration, there is a significant risk of bacterial infiltration and reinfection of the root canal system between appointments.
- Placing the calcium hydroxide dressings can be technically difficult, particularly in the apical regions where the canal walls may be parallel or even divergent. Repeated and prolonged extrusion of the calcium hydroxide in the periapical region means its alkaline pH could provoke an inflammatory response in the adjacent tissues.

Recent publications (Andreasen et al, 2002; Doyon et al, 2005), have suggested that the mechanical properties of dentin may be impaired by continued exposure to calcium hydroxide. This is particularly significant because of the increased risk to teeth already predisposed to having thin, fragile dentinal walls.

Teeth undergoing such treatment are therefore at risk of fracturing; this may result in loss of the tooth, especially in the case of immature anterior teeth.

Apexification with mineral trioxide aggregate

To overcome these difficulties and risks, clinicians have long sought a material that could provide an immediate and impermeable apical plug. Different materials, namely those used for periodontal surgery, have been proposed. Despite the biocompatibility of these materials, they provide only a poor seal because they do not adhere to dentin, which limits their use in endodontics considerably. Studies on ProRoot MTA over the past 10 years have demonstrated its perfect biocompatibility and its excellent sealing properties. It is currently the material of choice for apexification.

The aim is to create an apical barrier by placing a plug of ProRoot MTA, which then hardens (Box 5-1). The endodontic treatment can be completed at a second visit, and the tooth is then restored. Apical closure and the development of a hard tissue layer occur physiologically over time and are accompanied by the formation of a relatively normal periodontium (Shabahang et al, 1999; Felippe et al, 2006). The advantage of this technique is being able to complete treatment in two visits without a delay—it avoids the need for calcium hydroxide changes and multiple appointments. Furthermore, the coronal restoration can be placed almost immediately, limiting the risk of root fracture.

Box 5-1 Technique for placement of an apical plug of ProRoot MTA

1. Preoperative radiographs are necessary to estimate the length of the tooth and the diameter of the apical opening. A good quality radiograph is essential so that treatment can be completed as well as possible (Fig 5-4a).
2. After anesthesia has been administered, any missing walls of the tooth are restored before rubber dam is fitted.
3. During access cavity preparation, overhanging enamel and dentin should be removed, and all canal orifices should be assessed for visibility. Straight-line access to the apical third of the canal should be created where possible. In maxillary central incisors, for example, once the palatal extent of the pulp roof has been removed, the large straight canal often allows direct vision of the apical third (Figs 5-4b and 5-4c).
4. Large-diameter H-files are used to instrument the canal walls, thus removing predentin and the superficial layer of infected dentin. Apex locators cannot be used for wide canals with a large open apex; working length must therefore be determined by taking a radiograph with a large-diameter file in situ.
5. As in conventional endodontic treatment, the canal is disinfected by copious irrigation with 2.5% or 3% sodium hypochlorite (Fig 5-4d). The irrigating solution will visibly effervesce as organic debris dissolves (known as the *champagne effect*), and irrigation of the canal must continue until the effervescence ceases.
6. If there is a calcium hydroxide dressing in place, ultrasonic tips or files are used to eliminate any traces of it from the canal (Fig 5-4e). Once the disinfection is complete, the canal is dried with large-diameter paper points.
7. A dedicated MTA carrier, the MTA Gun, is needed to deposit the material into the canal. Designed with a straight tip and available with tips of varying sizes, it allows precise placement of ProRoot MTA directly into the apical third of the canal. A radiograph is taken with the MTA carrier in the canal to determine how far the tip penetrates (Fig 5-4f). It should lie 1-2 mm short of the apex, leaving space for the apical plug to be placed (Fig 5-4g).

Box 5-1 Technique for placement of an apical plug of ProRoot MTA *(continued)*

8. The ProRoot MTA is mixed on a glass slab and loaded into the MTA carrier before being placed at the apex (Fig 5-4h). Unlike other traditional materials used in dentistry, ProRoot MTA is a material that does not need to be condensed. With the butt of a paper point or a plugger the material is gently packed into place and thereby brought into contact with the adjacent tissues (Fig 5-4i).
9. To ensure the material is evenly dispensed, an ultrasonic tip can be vibrated against the crown of the tooth; this will also cause any excess water in the mix to rise to the surface where it can be absorbed with paper points.
10. A radiograph at this stage allows assessment of the position of the apical plug (Fig 5-4j). If it is too far from the apical foramen, it can be adjusted with a large-diameter endodontic plugger.
11. More MTA is added until a 5-mm plug is created apically; this thickness of material ensures a good apical seal (Figs 5-4k and 5-4l).

ProRoot MTA will reach a full set only after a minimum of 4 hours in a damp environment. A moist cotton pledget is placed into the canal, and the access cavity is sealed temporarily. Treatment cannot be completed in one visit since a definitive restoration can be placed only after the ProRoot MTA is fully set. The canal should not be entirely filled with ProRoot MTA in case the tooth might need to be prepared for a post-retained crown in the future. It should be kept in mind that, once set, the material is very difficult to remove.

At the next appointment, which may be the following day, the temporary dressing is removed and a right-angled probe is used to check that the ProRoot MTA has set fully. If a post-retained crown is not necessary, the rest of the canal is filled conventionally with gutta-percha and a sealer (Figs 5-4m and 5-4n). In immature anterior teeth, it is preferable not to extend the gutta-percha obturation to the level of the cementoenamel junction. Indeed, thin dentinal walls render these teeth particularly susceptible to fracture. To reinforce the treated tooth, it is advisable to restore the coronal part of the canal (to the level of crestal bone) and the access cavity with composite. If the root is particularly short (relatively common in immature teeth), there may not be sufficient space for gutta-percha interposition between the post and the MTA plug.

Some authors recommend the use of a calcium hydroxide dressing prior to placement of the ProRoot MTA apical plug. Recent studies have shown that this confers no therapeutic advantage. Furthermore, the seal resulting from this technique is inferior to that obtained with immediate placement of ProRoot MTA (Hachmeister et al, 2002; Felippe et al, 2006).

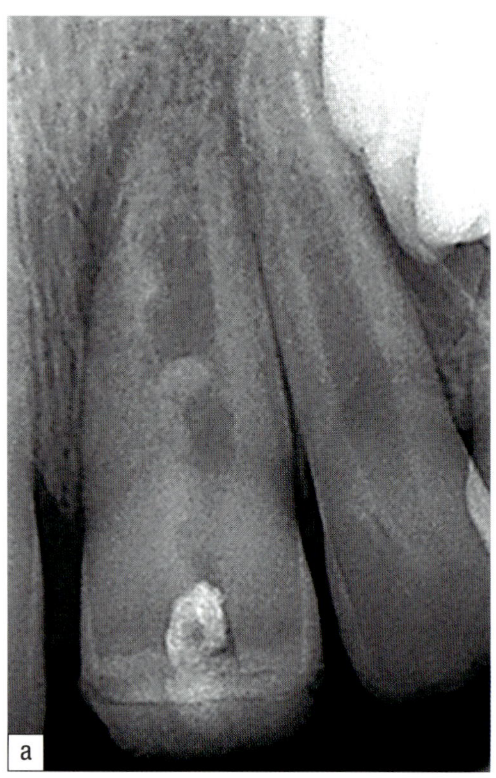

5-4a Preoperative radiograph of a maxillary left central incisor. The tooth has been treated with calcium hydroxide for several months in an attempt to induce apexification, but there has been no improvement. It has been decided to treat the tooth with MTA over two visits.

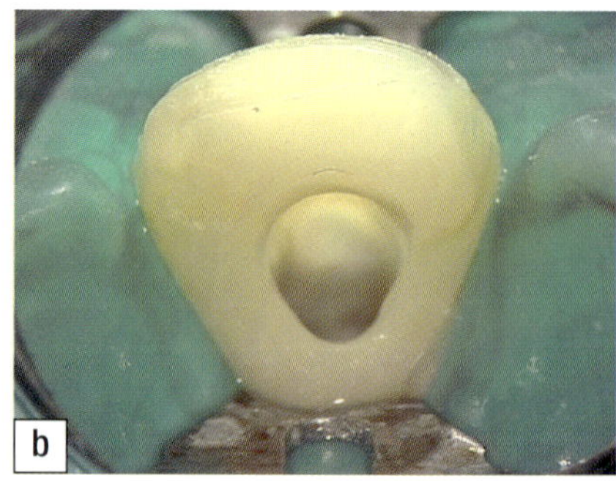

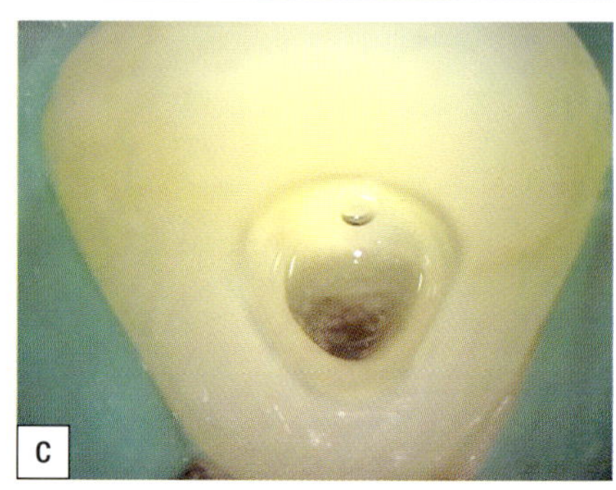

5-4b and 5-4c The access cavity is adjusted to ensure good access for instrumentation and irrigation. Once the palatal extent of the pulp roof has been removed, the large straight canal allows for good control of instruments, even in the apical third.

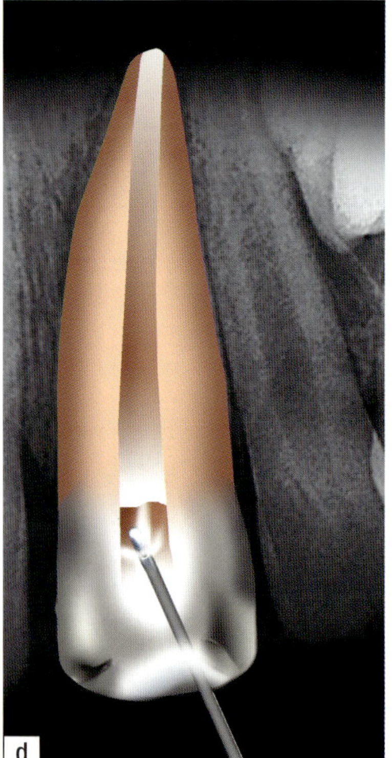

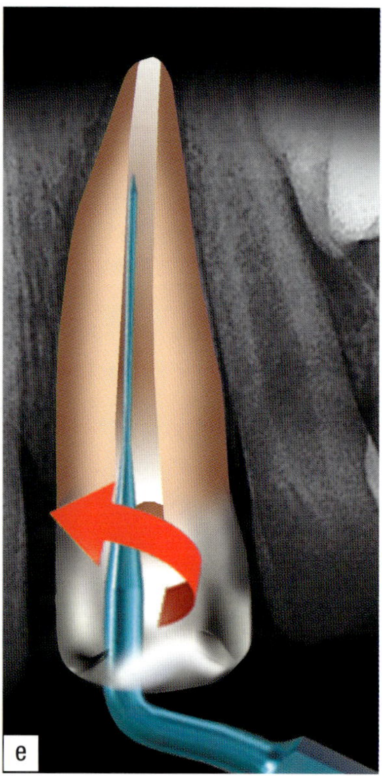

5-4d and 5-4e The canal is disinfected by copious irrigation with sodium hypochlorite. H-files are used to remove the superficial layer of infected predentin. Ultrasonic instruments ensure optimum cleaning: all traces of calcium hydroxide must be eliminated before the canal is obturated.

5-4f and 5-4g The tip of the MTA Gun is placed into the canal, and a radiograph is taken to confirm the working length. The carrier lies 1 to 2 mm short of the apex, leaving space for placement of the apical plug. A rubber stop on the MTA Gun marks the working length.

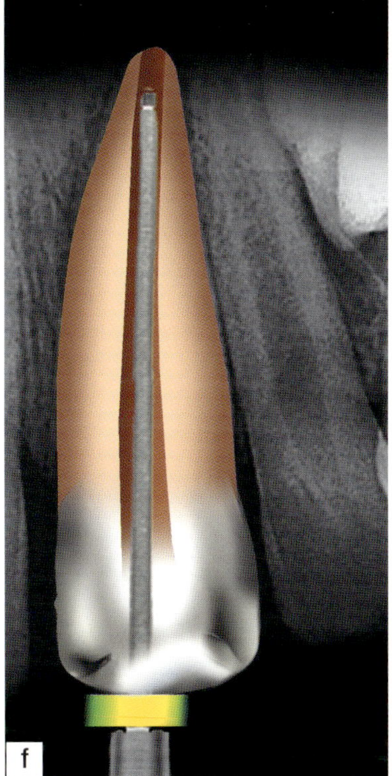

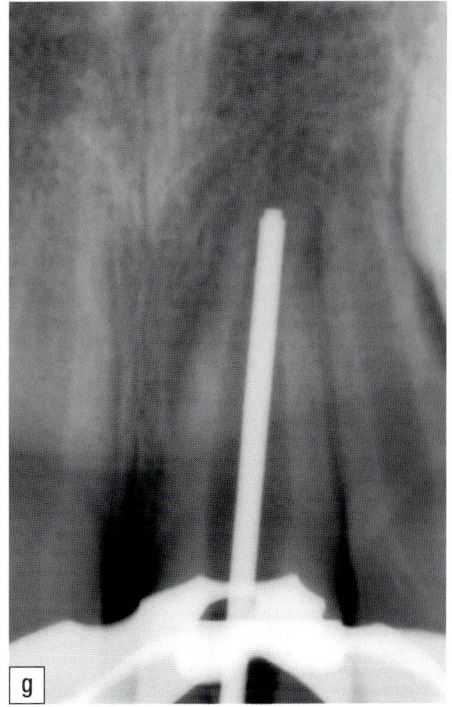

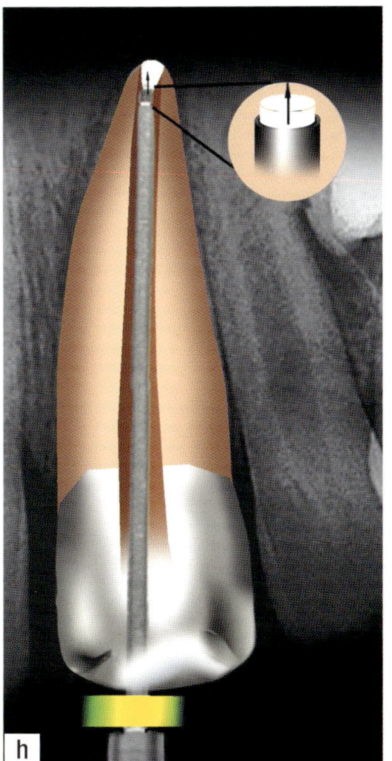

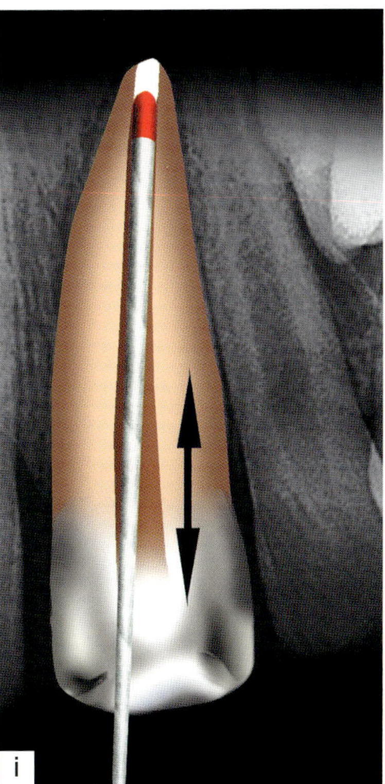

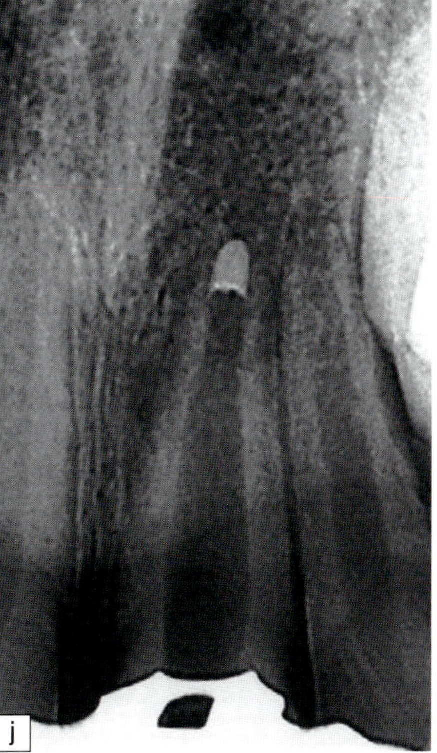

5-4h, 5-4i, 5-4j The ProRoot MTA is *(h)* deposited at the apex and *(i)* gently packed into place with the butt of a paper point; *(j)* this first stage is checked by taking a radiograph.

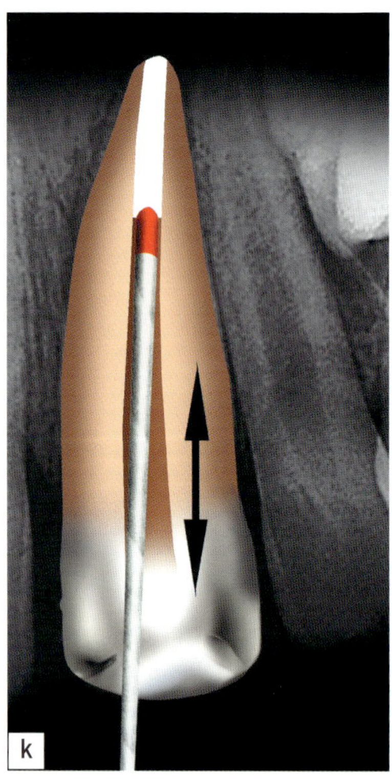

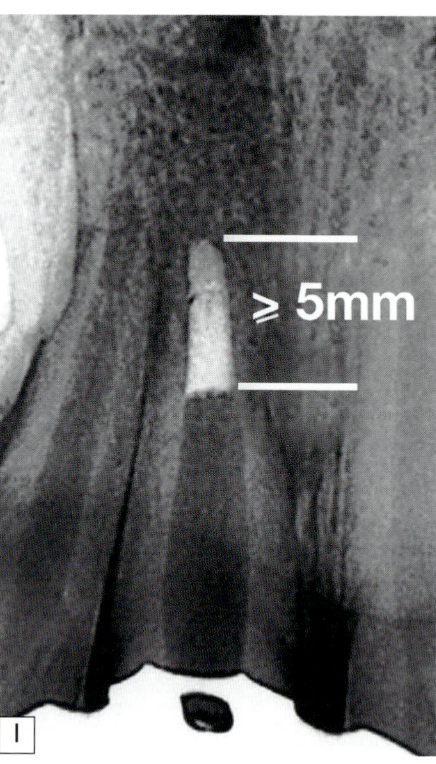

5-4k and 5-4l Further additions of MTA complete the obturation and create an apical plug of 4 to 5 mm. The plug is covered with a moist cotton pledget, and a provisional restoration is placed for 24 hours.

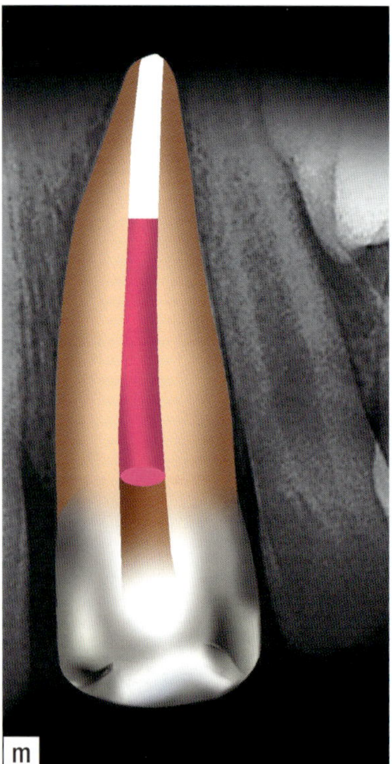

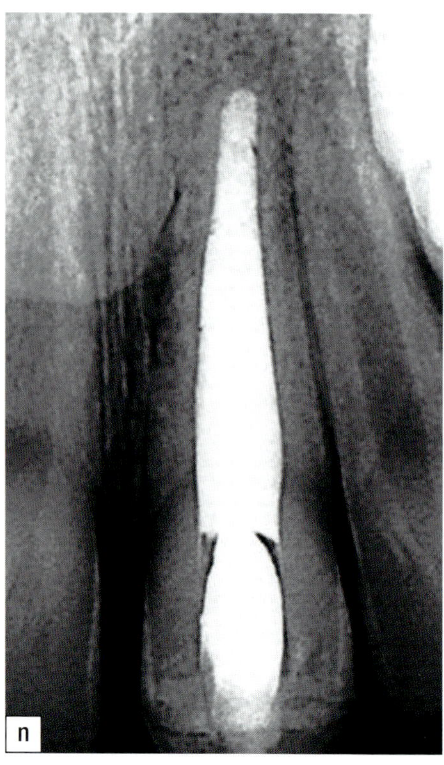

5-4m and 5-4n At the second visit, a right-angled probe is used to check that the MTA has reached a full set. The remainder of the canal is obturated with gutta-percha. A coronal restoration can be placed immediately.

Intermediate calcium hydroxide dressings are necessary only in certain situations. Whether a canal is to be obturated with MTA or conventionally with gutta-percha, the decision of when to obturate is based on the same criteria. If an inflammatory exudate persists or the tooth is symptomatic, obturation with ProRoot MTA should be postponed; otherwise its setting reaction may be compromised. A dry canal is a prerequisite for obturation. In the presence of an inflammatory exudate, the tooth is dressed with calcium hydroxide for several days (or even weeks) until an dry environment has been established (Figs 5-5a to 5-5e).

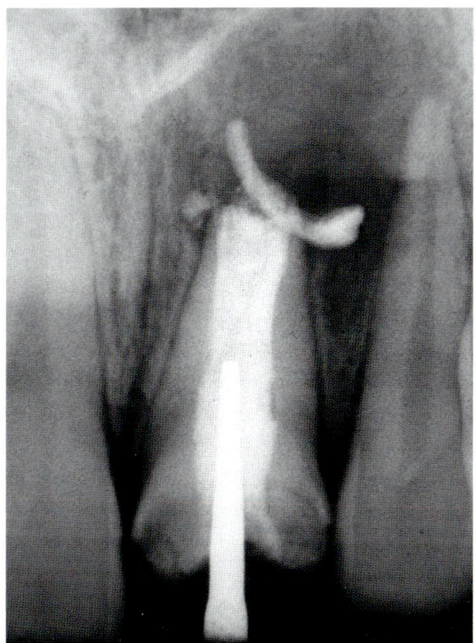

5-5a Preoperative radiograph of a central incisor with an acute apical abscess.

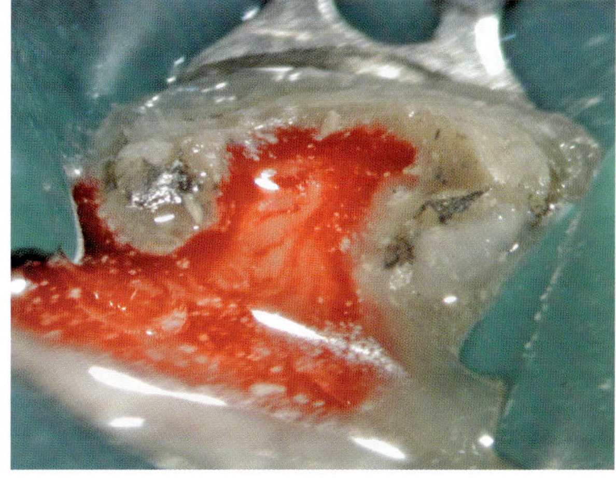

5-5b Coronal access and drainage of the abscess.

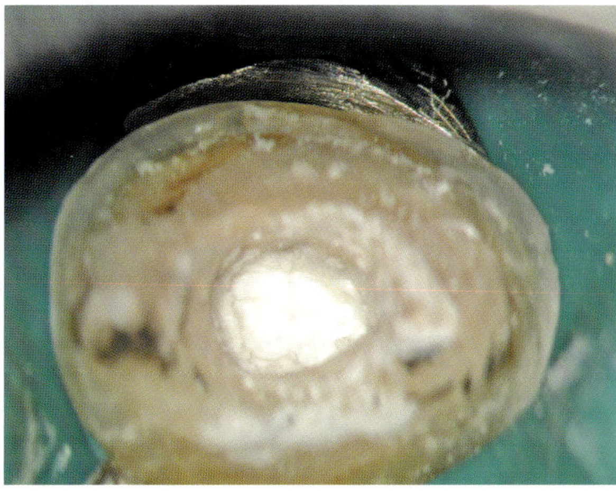

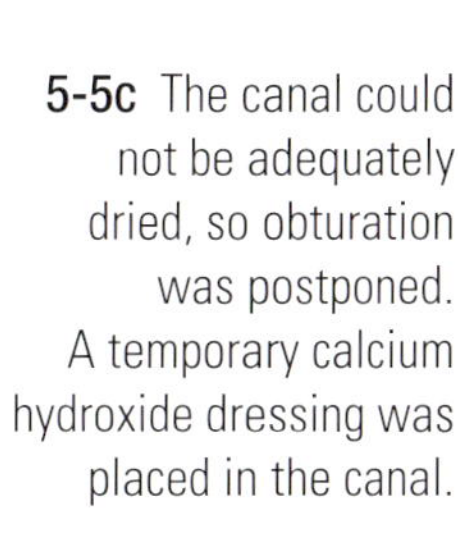

5-5c The canal could not be adequately dried, so obturation was postponed. A temporary calcium hydroxide dressing was placed in the canal.

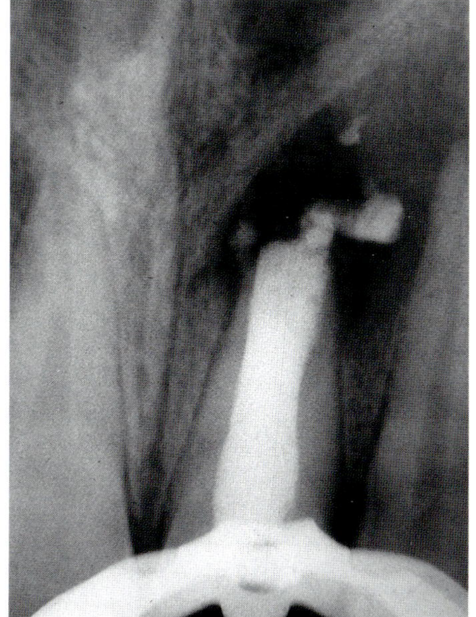

5-5d At the next visit, good conditions enabled successful placement of an apical plug of MTA.

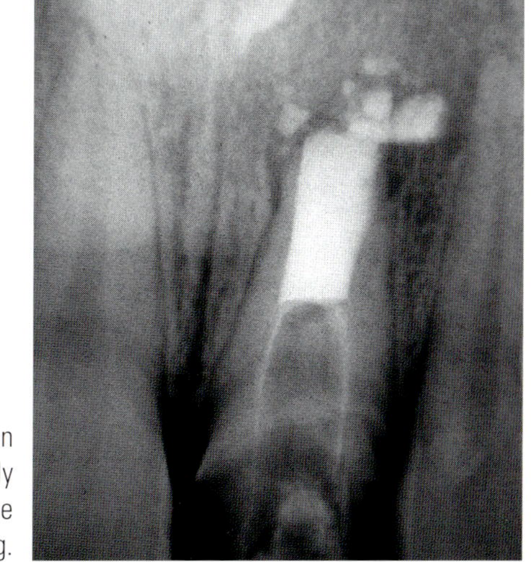

5-5e Radiograph taken 18 months postoperatively shows evidence of bony healing.

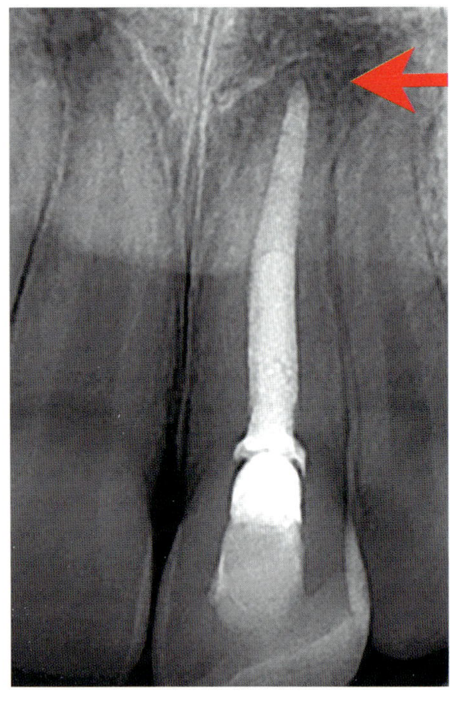

5-6 Radiograph taken 10 months after placement of an MTA plug. Apical closure (*red arrow*) can be seen.

Postoperative follow-up: Endodontic treatment of the tooth is completed over the course of two visits. Regular clinical and radiographic follow-up allows healing to be monitored and apical closure to be assessed (Fig 5-6).

Management of Other Cases with Open Apices

Management of teeth with wide-open apices often involves the treatment of immature maxillary incisors. There are, however, other situations when similar management is required.

Horizontal root fracture

Endodontic treatment is not always necessary following a horizontal root fracture, particularly if the fracture line lies below the level of the bony crest. Nevertheless, if the coronal fragment becomes necrotic, endodontic treatment must be performed. The apical fragment, however, is left untreated; it can be removed surgically if a lesion develops. If the portion of the root to be treated is large at the level of the fracture line, obturation with ProRoot MTA as described previously is the treatment of choice (Figs 5-7a to 5-7d).

Failure of apical surgery

When apical surgery has failed, subsequent orthograde endodontic retreatment may be indicated even though this does not follow the normal, logical order of treatment.
Endodontic surgery with root-end resection often leaves a canal with an apex that is large in diameter. If a canal is to be obturated postoperatively, it may therefore present with an abnormally large or misshapen apical foramen due to the retrograde preparation that has previously been completed. In these cases, placement of an apical plug of ProRoot MTA and conventional obturation is the treatment of choice (Figs 5-8a to 5-8d).

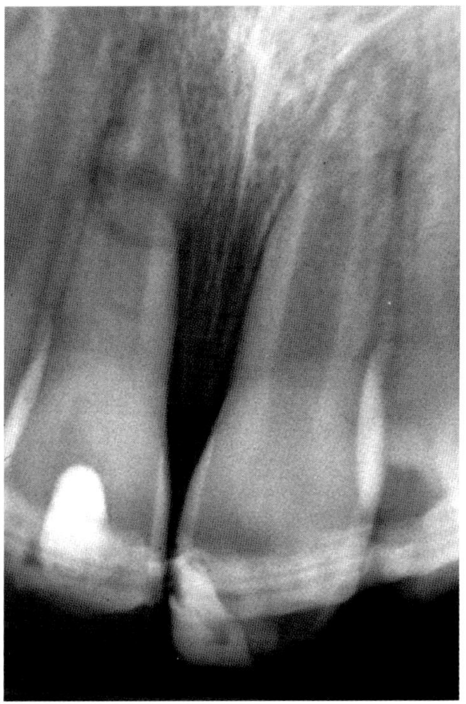

5-7a Preoperative radiograph of an incisor with a horizontal fracture in the apical third.

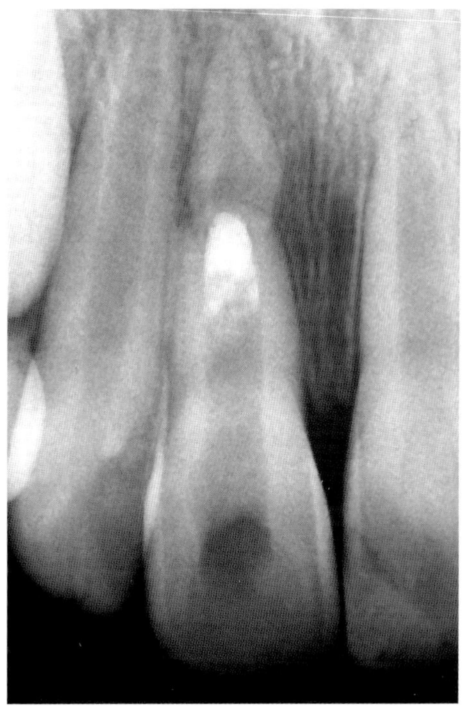

5-7b Following pulp necrosis, the coronal fragment was cleaned and obturated. The apical fragment was left untreated. A radiograph was taken to assess the adequacy of the MTA plug.

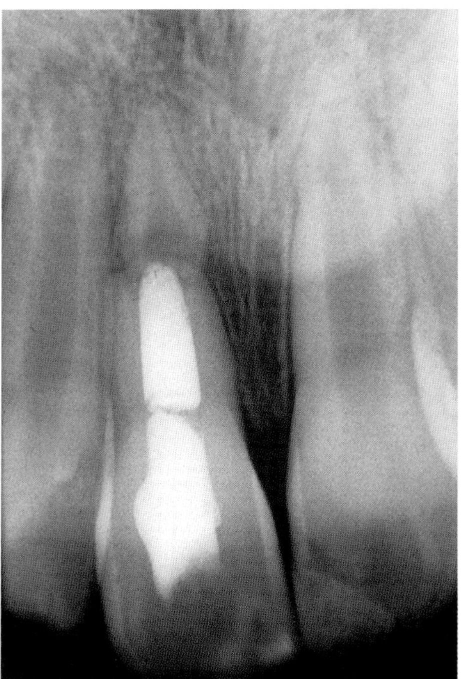

5-7c Immediate postoperative radiograph.

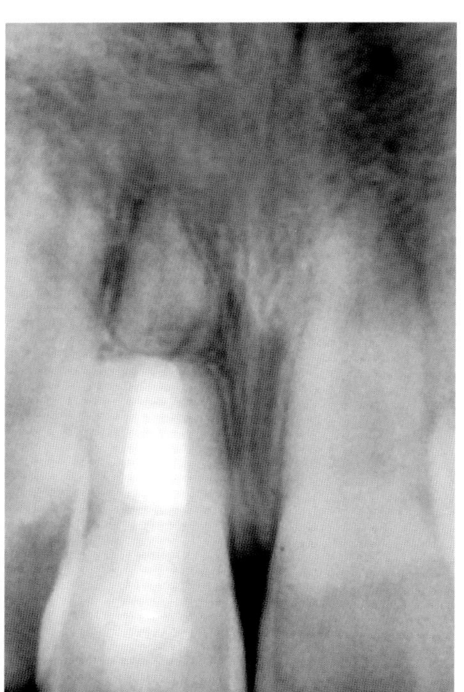

5-7d Radiograph taken 1 year postoperatively. There is no sign of infection, and a bony callus has formed at the fracture site. Mobility of the tooth is within physiologic limits.

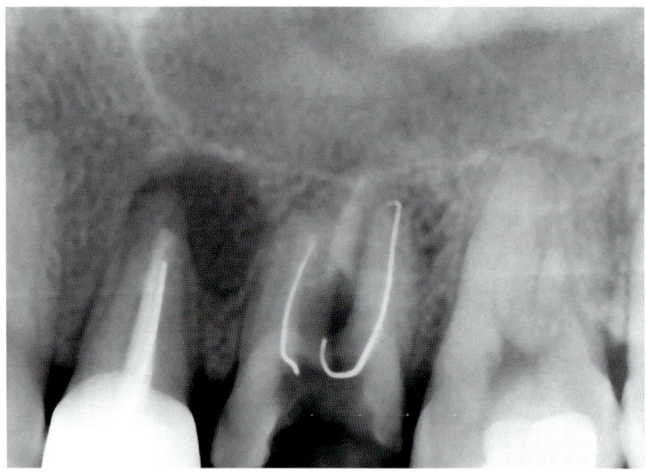

5-8a Despite apical surgery, a lesion of endodontic origin persists at the apex of this premolar.

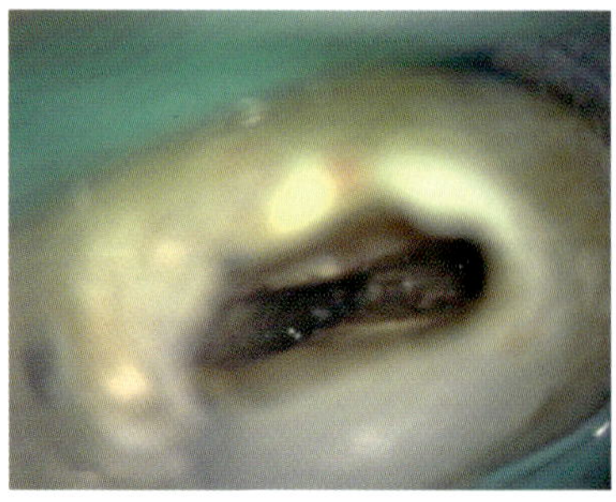

5-8b Root-end resection and retrograde preparation with ultrasonic instruments have transformed the narrow, circular foramen into an elongated opening.

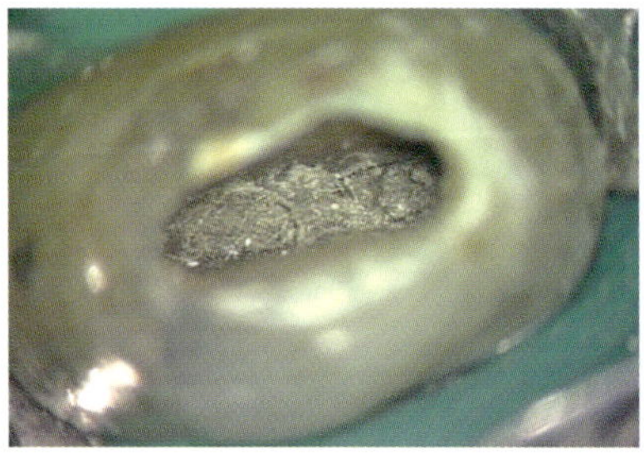

5-8c Obturating this canal with gutta-percha would be technically very difficult to do. Apical obturation with MTA is the preferred treatment.

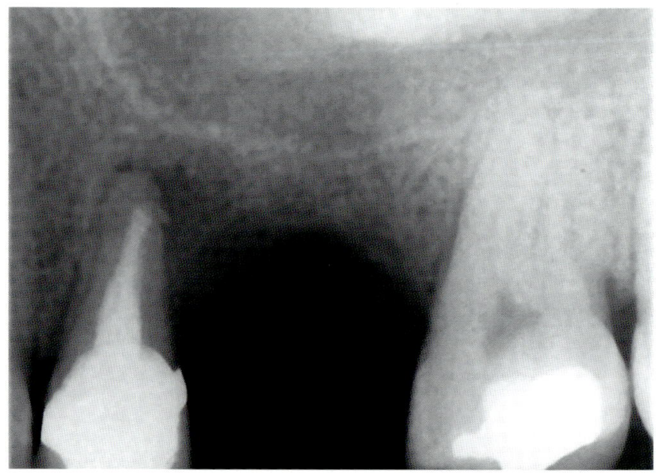

5-8d Radiograph taken 18 months postoperatively demonstrates almost total healing of the lesion.

Alternative Treatment Options

Although apexification is the treatment of choice for teeth with open apices, there are alternative treatment options.

Placement of an apical plug of gutta-percha

The quality of endodontic obturation is directly related to the quality of the canal preparation. The first step during obturation is to adapt the master cone in the apical third of the canal. In a tooth with an open apex, a tapered preparation is almost impossible to achieve for the reasons described previously (Fig 5-9a). The "customized cone" technique involves taking an impression of the apical third with gutta-percha to create a customized apical plug. This technique is also used to fill the coronal part of large canals after apexification with calcium hydroxide or after placement of an MTA plug.

If the canal is very wide, an extra-large gutta-percha point is created by merging several gutta-percha points together. The gutta-percha points are carefully softened in a flame and then fused together by being rolled between two glass slabs or manipulated with a large spatula. The size and diameter of the new gutta-percha point are adapted to the dimensions of the canal (Fig 5-9b). The larger end of the gutta-percha point is dipped in chloroform for 2 or 3 seconds to soften the surface. The softened point is then placed into the canal, which has been filled with hypochlorite. The gutta-percha point is placed a little shorter than working length and moved up and down for a few seconds to allow molding it to the shape of the apical third of the canal. It is then removed and dipped in sodium hypochlorite (Fig 5-9c). Once the canal has been dried, the gutta-percha point is also dried and covered with sealer, placed into the canal, and delicately condensed (Fig 5-9d). Obturation with the customized cone technique is technically difficult and may pose cer-

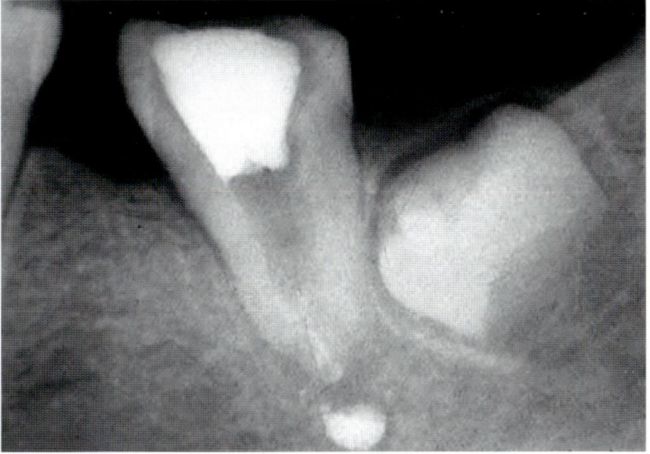

5-9a Preoperative radiograph of a mandibular molar with a large apex.

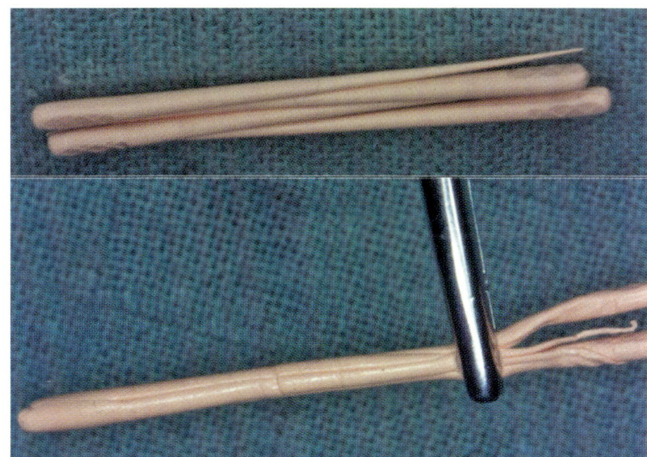

5-9b An extra-large gutta-percha point is prepared by placing several gutta-percha points top to bottom alongside each other. After the gutta-percha points have been softened in a flame, they are rolled between two glass slabs or manipulated with a large spatula, which fuses them together.

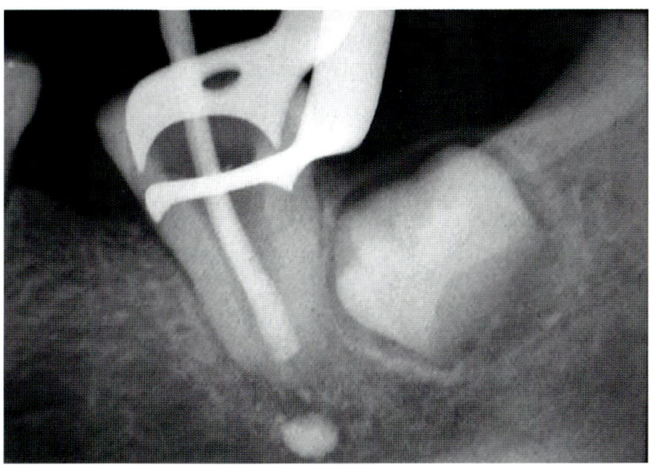

5-9c A radiograph is taken to check the fit of the gutta-percha point. The end of the extra-large gutta-percha point is dipped in chloroform for 2 to 3 seconds and placed into the canal. The gutta-percha molds itself to the shape of the canal walls.

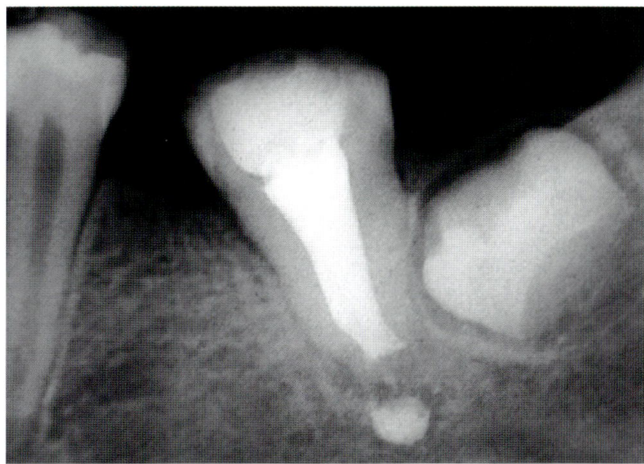

5-9d Postoperative radiograph.

tain problems:

- In canals with divergent walls where preparation is impossible (eg, blunderbuss apex), the molded gutta-percha point cannot be removed from the canal without becoming deformed and distorted.
- The end of the gutta-percha point is softened with a solvent to allow it to mold to the shape of the canal; the action of this solvent cannot be controlled and may continue even after obturation has been completed. A good long-term seal cannot therefore be guaranteed.
- Clinicians need to be experienced with this technique to produce a good result.

For these reasons, and because of the availability of new materials such as MTA, the customized cone technique is now rarely used to treat teeth with open apices.

Apical surgery

Given the difficulties of obturating large canals, apical surgery and retrograde obturation with amalgam or glass ionomer was often proposed as the treatment of choice. However, apical surgery is no longer considered as first-line treatment because of the simplicity and the reproducibility of apexification treatment with MTA. Similarly to endodontic retreatment, surgery is second-line treatment to deal with failing conventional endodontic treatment and should be considered in the following situations: long-term failure of treatment, persistent symptoms, a tooth that proves impossible to obturate well in the apical third, or an abscess that indicates a recurrent problem of endodontic origin.

During the surgical procedure, the lesion is curetted and the existing obturation material is assessed to determine if it reached a full set. If the material is not fully set, it is removed and retrograde obturation is completed. If the material appears to have set and hardened, there is no reason to replace it; the lesion is simply curetted and the surface of the obturation material is smoothed (Figs 5-10a to 5-10d).

Management of teeth with open apices often involves treating traumatized immature teeth in young patients. It is clear that surgery should be avoided if possible. On the other hand, if surgery is necessary, good orthograde obturation may avoid the need for retrograde obturation at the time of surgery.

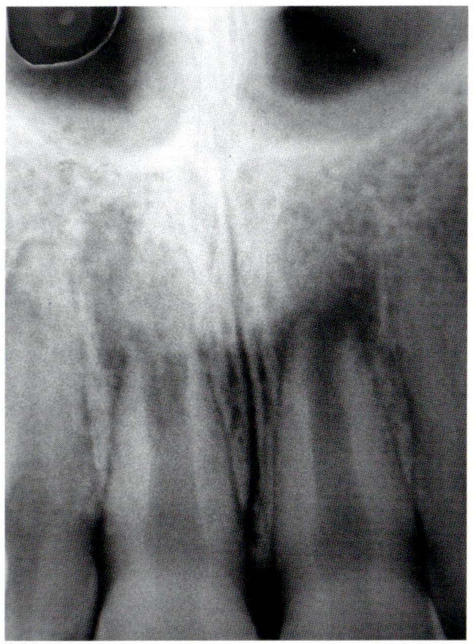

5-10a Both maxillary central incisors presented with periapical lesions of endodontic origin.

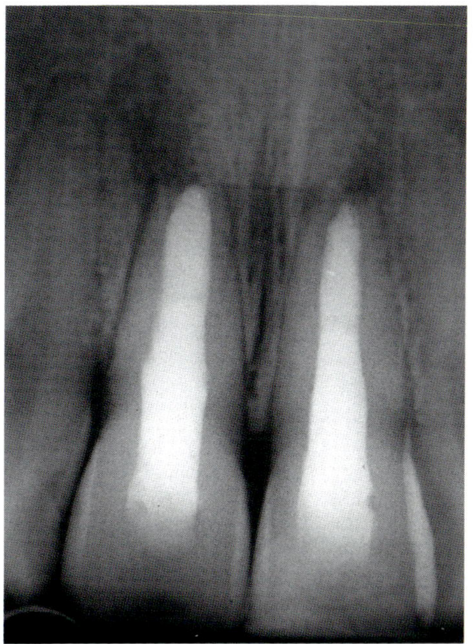

5-10b Radiograph showing favorable progress and the formation of an apical barrier at the apex of the maxillary right central incisor. However, the absence of any signs of healing at the apex of the maxillary left central incisor indicates the need for surgery.

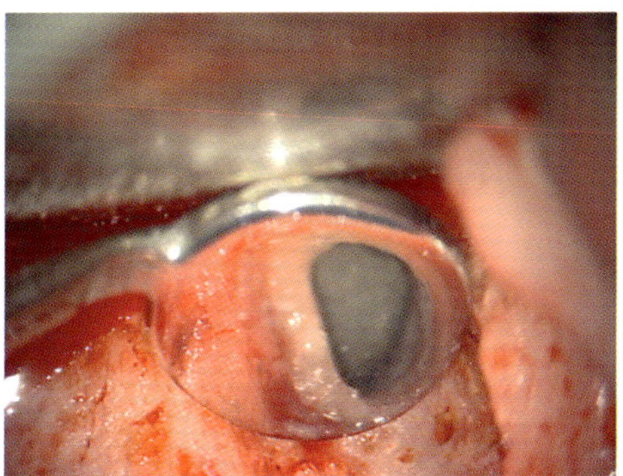

5-10c Once the lesion had been curetted, it became apparent that the MTA had never set fully; an inadequate seal was therefore the reason for the failure. Retrograde preparation was completed and the canal was re-obturated with MTA to ensure a good seal.

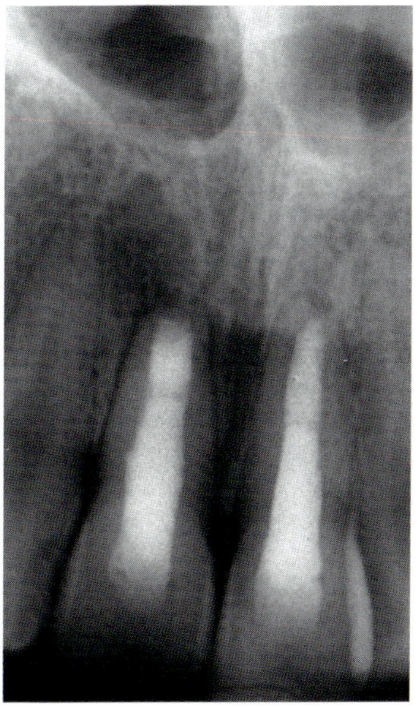

5-10d Radiograph taken 9 months postoperatively shows that the lesion is healing and apical closure has occurred.

Prognosis and Retreatment

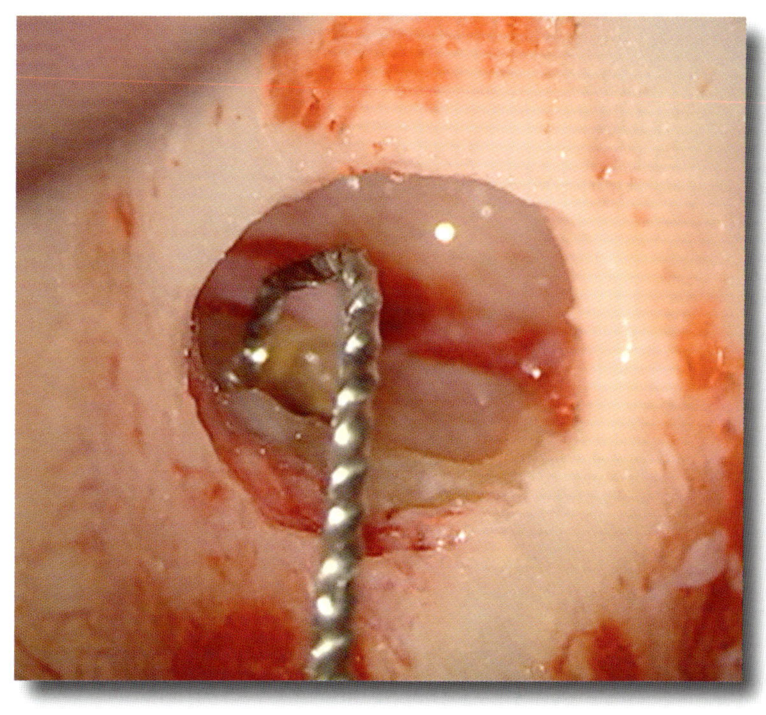

Thirty years ago, extraction was considered the treatment of choice whenever endodontic failure occurred. Greater understanding, new technologies, improvements in pain control, advances in restorative techniques, and above all, better information for the public have led to high expectations and demands. Patients nowadays hope to maintain their natural dentition for as long as possible. This explains why, although it is a difficult procedure to perform, endodontic retreatment is now undertaken on almost a daily basis in dental practices. Furthermore, with an aging population, it is likely that more and more teeth will need retreatment in future years.

Many authors have looked at the prognosis of endodontic treatment. Epidemiologic studies show that 1.4% to 10.0% of examined teeth (treated or untreated) carry an apical lesion that is evident radiographically. The same studies conclude that 24.5% to 46.0% of these lesions are associated with teeth that have already been endodontically treated. Numerous epidemiologic studies have analyzed the prognosis of endodontic treatment and retreatment. To date, 21 studies looking at between 50 and 1,462,936 teeth report a success rate ranging from 58% to 88%. *Can endodontic retreatment therefore be considered a predictable procedure?* Despite adopting a rational approach to endodontic retreatment, practitioners rarely reach a unanimous decision on whether a tooth needs to be retreated.

Finally, does the longevity of a tooth depend solely on the success or failure of endodontic treatment? Approaching the problem from this angle suggests that the practitioner alone is responsible for an unfavorable treatment outcome. It does not take into account extrinsic factors that may directly or indirectly influence the appearance of an inflammatory periapical lesion, such as extraradicular infection, anatomic complexities, complications related to the initial endodontic treatment, or fractures. A recent tendency discourages use of the somewhat restrictive terms *success* and *failure* in favor of the terms *healing* and *nonhealing* to more appropriately reflect the overall state of health of the periradicular tissues (Friedman, 2002).

Endodontic Disease and Its Management

Endodontic disease is caused by infection of the root canal system. The presence of bacteria and their toxins in the canal causes irritation of the surrounding bone at the apical foramen and any other portals of exit (apical or lateral). The periapical lesion is therefore the host's response to bacterial assault; it appears radiographically as a radiolucent area.

Several terms are used to describe this type of lesion. The most common phrase is *apical periodontitis*. More recently, the term *lesion of endodontic origin (LEO)* has been proposed to imply the inflammatory rather than infectious nature of the lesion as well as its location in the periodontium, which is not necessarily apical; above all, it reflects the endodontic origin of such a lesion.

The development of a radiographic lesion and the appearance of symptoms are the only criteria for determining if disease is present. Often the tooth is asymptomatic, since the majority of these lesions are of a chronic nature. Destruction of bone indirectly confirms the presence of bacteria in the root canal system. The disappearance of the radiolucent area following treatment indicates bone remineralization and therefore healing of the lesion. It is the only clinical means of confirming the efficacy of the canal disinfection and the adequacy of the seal provided by the root filling.

The practitioner must consider endodontic infection a disease and the periapical lesion a consequence of the disease. Thus, treatment should be focused on dealing with the root canal system and not on eradicating the lesion seen within the bone. Simple surgical enucleation of granulation tissue or a cyst does not therefore treat the disease. Recurrence of the infection is inevitable, as bacteria may persist and multiply in the root canal system.

Assessment of Periodontal Health

The appearance of a radiolucency on a radiograph indicates the presence of an inflammatory lesion within the bone but reveals no further information regarding the histologic nature of the lesion or its development over time. The chronology of disease is important.

Limiting the term *healthy* to teeth without periapical lesions and referring to a tooth with a radiolucency as having *associated pathology* is extremely simplistic. Lesions do not appear and disappear immediately; bone destruction and remineralization happens over months or even years. A tooth that has recently had inadequate endodontic treatment performed on it should be considered potentially diseased. If a radiograph is taken and the lesion is not visible, it may appear that the treatment was successful. Similarly, a tooth that has recently had a good quality root filling placed but has an associated radiolucency should still be considered potentially healing despite the radiolucency visible at this stage. These situations demonstrate the complexity of endodontic disease and its treatment. A series of radiographs taken at different time intervals after retreatment is necessary to allow the quality of the treatment to be assessed.

As with all diseases, it is essential to take into consideration the development and progression of the pathology. An increase or decrease in size of a lesion over time has long been considered the only method of assessing healing. Ørstavik, in proposing the Periapical Index (PAI), suggested evaluating the bone trabeculae in the inflammatory zone and scoring it on a scale of 1 to 5 (Ørstavik et al, 1986). In this way, by comparing radiographs taken at different intervals (approximately every 3 to 6 months), any changes in the lesion can be monitored. Ørstavik also recommended a monitoring period of 12 months to fully understand the progression of the lesion; in his prospective studies he showed that 90% of teeth with signs of healing at 12 months eventually underwent complete healing. For large lesions, complete healing can take up to 8 years. If treatment has been completed well and the coronal seal is maintained, the healing process rarely reverses.

Prognosis of Endodontic Treatment and Retreatment

Epidemiologic studies performed in various countries show that the percentage of inadequate endodontic treatment ranges from 33% to 79%, and the prevalence of radiographic lesions of endodontic origin varies from 20% to 65% (Friedman, 1998).

Initial treatment

- *In the absence of a radiographic lesion*, the success rate of initial endodontic treatment varies from 83% to 100%, with no significant difference seen between treatment on vital pulps and treatment on nonvital teeth. More than 75% of all failures (with lesions appearing after treatment) were identified in the first year after treatment. Thus a follow-up appointment 1 year postoperatively is generally predictive of the final outcome.

- *In cases where a radiographic lesion exists preoperatively*, the success rate for initial treatment varies from 46% to 93%. This variability is due to different methodologies employed in study protocols and different criteria used to evaluate results. Almost 89% of lesions that will eventually heal show signs of healing during the course of the first year after treatment. If treatment has been performed properly, the healing process rarely reverses.

However, teeth that have undergone apexification treatment with calcium hydroxide have a relapse rate of 8%; this can occur 2 to 3 years after definitive obturation has been performed, despite initial signs of healing. These delayed failures are thought to be related to porosity of the apical barrier associated with a defective coronal seal.

Retreatment
- *In the absence of a radiographic lesion*, reported success rates of endodontic retreatment are high, between 89% and 100%.
- *In cases where a radiographic lesion exists preoperatively*, however, the success rate varies between 56% and 84%, lower than the reported success rates for initial treatment. Obstructions and blockages encountered during endodontic retreatment prevent thorough cleaning and disinfection of the root canal system and therefore lower the success rates; obstructions include blockages, ledges, obturation material that adheres to the canal walls and harbors bacteria, fractured instruments, and calcified canals (Friedman, 1998; Gorni and Gagliani, 2004).

In one of the few prospective studies published (Farzaneh et al, 2004), two main factors were found to influence success rates in initial treatment and retreatment:
- Presence of a preoperative lesion: Success rates were negatively affected.
- Operative technique: Higher success rates were reported in teeth treated with the Schilder technique (canals prepared in a step-by-step manner and obturated with gutta-percha using a warm vertical condensation technique) than in teeth prepared with the step-back technique and obturated with cold lateral condensation.

In retreatment cases the presence of a perforation was also found to affect success rates significantly.

Factors That Can Interfere with Healing

Several possible causes of failure of good endodontic treatment and retreatment have been recognized (Siquiera, 2001; Nair, 2006). Several main factors have been identified as being responsible for the persistence of a periapical lesion despite completion of adequate endodontic retreatment.

Intracanal bacteria
Retreatment aims to eliminate bacteria and remove all necrotic debris from the root canal system, thereby cutting off the bacterial nutrient supply and preventing further proliferation of micro-organisms. Nevertheless, persistence of bacteria in the root canal system is often cited as the reason for lesions that persist months after retreatment. The organisms that persist after retreatment are different from those found in untreated canals; only a few species appear to survive. The dominant organisms seen are *Enterococcus* and *Streptococcus*, but *Actinomyces* and *Candida* have also been implicated. These micro-organisms survive in niches (eg, lateral canals, irregularities in dentin) that are inaccessible to the irrigating solutions (Nair, 2006).

Periradicular infection

During canal preparation and instrumentation, bacteria may be forced into the periapical region, where some species are capable of surviving (Nair, 2006). Furthermore, some bacteria appear to have the ability to migrate into the periapical area and form a biofilm on the root surface. These micro-organisms are resistant to the host's immune response and become a source of infection (Noiri et al, 2002). At this point the disease is no longer endodontic but periradicular, and thus cannot be treated by orthograde treatment alone; apical surgery is indicated. These resistant micro-organisms tend to be different than the normal intracanal species (eg, *Actinomyces israeli* and *Propionibacterium propionicum*).

Foreign body in the lesion

A foreign body in a periapical lesion, particularly sealer or gutta-percha, is often thought to cause disease. It appears, however, that the extruded material supports the micro-organisms instead of acting as a direct irritant itself. It is very difficult, if not impossible, to eliminate these foreign bodies with an orthograde approach. In such cases, apical surgery is indicated. Other substances, including cellulose fibers (from paper points) and starch particles (from powdered gloves), have been identified in refractory lesions (Nair, 2006).

Histologic nature of the lesion

It is a common misconception that periapical granulomas may heal after endodontic treatment but cystic lesions will not. Numerous studies (Nair, 2006) have shown that there are two types of cyst:

- "Bay" cysts communicate with the pulp of the tooth. These cysts respond like granulomas and disappear if irritants in the root canal system are eliminated. Nevertheless it is important to acknowledge that controlling moisture contamination in such circumstances may prove very difficult. A poorly dried canal may impair the quality of the obturation and therefore indirectly lead to failure.
- "True" cysts have an epithelial lining that renders the lesion a separate entity with no communication with the root canal system. In these cases, disinfection of the root canal will not bring about healing or bony infill because of the nature of the lesion. Supplemental surgery to enucleate the cyst is necessary.

It is impossible to determine the nature of the lesion preoperatively, so in each of these cases management starts with endodontic treatment or retreatment followed by a period of clinical and radiographic monitoring. Those cases that appear to be failing can then be treated surgically.

Poor coronal seal

The effect of a poor coronal seal on the prognosis of endodontic treatment is clearly demonstrated in the literature. Bacterial contamination, a result of a deficient coronal restoration, leads to reinfection of the root canal system and subsequent failure. To provide favorable conditions for healing, a definitive coronal restoration (cast restoration or post-retained crown) should be placed within 30 days after obturation. Meanwhile, a provisional restoration must be placed to bring the tooth back into occlusion; a functional tooth is preferred, if not essential, to stimulate healing of the periodontal tissues. *A provisional crown does not provide an adequate seal.*

Deciding when to place a definitive restoration can be difficult. Good retreatment ensures complete disinfection of the canal; this asepsis is then maintained by obturation of the canal and provision of a coronal seal. If the clinician is confident retreatment has been properly performed and yet pathology persists, the problem is likely to be an extraradicular rather than intracanal infection. Apical surgery should then be considered. This surgical procedure will not be affected by the presence of a coronal restoration.

Endodontic Surgery: An Adjunct to Treatment

Once orthograde retreatment has been completed and a coronal restoration provided, radiographs should be taken at 3, 6, and 12 months to assess the progress of the lesion and to monitor any changes. If the lesion does not reduce between two successive appointments and/or clinical symptoms arise, the persistence of infection is confirmed. There are two therapeutic alternatives at this point:

- In cases with a large lesion, or in the absence of any clinical symptoms, a period of further monitoring may be considered. A monitoring period of just 1 year may not be indicative of definitive long-term prognosis.
- In cases with small or moderately sized lesions, if there is no sign of healing, if the PAI is unfavorable, or if clinical signs and symptoms have appeared (eg, pain, abscess, sinus tract), a surgical approach should be considered (Box 6-1).

Surgery, in the majority of cases, is adjunctive treatment to complement the orthograde treatment and should not be seen as a substitute.

Box 6-1	**Main indications for surgery**
Recurrent clinical signs or symptoms appear or persist after retreatment	
Signs of healing (or other favorable changes) are absent 12 months after retreatment (Figs 6-1a to 6-1e)	
Obstructions (eg, blockages, calcified canals, fractured instruments) that cannot be bypassed render it technically impossible to complete satisfactory endodontic treatment from an orthograde approach. If these blockages prevent disinfection of the apical part of the canal, surgical intervention is justified.	
Removal of the coronal restoration is likely to cause significant harm to the underlying tooth. This is the only indication for surgery as an alternative to orthograde treatment rather than as complementary to orthograde treatment.	

Regardless of indication, the advantages and disadvantages of each course of treatment (retreatment or surgery) should be taken into consideration and evaluated (Box 6-2). *If there is any doubt whether to perform conventional orthograde or surgical retrograde retreatment, orthograde retreatment should be attempted first.*

The main goal of apical surgery is exactly the same as that of orthograde treatment: to eliminate bacterial irritants. The two treatments differ only in technique. In endodontic surgery a full-thickness flap is raised, a window is created in the overlying bone, and the inflammatory tissue is curetted away. After the apical third is prepared with ultrasonic tips, the canal is dried and a retrograde root filling is placed.

A retrograde root filling is necessary even if the canal has previously been obturated. Root-end resection and curettage eliminate the lesion but do not address the source of infection, namely bacteria within the canal. Root-end resection and curettage alone lead to reinfection, since bacteria remain within the root canal system. Furthermore, even if the main

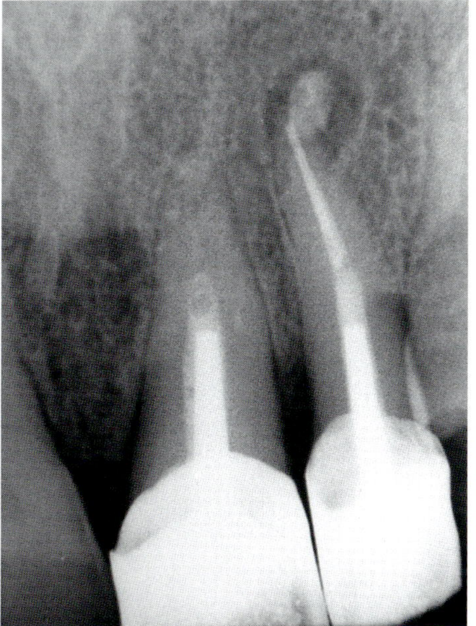

6-1a Preoperative radiograph of a maxillary lateral incisor shows a periapical lesion and extrusion of material through the apex.

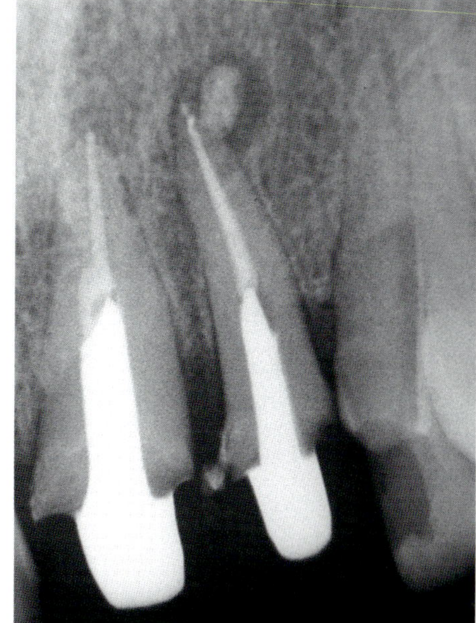

6-1b Radiograph taken 12 months postoperatively demonstrates the persistence of the lesion despite the endodontic retreatment.

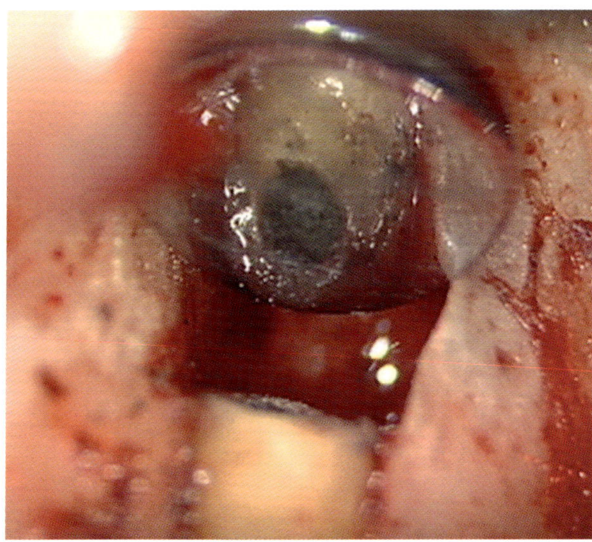

6-1c A surgical approach is adopted. The lesion is curetted, the apex of the root is sectioned, and the last few millimeters of the root are prepared and obturated with ProRoot MTA.

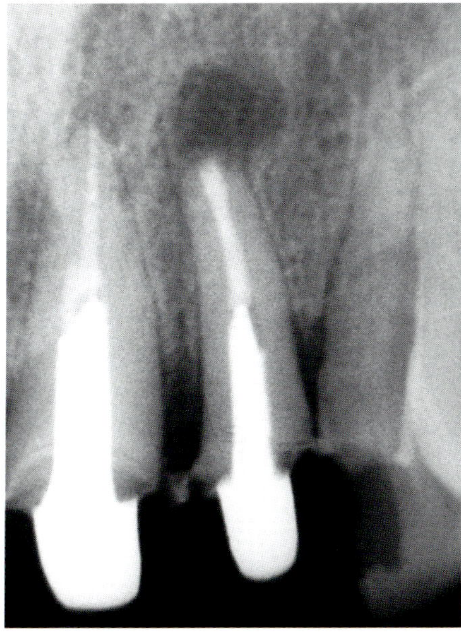

6-1d Postoperative radiograph.

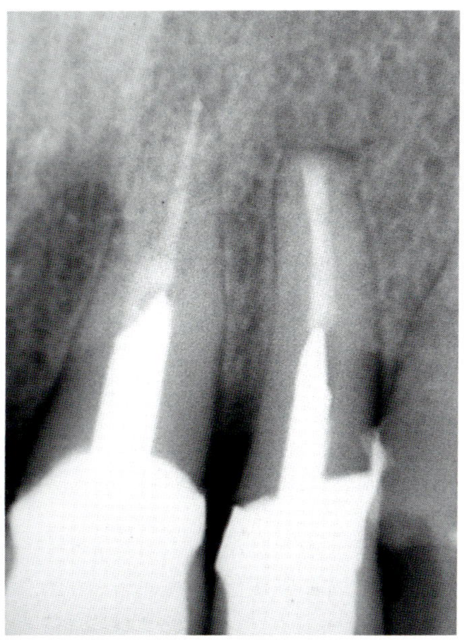

6-1e Radiograph taken 10 months postoperatively demonstrates healing and bony infill.

canal has been prepared and obturated via an orthograde approach, root-end resection often exposes an isthmus that has not been prepared or obturated; this must therefore be included in the retrograde preparation (Figs 6-2a to 6-2e).

In certain situations, retrograde endodontic treatment can be considered a first-line treatment. This is particularly true when removal of a post runs a high risk of fracturing the root or causing a perforation. In such cases, every effort should be made to clean and prepare as much of the root canal as possible from a retrograde approach (Figs 6-3a to 6-3f). Unfortunately, limited access in the posterior regions, the anatomy and location of some roots, and a lack of suitable instruments often prevents deep enough obturation into the canals. In the majority of cases, it is technically difficult to retreat a canal along its full length from a surgical approach. If a simple apical plug of 2 to 3 mm is placed in an unfilled, infected canal, residual bacteria will inevitably, over time, migrate into the periapical tissues. Even if favorable signs appear in the first few months after treatment, these remaining bacteria will eventually cause a recurrence of periapical pathology. For this reason, the length of the canal to be treated via a retrograde approach should be as short as possible. Conventional orthograde endodontic treatment is performed on the accessible portion of the canal; after a monitoring period, a surgical approach is adopted to allow preparation and obturation of the apical part of the canal that was impossible to disinfect in the conventional way (Friedman, 2005).

Box 6-2 Factors influencing the success of surgery

Orthograde retreatment prior to surgery. Success rates for apical surgery performed after failure of retreatment are higher (84% to 91%) than success rates for surgery performed directly after failure of initial treatment. This is probably because if initial treatment fails, the bacteria responsible for the failure remain within the canal and retrograde obturation is not sufficient to isolate and protect the periapical region. However, if retreatment is performed well yet still fails, the bacteria responsible for failure are likely extraradicular and will be eliminated by root-end resection and curettage.

Use of a biocompatible material to create a good seal for retrograde obturation. To create conditions favorable for healing, it is necessary to eliminate bacteria from within the canal and prevent any residual bacteria or their toxins from migrating into the periapical area. A root-end filling is therefore essential to maintain the seal provided by the gutta-percha.

Surgical method and technique. Current techniques complemented by the use of magnification devices and specially designed equipment (eg, micro-mirrors, ultrasonic instruments for retrograde preparation, biocompatible materials to provide a good seal [ProRoot MTA]) considerably improve the success rates.

Quality of the coronal restoration, which must provide a good seal and prevent reinfection.

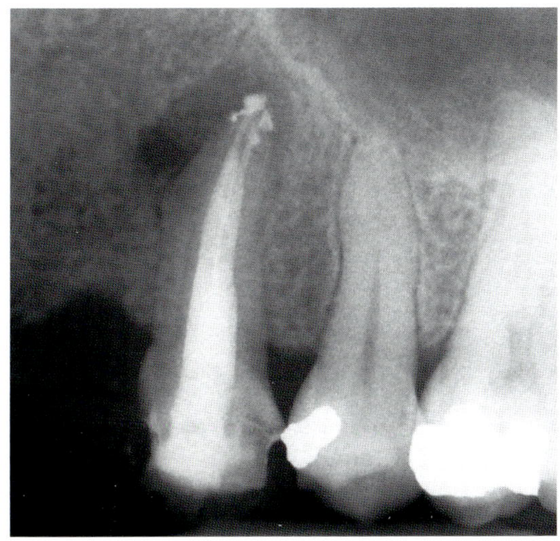

6-2a Preoperative radiograph of a symptomatic maxillary premolar with a persistent lesion several months after retreatment.

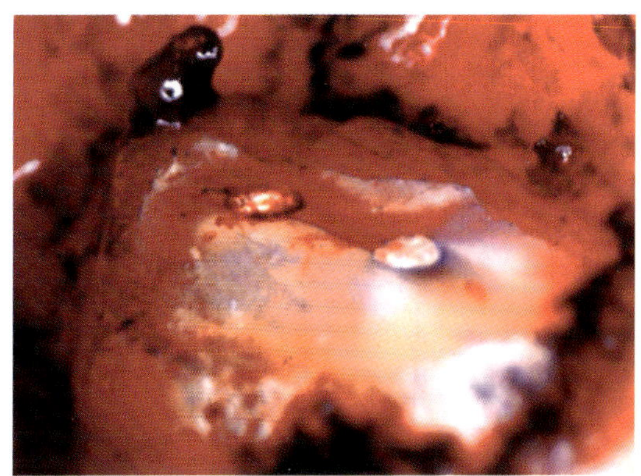

6-2b Root-end resection exposes the canals (obturated with gutta-percha) and reveals the isthmus connecting them.

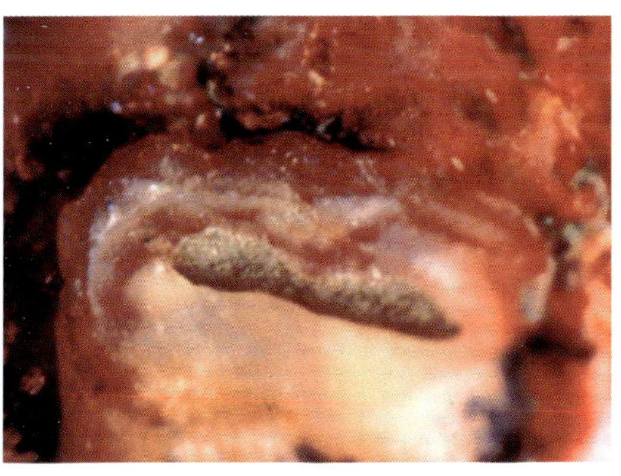

6-2c Retrograde cavity prepared with ultrasonic instruments. The canals and the isthmus can now be obturated with ProRoot MTA.

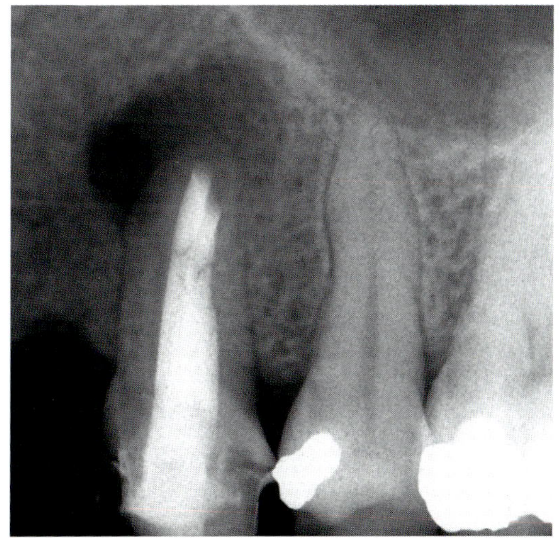

6-2d Immediate postoperative radiograph.

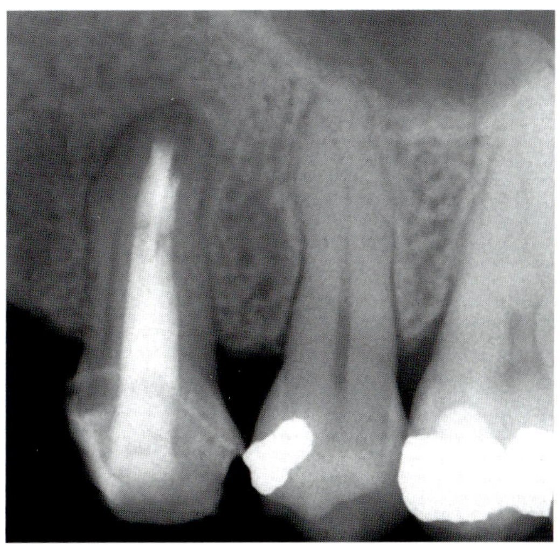

6-2e Radiograph taken 6 months postoperatively demonstrates almost complete healing.

In conclusion, recommended techniques for initial endodontic treatment are well documented; and if they are performed well, success rates are high. Endodontic retreatment is an attempt to manage an already compromised tooth. Compared to primary endodontic treatment, this procedure is technically more difficult to perform, has greater risks involved,

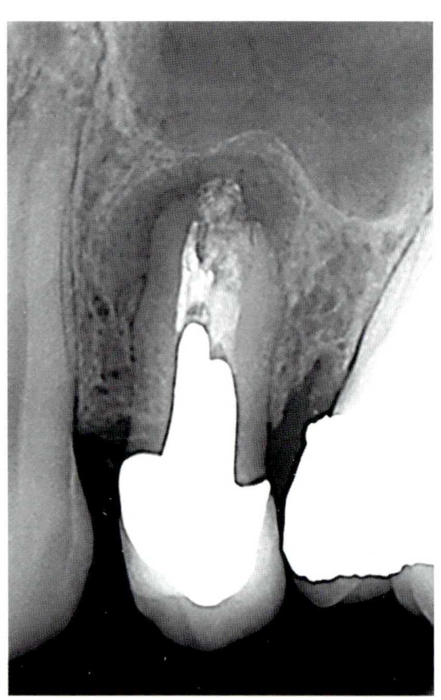

6-3a Given the shape of the post and the thin dentinal walls, removing the restoration from this maxillary premolar could endanger the underlying tooth. Surgical endodontic treatment is advised.

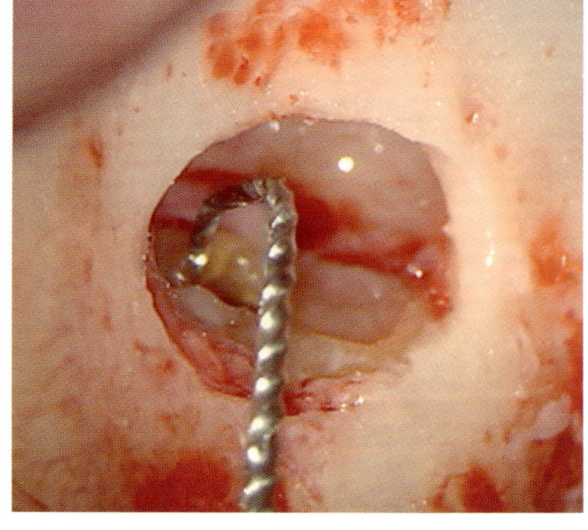

6-3b Obturation material is removed from the canal up to the level of the post using a precurved ultrasonic K-file.

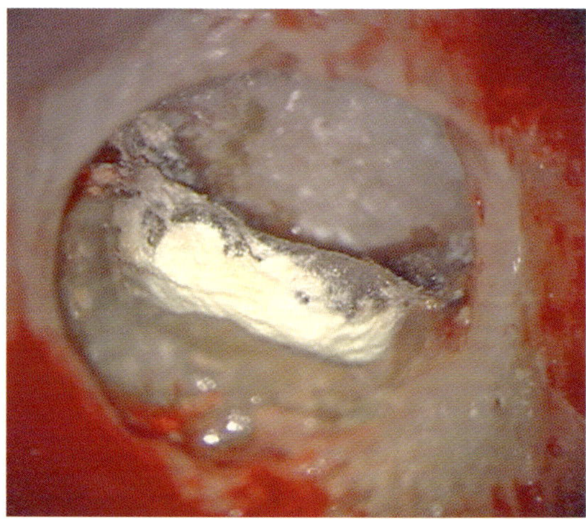

6-3d The canal is disinfected with 2% chlorhexidine, dried, and obturated with ProRoot MTA.

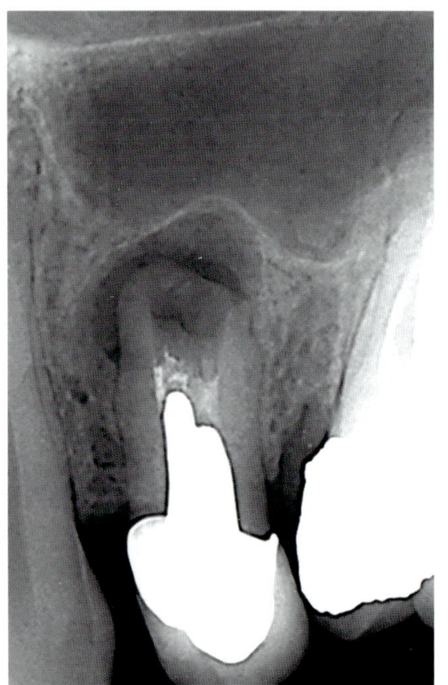

6-3c Radiograph taken during treatment to verify that all obturation material has been removed.

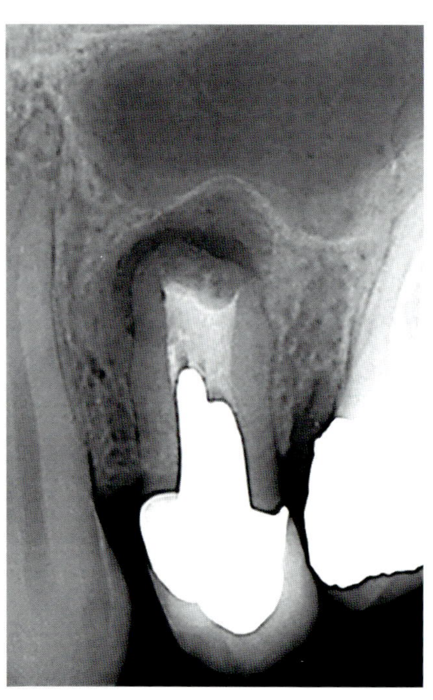

6-3e Immediate postoperative radiograph.

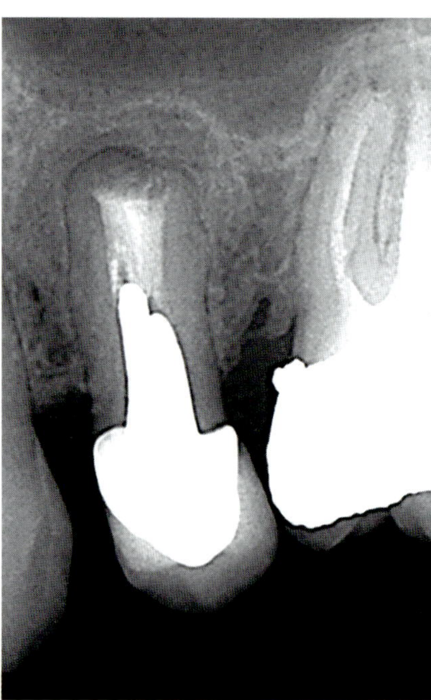

6-3f Radiograph taken 9 months postoperatively. Elimination of bacterial irritants and retrograde obturation have allowed healing to take place.

and is clinically more unpredictable. Clinicians should therefore endeavor to complete initial endodontic treatment to the best of their abilities so that retreatment, by definition more difficult and more risky, is avoided. When failures do present, successful retreatment depends on the clinician's knowledge of materials and techniques, experience, acknowledgment of ability, and patience.

In cases where orthograde treatment has been unsuccessful, endodontic surgery, performed diligently and methodically, is the only alternative and provides a potential means of saving the tooth.

Bibliography

Abbott PV. Incidence of root fractures and methods used for post removal. Int Endod J 2002;35:63–67.

Aeinehchi M, Eslami B, Ghanbariha M, Saffar AS. Mineral trioxide aggregate (MTA) and calcium hydroxide as pulp-capping agents in human teeth: A preliminary report. Int Endod J 2003;36:225–231.

Akerblöm A. The prognosis of endodontic treatment of obliterated root canals. J Endod 1984;14:565–567.

Andreasen JO, Farik B, Munksgaard EC. Long term calcium hydroxide as a root canal dressing may increase risk of fracture. Endod Dent Traumatol 2002;18:134–137.

Aryanpour S, Van Niewenhuisen JP, D'Hoore H. Endodontic retreatment decision: No consensus. Int Endod J 2000;33:208–218.

Boucher Y, Matossian L, Rilliard F, Machtou P. Radiographic evaluation of the prevalence and technical quality of root canal treatment in a French subpopulation. Inter Endod J 2002;35:229–238.

Doyon GE, Dumsha T, Von Fraunhofer JA. Fracture resistance of human root dentin exposed to intracanal calcium hydroxide. J Endod 2005;31:895-897.

Farzaneh M, Abitbol S, Friedman S. Treatment outcome in endodontics—The Toronto study. Phase I and II: Orthograde retreatment. J Endod 2004;30:627–633.

Farzaneh M, Abitbol S, Lawrence HP, Friedman S. Treatment outcome in endodontics—The Toronto study. Phase II:Initial treatment. J Endod 2004;30:302–309.

Felippe M, Felippe W, Marques M, Antoniazzi J. The effect of the renewal of calcium hydroxide paste on the apexification and periapical healing of teeth with incomplete root formation. Int Endod J 2005;38:436–442.

Felippe W, Felippe M, Rocha MJC. The effect of mineral trioxide aggregate on the apexification and periapical healing of teeth with incomplete root formation. Int Endod J 2006;39:2–9.

Friedman S. Considerations and concepts of case selection in the management of post-treatment endodontic disease (treatment failures). Endod Topics 2002;1:54–78.

Friedman S. The prognosis and expected outcome of apical surgery. Endod Topics 2005;11:219–262.

Friedman S. Treatment outcome and prognosis of endodontic therapy. In: Orstavik D, Pitt Ford TR (eds). Essential Endodontology. Oxford: Blackwell, 1998:367–401.

Fuss Z, Trope M. Root perforations:classifications and treatment choices based on prognostic factors. Endod Dent Traumatol 1996;12:255–264.

Gorni F, Gagliani M. The outcome of endodontic retreatment: A 2-yr Follow-up. J Endod 2004;30:1–4.

Hachmeister DR, Schindler WG, et al. The sealing ability and retention characteristics of mineral trioxide aggregate in a model of apexification. J Endod 2002;28:386–390.

Holland R, Filho JAO, de Souza V, Nery MJ. Mineral Trioxide repair of lateral perforations. J Endod 2001;27:281–284.

Hulsmann M. Retreatment decision making by a group of general practitioners in Germany. Int Endod J 1994;27:125–132.

Kvist T, Reit C. The perceived benefit of endodontic retreatment. Int Endod J 2002, 35:359–365.

Lee SJ, Monsef M, Torabinejad M. Sealing ability of a mineral trioxide aggregate for repair of lateral root perforations. J Endod 1993;11:541–544.

Machtou P. Guide clinique d'endodontie. Paris: Editions CdP, 1993.

Nair PNR. On the causes of persistance of apical periodontitis : A review. Int Endod J 2006;39:249–281.

Nakata TT, Bae KS, Baumgartner JC. Perforation repair comparing mineral trioxide aggregate and amalgam using anaerobic bacterial leakage model. J Endod 1998;24:184–186.

Noiri Y, Ehara A, Kawahara T, Takemura N, Ebisu S. Participation of bacterial biofilms in refractory and chronic periapical periodontitis. J Endod 2002;28:679–683.

Orstavik D, Kerekes K, Eriksen HM. The periapical index: A scoring system for radiographic assessment of apical periodontitis. Endod Dent Traumatol 1986;2:20–34.

Pagonis TC, Fong CD, Hasselgren G. Retreatment decisions—A comparison between general practitioners and endodontic postgraduates. J Endod 2000;26:240–241.

Pertot WJ, Simon S. Réussir Le Traitement Endodontique, Paris: Editions Quintessence International, 2003.

Pitt Ford T, Torabinejad M, McKendry D, Hong CU, Karyawasam S. Use of mineral trioxide aggregate for repair of furcal perforations. Oral Surg Oral Pathol Oral Med 1995;79:756–762.

Ruddle C. Nonsurgical retreatment. J Endod 2004;30:827–845.

Schilder H. Cleaning and shaping the root canal. Dent Clin North Am 1974;18:269–296.

Schilder H. Filling root canals in three dimension. Dent Clin North Am 1967;11:723–744.

Shabahang S, Torabinejad M, Boyne PP, Abedi H, McMillan P. A comparative study of root-end induction using osteogenic protein-1, calcium hydroxide, and mineral trioxide aggregate in dogs. J Endod 1993;25:1–5.

Siquiera JF. Aetiology of root canal treatment failure : Why well-treated teeth can fail. Int Endod J 2001;34:1–10.

Sjögren U, Happonen RP, Kahnberg KE, Sundqvist G. Survival of *Arachnia propionica* in periapical tissue. Int Endod J 1988;21:277–282.

Spili P, Parashos P, Messer H. The impact of instrument fracture on outcome of endodontic treatment. J Endod 2005;31: 845–850.

Suter B, Lussi A, Sequeira P. Probability of removing fractured instruments from root canals. Int Endod J 2005;38:112–123.

Torabinejad M, Higa R, Mc Kendry DJ, Pitt Ford T. Dye leakage of root-end filling materials: Effects of blood contamination. J Endod 1994;20:159–163.

Torabinejad M, Pitt Ford TR, Mc Kendry DJ, Abedi HR, Miller DA, Kariyawasam SP. Histologic assessment of mineral trioxide aggregate as a root-end filling in monkeys. J Endod 1997;23:225–228.

Webber RT. Apexogenesis versus apexification. Dent Clin North Am 1984;28:669–697.

Index

Page numbers followed by "f" denote figures; those followed by "t" denote tables; those followed by "b" denote boxes

A

Algorithms, 87t–89t
Amalgam restorations, 26
Angled radiographs, 19, 20f, 50f
Anterior teeth, perforations in, 96–100, 97f–100f
Apex
- extrusion of material through, 21–22, 22f
- open. *See* Open apices.

Apexification
- with calcium hydroxide
  - commercial preparations, 115–116
  - difficulties associated with, 117
  - follow-up, 116–117
  - relapse rate for, 134
  - temporary, 116, 117f
- description of, 114–115
- with mineral trioxide aggregate, 118–119, 120f–123f

Apexogenesis, 113, 114f
Apical abscess, 123f
Apical foramen, 21f
Apical periodontitis, 132
Apical plug
- description of, 115
- gutta-percha, 126–128, 127f
- mineral trioxide aggregate, 118, 118b, 121f, 124, 126f

Apical surgery, 124, 126f, 128, 129f

B

Bacteria
- canal contamination by, 14, 15f
- coronal seal deficiency and, 15
- healing affected by, 134
- perforation contamination by, 92–93, 93f, 103
- reinfection caused by, 135

Buccal perforations, 94, 97f

C

C+ file, 61f, 70f
Calcium hydroxide
- apexification with. *See* Apexification, with calcium hydroxide.
- for pulp capping, 113

Canals
- access to
  - blockage risks, 55, 56f
  - coronal, 79, 79f
  - factors that affect, 24
  - improvements in, 46
  - obstruction during, 56, 63, 64, 134
  - resistance during, 56
  - straight-line, 55, 56f, 76
  - through crown, 25
- anatomy of, 46–55, 47f–55f
- apical portion of. *See also* Open apices.
  - inability to negotiate through, 73–75
  - untreatment of, 84, 86f
- bacterial contamination of, 14, 15f
- equipment and tools for identifying, 53–54, 54f
- fractured instrument removal affected by anatomy of, 76
- inadequate preparation of, failures secondary to, 22
- in incisors
  - mandibular, 51, 51f
  - maxillary, 46, 47f
  - ledges in, 56, 63, 64f, 68, 72, 83f
  - in mandibular canines, 49, 50f
  - in molars
  - mandibular. *See* Mandibular molars, canals of.
  - maxillary, 49, 50f, 55f
- in premolars
  - mandibular, 51, 51f–52f
  - maxillary, 47–49, 48f–49f
- radiographic assessment of, 20
- untreated part of, 68, 73–75
- widening of, using Gates Glidden drill, 82f

Ceramic posts, 43, 43f
"Champagne effect," 54
Chewing-related pain, 12
Clinical examination, 24b
Cold lateral condensation technique, 65
Composite restorations, 26
Cone technique, 128
Coronal restorations
- definitive, 74
- existing, removal of, 26–32
- new, 14, 14f–15f
- radiographic assessment of, 20

Coronal seal
- crown lengthening used to improve, 18
- deficient, 15
- healing success affected by, 135–136

Cracked tooth, 12
Crown(s)
- decementing of, 26–30
- intact, 26–30
- metal, 29b
- porcelain-fused-to-metal, 27, 28b, 29f
- post-retained, 38
- provisional restoration use of, 25, 135
- removal of, 25–30, 26f–30f
- resin-bonded, 30
- sectioning of, 30, 30f

Crown lengthening, 18
Crown removers, 26f–27f, 26–28
Cysts, periapical, 135

D

Decision-making factors
- cost-benefit ratio, 19
- operator skill and experience, 19
- patient cooperation, 19
- periodontal assessment, 16–17, 17f–18f
- restorability of the tooth, 18
- surgery time required, 19
- tooth importance, 16
- treatment alternatives, 16

Dentin, 112, 117
DG-16 probe, 58
Dyes, 54

E

Electric crown remover, 27, 31
Endo-Bender pliers, 69
Endodontic disease, 132–133
Endodontic surgery, 136–141, 137f, 139f–140f
Endodontic treatment
- failure of, 10–11, 133
- inflammation after, 12
- objectives of, 10, 14, 18
- prognosis of, 132–134
- success rate for, 11, 84, 133–134

Existing restoration removal
- amalgam, 26
- composite, 26
- coronal restorations, 26–32
- crowns
  - core material used with, 25, 25f
  - decementing of, 26–30
  - intact, 26–30

provisional restoration use of, 25
sectioning of, 30, 30f
direct restorations, 26
fixed partial dentures, 31f, 31–32
posts
ceramic, 43, 43f
fiber, 41, 42f
indirect casted, 35
passive, 32
split-pin, 39–40, 40f–42f
threaded, 33, 33f–34f
reasons for, 25

F
Failure
inadequate canal preparation as cause of, 22
of endodontic treatment, 10–11, 133
of retreatment, 20
Fiber posts, 41, 42f
Fistula, 17
Fixed partial dentures
maxillary incisor replaced with, 100f
removal of, 31f, 31–32
Fracture
post, 33, 34f, 109
root. *See* Root fracture.
tooth. *See* Tooth fracture.
Fractured instrument removal
advances in, 75
canal anatomy effects on, 76
chemically cured composite technique for, 81, 82f
determinations before beginning, 76
factors that affect, 75–76
fragment
gutter created around, 79, 80f
location of, 76
negotiating hand files past, 78f
Gates Glidden drill used in, 79, 80f
healing after, 78f
IRS method, 81, 82f, 85f
Lenticulo spiral filler, 77f, 82, 84, 85f
Masseran kit for, 81, 82f
placement of cotton wool pledgets in other canals before, 77, 78f
radiographic evaluations, 78f
success rates of retreatment and, 87, 88t–89t
systems for, 81, 82f
techniques for, 76–84, 77f–84f
thermocompaction devices, 84
ultrasonic tips used in, 79, 80f, 83f
ultrasonic vibration for, 77
Furcation lesions, 16–17, 17f
Furcation perforations, 102, 102f, 108f

G
Gates Glidden drill, 41, 42f, 55, 60, 65f, 79, 80f, 82f–83f
Gutta-percha
apical plug, for open apices, 126–128, 127f, 139f
for maxillary lateral incisor perforations, 97f
removal of, 65–66, 66f, 88f

H
Hand files, 60, 61f, 63, 64f
Healing
factors that interfere with, 134–136
after fractured instrument removal, 78f
H-file, 60, 61f, 65f, 68, 101f, 115
History-taking, 19

I
Iatrogenic perforations, 92, 109–110
Immature teeth, 112–114, 119
Incisors
mandibular, 51, 51f
maxillary. *See* Maxillary central incisor; Maxillary lateral incisor.
Indications
clinical symptoms, 12
coronal seal deficiency, 15
new coronal restorations are planned, 14, 14f–15f
periapical lesions, 13, 13f
radiographic evidence, 13
Indirect casted posts, 35
Inflammation, 12
Infrabony perforations, 96–100, 97f–100f
Instruments
fractured. *See* Fractured instrument removal.
obturation material removal. *See* Obturation material removal, instruments for.
rotary nickel-titanium. *See* Rotary nickel-titanium instruments.
IRS, 81, 82f, 85f

K
K-file, 140f

L
Ledges
in fractured instrument removal, 80f, 83f
during obturation material removal, 56, 63, 64f, 68, 72
Lenticulo spiral filler, fractured, 77f, 82, 84, 85f
Lesion of endodontic origin, 132
Lesions. *See* Periapical lesions.
Long-shank tungsten carbide burs, 54, 54f

M
Mandibular canines, 49, 50f
Mandibular incisors, 51, 51f
Mandibular molars
apex of, 127f
canals of
anatomy of, 52, 52f
distal, 70, 71f–72f
mesial, 69, 70f, 86f, 102
periapical lesions, 86f
pulp chamber floor perforations, 104f
retreatment of, 11f–12f
Mandibular premolars, 51, 51f–52f
Masseran kit, 81, 82f, 84
Maxillary central incisor, 123f, 129f
Maxillary lateral incisor
apexification in, 120f
canals of, 46, 47f

fixed partial denture abutment use of, 21f
fractured instruments in, 82f
perforation in, 96–100, 97f–100f, 110f
periapical lesion in, 137
post and core restoration of, 36f
Maxillary molars
canals of
anatomy of, 49, 50f, 55f
palatal, 72
mesial root of, 74f
perforations in, 100, 101f
periapical radiograph of, 22f
Maxillary premolars, 47–49, 48f–49f, 139f
Medicolegal record, 20
Mesial canals, 69, 70f, 86f, 102
Metal crowns, 29b
Metalift crown removal system, 27, 27f
Methyl cellulose, 115
Mineral trioxide aggregate
apexification with, 118–119, 120f–123f
apical plug, 118, 118b, 121f, 124, 126f
canal obturation with, 122
for perforations, 94–96, 98f, 100, 107, 109f, 113
Molars. *See* Mandibular molars; Maxillary molars.

O

Obturation
cone technique for, 128
gutta-percha apical plug, 126–128, 127f, 139f
retrograde, 138b
Obturation material removal
canal access affected by, 56
carrier-based material, 68
cleaning of canal after, 73
factors that affect, 56, 58
guidelines for, 55–56
gutta-percha, 65–66, 66f, 88f
H-file for, 60, 61f
identifying of material, 56–58, 57f
instruments for
forcing of, 56, 61f, 66
fractured. *See* Fractured instrument removal.
hand files, 60, 61f
Pro-Taper Universal system, 62, 62f–64f
R-Endo System, 62, 62f
rotary nickel-titanium, 62f–64f, 62–63
technique, 63
ledges encountered during, 56, 63, 64f, 68, 72
negotiating the untreated part of the canal after, 68
obstruction during, 56, 63, 64, 70f–71f
pastes, 58–60, 59f, 88f
radiographic confirmation of, 140f
silver points, 66–68, 67f, 87t
solvents, 63
Occlusion, sensitivity in, 12
Open apices
apexification for. *See* Apexification.
apexogenesis, 113, 114f
apical surgery failure, 124, 126f
gutta-percha apical plug for, 126–128, 127f
horizontal root fracture, 124, 125f
immature teeth, 112–114

P

Pain
differential diagnosis of, 12
referred, 12
Parachute technique, 31, 31f
Passive posts, 32
Pastes, 58–60, 59f, 88f
Perforations
in anterior teeth, 96–100, 97f–100f
apical third of canal, 105–110
bacterial contamination, 92–93, 93f, 103
buccal, 94, 97f
causes of, 53, 56
in coronal third, 95–101
cortical bone and, 93
definition of, 92
etiologies of, 92
furcation, 102, 102f, 108f
iatrogenic, 92, 109–110
infrabony, 96–100, 97f–100f
large, 107–110
in maxillary incisors and canines, 96–100, 97f–100f, 110f
in maxillary molars, 100, 101f
middle third of canal, 105–110
mineral trioxide aggregate for, 94–96, 98f, 100
obturation of, 105, 106f, 108b
in posterior teeth, 100, 101f
prevention of, 43
prognostic factors, 92–93, 93f–94f
pulp chamber floor, 93f–94f, 103, 104f
repair of
description of, 93–94
materials used in, 94–95
radiographs after, 104f
root, 94
rotary instruments as cause of, 53, 95
sealing of, 99, 99f
site of, 92–93, 93f
size and shape of, 93, 94f
small, 105, 106f–107f
strip, 102, 102f
suprabony, 95–96
treatment of, 92–93, 93f–94f
Periapical cysts, 135
Periapical index, 133
Periapical lesions
foreign body in, 135
illustration of, 13f, 86f
maxillary lateral incisor, 137
Periodontal assessment, 16–17, 17f–18f, 133
Periodontal pocket, 17, 18f
Periodontal probing, 16–17, 17f
Periradicular infection, 135
Porcelain-fused-to-metal crowns, 27, 28b, 29f
Post(s)
ceramic, 43, 43f
fiber, 41, 42f

fracture of, 33, 34f, 109
indirect casted, 35
passive, 32
removal of, 32–43, 109
split-pin, 39–40, 40f–42f
threaded, 33, 33f–34f
universal post remover, 35, 35f–37f
WAM X removal system, 38, 38f–39f
Posterior teeth, perforations in, 100, 101f
Premolars
mandibular, 51, 51f–52f
maxillary, 47–49, 48f–49f, 139f
Preoperative considerations. *See* Decision-making factors.
ProRoot mineral trioxide aggregate
apexification with, 118b–119b, 120f–123f
for perforations, 94–96, 98f, 100, 107, 109f, 113
Pro-Taper Universal system, 62, 62f–64f
Provisional restorations, 25, 135
Pulp capping, 113
Pulp chamber floor perforations, 93f–94f, 103, 104f
Pulpal shock, 112
Pulpectomy, 112
Pulpotomy, 113

R
Radiographs
angled, 19, 20f, 50f
calcium hydroxide, 116f
information derived from, 20, 24b
maxillary molars, 22f
obstruction evaluations using, 63, 64f
obturation material, 140f
perforation repair, 104f
periapical lesion detection on, 13f
pretreatment uses of, 19, 20f
Referred pain, 12
Removal techniques
existing restorations. *See* Existing restoration removal.
fractured instrument. *See* Fractured instrument removal.
R-Endo System, 62, 62f
Resin-bonded crowns, 30
Restorations
coronal. *See* Coronal restorations.
existing, removal of. *See* Existing restoration removal.
provisional, 25, 135
Retreatment
actions before starting, 19
algorithms, 87t–89t
conventional, surgical approach vs, 21f–22f, 21–22
coronal approach, 105
decision making regarding. *See* Decision-making factors.
definition of, 10
failure of, 20
goals of, 10, 14, 22
indications for. *See* Indications.
prognosis of, 132–134
risks associated with, 84
success rates for, 134
Retrograde endodontic treatment, 138, 140f
Retrograde obturation, 21f
Root fillings
inadequate, 14, 15f
resin-based, 58
retrograde, 136
Root fracture. *See also* Tooth fracture.
differential diagnosis of, 17, 18f
horizontal, 124, 125f
pain and, 12
Root perforation, 94
Rotary nickel-titanium instruments
gutta-percha removal using, 66
paste removal using, 62f–64f, 62–63
perforations caused by, 95

S
Screwdrivers, 33, 34f
Sectioning of crowns, 30, 30f
Silver points, 66–68, 67f, 87t
Smooth-sided posts, 32
Sodium hypochlorite, 54, 113, 120f
Solvents, 63, 85f
Split-pin posts, 39–40, 40f–42f
Stainless steel hand files, 60, 61f, 63, 64f
Strip perforations, 102, 102f
Suprabony perforations, 95–96
Surgery
apical, 124, 126f, 128, 129f
endodontic, 136–141, 137f, 139f–140f
retreatment, 21f–22f, 21–22

T
Teeth
angulation of, 110b
anterior, 96–100, 97f–100f
immature, 112–114, 119
posterior, 100, 101f
restorability of, 18
strategic importance of, 16
Temperature-related pain, 12
Thermocompaction devices, 84
Threaded posts, 33, 33f–34f
Tooth fracture. *See also* Root fracture.
calcium hydroxide exposure and, 117
during crown removal, 26f

U
Ultrasonic tips
canal identification using, 54
in fractured instrument removal, 79, 80f, 83f
obturation material removal using, 56
post removal using, 33, 33f, 41
Universal post remover, 35, 35f–37f

W
WAM X, 38, 38f–39f
WAMkey, 28b–29b, 28f–29f, 28–30

Imprimé en France par EUROPE MEDIA DUPLICATION S.A.S.
53110 Lassay-les-Châteaux
N° 20962 - Dépôt légal : avril 2009

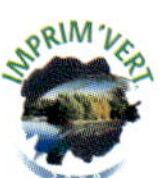